Perinatal Asphyxia: Moving the Needle

Editor

LINA F. CHALAK

CLINICS IN PERINATOLOGY

www.perinatology.theclinics.com

Consulting Editor
LUCKY JAIN

September 2024 • Volume 51 • Number 3

ELSEVIER

1600 John F. Kennedy Boulevard • Suite 1800 • Philadelphia, Pennsylvania, 19103-2899

http://www.theclinics.com

CLINICS IN PERINATOLOGY Volume 51, Number 3
September 2024 ISSN 0095-5108, ISBN-13: 978-0-443-13009-0

Editor: Kerry Holland
Developmental Editor: Nitesh Barthwal

Clinics in Perinatology (ISSN 0095-5108) is published quarterly by Elsevier Inc., 360 Park Avenue South, New York, NY 10010-1710. Months of issue are March, June, September, and December. Business and Editorial Offices: 1600 John F. Kennedy Blvd., Ste. 1800, Philadelphia, PA 19103-2899. Customer Service Office: 3251 Riverport Lane, Maryland Heights, MO 63043. Periodicals postage paid at New York, NY and additional mailing offices. Subscription prices are $351.00 per year (US individuals), $398.00 per year (Canadian individuals), $475.00 per year (international individuals), $100.00 per year (US and Canadian students), and $195.00 per year (International students). For institutional access pricing please contact Customer Service via the contact information below. International air speed delivery is included in all Clinics subscription prices. All prices are subject to change without notice. Orders, claims, and journal inquiries: Please visit our Support Hub page https://service.elsevier.com for assistance.

Reprints. For copies of 100 or more, of articles in this publication, please contact the Commercial Reprints Department, Elsevier Inc., 360 Park Avenue South, New York, NY 10010-1710. Tel. 212-633-3874; Fax: 212-633-3820; E-mail: reprints@elsevier.com.

Clinics in Perinatology is also published in Spanish by McGraw-Hill Interamericana Editores S.A., P.O. Box 5-237, 06500 Mexico D.F., Mexico.

Clinics in Perinatology is covered in *MEDLINE/PubMed (Index Medicus) Current Contents, Excepta Medica, BIOSIS and ISI/BIOMED.*

Contributors

CONSULTING EDITOR

LUCKY JAIN, MD, MBA
George W. Brumley Jr Professor and Chairman, Department of Pediatrics, Emory University School of Medicine, Pediatrician-in-Chief, Children's Healthcare of Atlanta, Atlanta, Georgia, USA

EDITOR

LINA F. CHALAK, MD, MSCS
Professor, Department of Pediatrics, William Buchanan Endowed Chair Professor of Pediatrics and Psychiatry, Division Chief Interim, Neonatal-Perinatal Medicine, Director, Fetal and Neonatal Neurological Intensive Care Unit, Neurological Neonatal Intensive Care Fetal and Neonatal Neurology Fellowship Program, University of Texas Southwestern Medical School, UT Southwestern Medical Center, Dallas, Texas, USA

AUTHORS

AFAF AHMED, MBBS
Resident Physician, Division of Pediatric and Developmental Neurology, Department of Neurology, Washington University in St Louis, St Louis, Missouri, USA

TAYYBA ANWAR, MD
Neurophysiologist, Department of Neurology, Children's National Hospital, Washington, DC, USA

NADIA BADAWI, AM, MB, PhD
Professor, Cerebral Palsy Alliance Research Institute, Specialty of Child and Adolescent Health, Sydney Medical School, Camperdown, Faculty of Medicine and Health, Department of Paediatrics, The University of Sydney, Allambie Heights, Sydney, Medical Director and Co-Head, Grace Centre for Newborn Intensive Care, The Children's Hospital at Westmead, Sydney Children's Hospital Network, The University of Sydney, Westmead, New South Wales, Australia

ALICE C. BAKER, MD, MPH
Neonatal Perinatal Medicine Fellow, Department of Pediatrics, Yale University School of Medicine, New Haven, Connecticut, USA

JOHN BARKS, MD, PhD
Professor, Division Director, Department of Pediatrics and Communicable Diseases, The University of Michigan, Ann Arbor, Michigan, USA

LYNN BITAR, MD, MSc
Post Doctoral Research Fellow, Division of Neonatal-Perinatal Medicine, Department of Pediatrics, University of Texas Southwestern Medical Center, Dallas, Texas, USA

STEPHANIE M. BOYD, MBBS (Hons), BSc (Med), MPHTM, FRACP
Staff Specialist Neonatologist, Grace Centre for Newborn Intensive Care, The Children's Hospital at Westmead, Westmead, New South Wales, Australia; Faculty of Medicine and Health, University of Sydney, Campderdown, New South Wales, Australia

GERALDINE B. BOYLAN, PhD
Director, INFANT Research Centre, University College Cork, Department of Paediatrics and Child Health, University College Cork, Paediatric Academic Unit, Cork University Hospital, Wilton, Cork, Ireland

AOIFE BRANAGAN, MB, MSc
Discipline of Paediatrics, Trinity College Dublin, The University of Dublin, Trinity Translational Medicine Institute (TTMI), St James Hospital and Trinity Research in Childhood Centre (TRiCC), Neonatal Fellow, Department of Paediatrics, The Coombe Hospital, Health Research Board Neonatal Encephalopathy PhD Training Network (NEPTuNE), Dublin, Ireland

CONSTANCE BURGOD, MRes, PhD
Research Associate, Department of Brain Sciences, Centre for Perinatal Neuroscience, Imperial College London, London, United Kingdom

LINA F. CHALAK, MD, MSCS
Professor, Department of Pediatrics, William Buchanan Endowed Chair Professor of Pediatrics and Psychiatry, Division Chief Interim, Neonatal-Perinatal Medicine, Director, Fetal and Neonatal Neurological Intensive Care Unit, Neurological Neonatal Intensive Care Fetal and Neonatal Neurology Fellowship Program, University of Texas Southwestern Medical School, UT Southwestern Medical Center, Dallas, Texas, USA

ALEXA K. CRAIG, MD
Associate Professor, Department of Pediatrics, Tufts University School of Medicine, Boston, Massachusetts; Division of Pediatric Neurology, Department of Pediatrics, The Barbara Bush Children's Hospital at Maine Medical Center, Portland, Maine, USA

JOANNE O. DAVIDSON, PhD
Associate Professor, Departments of Physiology and Paediatrics, University of Auckland, Auckland, New Zealand

LINDA S. DE VRIES, MD, PhD
Emeritus Professor, Department of Neonatology, Leiden University Medical Center, Leiden, The Netherlands

SIMERDEEP K. DHILLON, PhD
Post Doctoral Researcher, Department of Physiology, The University of Auckland, Auckland, New Zealand

STEVEN M. DONN, MD, FAAP, FAARC
Professor Emeritus, Division of Neonatal-Perinatal Medicine, Department of Pediatrics, C.S. Mott Children's Hospital, Michigan Medicine, Ann Arbor, Michigan, USA

ROGER G. FAIX, MD
Professor Emeritus, Department of Pediatrics, University of Utah School of Medicine, Salt Lake City, Utah, USA

JONATHAN M. FANAROFF, MD, JD
Professor, Department of Pediatrics, Case Western Reserve University School of Medicine, Director, Rainbow Center for Pediatric Ethics, Rainbow Babies & Children's Hospital, Cleveland, Ohio, USA

REEMA GAREGRAT, MD, DNB, MRCPCH
Neonatal Neurology Fellow, Department of Brain Sciences, Centre for Perinatal Neuroscience, Imperial College London, London, United Kingdom

HANNAH C. GLASS, MDCM, MAS
Professor, Department of Neurology, University of California San Francisco, San Francisco, California, USA

SHONA C. GOLDSMITH, PhD, BPhty(Hons)
Senior Research Fellow, CP Alliance Research Institute, Specialty of Child and Adolescent Health, Sydney Medical School, Faculty of Medicine and Health, The University of Sydney, Sydney, New South Wales, Australia

PIERRE GRESSENS, MD, PhD
Director, Université Paris Cité, NeuroDiderot, Inserm, Paris, France

ALISTAIR J. GUNN, MBChB, PhD
Professor, Department of Physiology, Faculty of Medical and Health Sciences, The University of Auckland, Auckland, New Zealand

ROD W. HUNT, PhD, FRACP, FRCP(UK)
Professor, Department of Paediatrics, Monash Newborn, Monash Health, Monash University, Clayton, Victoria, Australia; CP Alliance Research Institute, Specialty of Child and Adolescent Health, Sydney Medical School, Faculty of Medicine and Health, The University of Sydney, Sydney, New South Wales, Australia

Dr SIMONE L. HUNTINGFORD, BComm, BSc, MBBS, FRACP
Neonatal Neurology Fellow, Department of Paediatrics, Monash Newborn, Monash Health, Monash University, Clayton, Victoria, Australia; Staff Specialist Neonatologist, Paediatric Infant Perinatal Emergency Retrieval, Royal Children's Hospital, Parkville, Victoria, Australia

TERRIE INDER, MBChB, MD
Director for Neonatal Research, Neonatologist and Child Neurologist, Children's Hospital of Orange County, University of California, Irvine, California, USA

SANDRA E. JUUL, MD, PhD
Director and Professor, Institute on Human Development and Disability, Division of Neonatology, Department of Pediatrics, University of Washington, Seattle, Washington, USA

WENDY C. KING, PhD
Professor, Department of Epidemiology, School of Public Health, University of Pittsburgh, Pittsburgh, Pennsylvania, USA

ABBOT R. LAPTOOK, MD
Professor, Department of Pediatrics, Warren Alpert School of Medicine, Women and Infants Hospital of Rhode Island, Providence, Rhode Island, USA

MONICA LEMMON, MD
Associate Professor, Division of Pediatric Neurology and Developmental Medicine, Departments of Pediatrics and Population Health Sciences, Duke University School of Medicine, Durham, North California, USA

MICHELLE MACHIE, MD
Assistant Professor, Division of Pediatric Neurology, Department of Pediatrics, Neurology and Neurotherapeutics, University of Texas Southwestern Medical Center, Dallas, Texas, USA

SARAH J. McINTYRE, PhD, MPS, BAppSc (OT) Hons
Senior Research Fellow, CP Alliance Research Institute, Specialty of Child and Adolescent Health, Sydney Medical School, Faculty of Medicine and Health, The University of Sydney, Sydney, New South Wales, Australia

MARK R. MERCURIO, MD, MA
Professor, Director, Program for Biomedical Ethics, Department of Pediatrics, Yale University School of Medicine, New Haven, Connecticut, USA

ELEANOR J. MOLLOY, MB, PhD
Discipline of Paediatrics, Trinity College Dublin, The University of Dublin, Trinity Translational Medicine Institute (TTMI), St James Hospital and Trinity Research in Childhood Centre (TRiCC), Department of Paediatrics, The Coombe Hospital, Health Research Board Neonatal Encephalopathy PhD Training Network (NEPTuNE), Ireland, Department of Neonatology, Children's Health Ireland, Neurodisability, Children's Health Ireland (CHI) at Tallaght, Consultant Neonatologist and Paediatrician, Department of Paediatrics, Trinity Centre for Health Sciences, Tallaght University Hospital, Dublin, Ireland

SARA MUNOZ-BLANCO, MD
Assistant Professor, Department of Pediatrics, Johns Hopkins School of Medicine, Divisions of Perinatal-Neonatal Medicine, and Pediatric Palliative Care, Department of Pediatrics, Johns Hopkins Children's Center, Baltimore, Maryland, USA

PALLAVI MURALEEDHARAN, MHA, PhD
Research Associate, Department of Brain Sciences, Centre for Perinatal Neuroscience, Imperial College London, London, United Kingdom

DEIRDRE M. MURRAY, MD, PhD
INFANT Research Centre, University College Cork, CPF Chair in Early Brain Injury and Cerebral Palsy, Department of Paediatrics and Child Health, University College Cork, Paediatric Academic Unit, Cork University Hospital, Wilton, Cork, Ireland

KARIN B. NELSON, MD
Scientist Emeritus, National Institutes of Health, National Institute of Neurological Diseases and Stroke, Washington, DC, USA

JOHN M. O'TOOLE, PhD
INFANT Research Centre, University College Cork, Ireland; Cergenx Ltd., Dublin, Ireland

BETSY PILON, BA
Hope for HIE, West Bloomfield, Michigan, USA

JACOPO PROIETTI, MD
Assistant Professor, Department of Engineering for Innovation Medicine, University of Verona, Verona, Italy; Visiting Fellow, INFANT Research Centre, University College Cork, Cork, Ireland

MARK S. SCHER, MD
Emeritus Scholar and Professor, Division of Pediatric Neurology, Department of Pediatrics, Fetal/Neonatal Neurology Program, Case Western Reserve University School

of Medicine, Rainbow Babies and Children's Hospital, MacDonald Hospital for Women, University Hospitals Cleveland Medical Center, Shaker Heights, Ohio, USA

POLLIEANNA SEPULVEDA, BS, MSN
Research Program Manager, Department of Pediatrics, Neonatal-Perinatal Medicine, University of Texas Southwestern Medical School, Dallas, Texas, USA

SEETHA SHANKARAN, MD
Professor, Department of Pediatrics, University of Texas at Austin an Dell Medical School, Austin, Texas; Department of Neonatal-Perinatal Medicine, Wayne State University, Detroit, Michigan

RENÉE A. SHELLHAAS, MD, MS
Professor of Neurology, Senior Associate Dean for Faculty Promotions and Career Development, Washington University in St Louis, St Louis, Missouri, USA

JONATHAN L. SLAUGHTER, MD, MPH
Associate Professor, Department of Pediatrics and Epidemiology, Center for Perinatal Research, Nationwide Children's Hospital, Colleges of Medicine and Public Health, The Ohio State University, Columbus, Ohio, USA

BARBARA S. STONESTREET, MD
Professor (Emeritus), Department of Pediatrics, Women & Infants Hospital of Rhode Island, Providence, Adjunct Professor of Molecular Biology, Cell Biology and Biochemistry, The Alpert Medical School of Brown University, Barrington, Rhode Island, USA

SUDHIN THAYYIL, MD, FRCPCH, PhD
Professor of Perinatal Neuroscience, Department of Brain Sciences, Centre for Perinatal Neuroscience, Imperial College London, London, United Kingdom

REGINA L. TRIPLETT, MD, MS
Clinical Instructor, Department of Neurology, Washington University in St Louis, Saint Louis, Missouri, USA

STEPHEN R. WISNIEWSKI, PhD
Professor, Department of Epidemiology, School of Public Health, Vice Provost for Budget and Analytics, University of Pittsburgh, Pittsburgh, Pennsylvania, USA

THOMAS R. WOOD, BM BCh, PhD
Associate Professor, Division of Neonatology, Department of Pediatrics, Institute on Human Development and Disability, University of Washington, Seattle, Washington, USA

Contents

Neurologic depression in term/near-term neonates (neonatal encephalopathy, NE) is uncommon with modern obstetric care. Asphyxial birth, with or without co-factors, accounts for a minority of NE, while maldevelopment (congenital malformations, growth aberrations, genetic, metabolic and placental abnormalities) plays an enlarging role in identifying etiologic subgroups of NE. The terms NE and hypoxic-ischemic encephalopathy (HIE) have not been employed uniformly, hampering research and clinical care. The authors propose the term NE as an early working-diagnosis, to be supplemented by a diagnosis of NE due to HIE or to other factors, as a final diagnosis once workup is complete.

Reproductive, pregnancy, and placental exposomes influence the fetal neural exposome through toxic stressor interplay, impairing the maternal-placental-fetal (MPF) triad. Neonatal encephalopathy represents different clinical presentations based on complex time-dependent etiopathogenetic mechanisms including hypoxia-ischemia that challenge diagnosis and prognosis. Reproductive, pregnancy, and placental exposomes impair the fetal neural exposome through toxic stressor interplay within the MPF triad. Long intervals often separate disease onset from phenotype. Interdisciplinary fetal-neonatal neurology training, practice, and research closes this knowledge gap. Maintaining reproductive health preserves MPF triad health with life-course benefits.

The etiology of perinatal brain injury is multifactorial, but exposure to perinatal hypoxiaischemia (HI) is a major underlying factor. This review discusses the role of exposure to infection/inflammation in the evolution of HI brain injury, changes in immune responsiveness to subsequent inflammatory challenges after HI and modulation of neural outcomes with interaction between perinatal HI and inflammatory insults. The authors critically

Mild Encephalopathy (COOLPRIME), which uses sites' existing mild hypoxic-ischemic encephalopathy (HIE) treatment preference (hypothermia or normothermia) to assess hypothermia effectiveness and safety. COOLPRIME's primary aim is to determine the safety and effectiveness of hypothermia compared to normothermia in mild HIE. Engagement of Families and Community Affected by Hypoxic-Ischemic Encephalopathy strongly favored Effectiveness over Efficacy Trials leading to COOL PRIME design.

Lynn Bitar, Barbara S. Stonestreet, and Lina F. Chalak

This article summarizes the current evidence regarding inflammatory biomarkers (placental and postnatal) and provides a comprehensive understanding of their roles: (1) diagnostic accuracy to predict the severity of hypoxic-ischemia encephalopathy (HIE), (2) value in assessing treatment responses, and (3) prediction of both short- and long-term neurodevelopmental outcomes. In the early critical stages of perinatal asphyxia, inflammatory biomarkers may guide clinical decision-making. Additional research is required to increase our understanding of the optimal utility of biomarkers to predict the severity, evolution, and developmental outcomes after exposure to HIE.

Michelle Machie, Linda S. de Vries, and Terrie Inder

MRI of the brain is a critical tool in the diagnosis, evaluation, and management of neonatal encephalopathy (NE). More than simply a diagnostic and prognostic tool, MRI informs the biology, nature, and timing of the disease process resulting in NE, of which the largest single etiology is hypoxic-ischemic encephalopathy (HIE). Historically, 2 major patterns of injury were seen in HIE: a basal ganglia/thalamus predominant pattern and a watershed pattern of injury. The advent of therapeutic hypothermia for NE/HIE, alongside improvements in the application of imaging technology in newborn infants, has resulted in progressively more advanced MRI scoring systems.

Jacopo Proietti, John M. O'Toole, Deirdre M. Murray, and Geraldine B. Boylan

Electroencephalography (EEG) is a key objective biomarker of newborn brain function, delivering critical, cotside insights to aid the management of encephalopathy. Access to continuous EEG is limited, forcing reliance on subjective clinical assessments. In hypoxia ischaemia, the primary cause of encephalopathy, alterations in EEG patterns correlate with. injury severity and evolution. As HIE evolves, causing secondary neuronal death, EEG can track injury progression, informing neuroprotective strategies, seizure management and prognosis. Despite its value, challenges with interpretation and lack of on site expertise has limited its broader adoption. Technological advances, particularly in digital EEG and machine learning, are enhancing real-time analysis. This will allow EEG to expand its role in HIE diagnosis, management and outcome prediction.

Hypoxic-ischemic encephalopathy in low resource settings is associated with low occurrence of perinatal sentinel events, growth restriction, short birth depression, early seizure onset, white matter injury, and non-acute hypoxia on whole genome expression profile suggesting that intra-partum hypoxia might be occurring from a normal or augmented labor process in an already compromised fetus. Induced hypothermia increases mortality and does not reduce brain injury. Strict adherence to the updated National Neonatology forum guidelines is essential to prevent harm from induced hypothermia in low resource settings.

Hypoxic ischemic encephalopathy (HIE) is the most common cause of neonatal encephalopathy and results in significant morbidity and mortality. Long-term outcomes of the condition encompass impairments across all developmental domains. While therapeutic hypothermia (TH) has improved outcomes for term and late preterm infants with moderate to severe HIE, trials are ongoing to investigate the use of TH for infants with mild or preterm HIE. There is no evidence that adjuvant therapies in combination with TH improve long-term outcomes. Numerous trials of various adjuvant therapies are underway in the quest to further improve outcomes for infants with HIE.

Parents of newborns with hypoxic ischemic encephalopathy (HIE) can face communication challenges in the neonatal intensive care unit. Both specialty palliative care and primary palliative care trained clinicians can assist parents as they navigate traumatic experiences and uncertain prognoses. Using evidence-based frameworks, the authors provide samples of how to communicate with parents and promote parent well-being across the care trajectory. The authors demonstrate how to involve parents in a shared decision-making process and give special consideration to the complexities of hospital discharge and the transition home. Sustained investment to guide the development of effective communication skills is crucial to support families of infants with HIE.

Hypoxic ischemic encephalopathy (HIE) in neonates can cause severe, life-long functional impairments or death. Treatment of these neonates can involve ethically challenging questions about if, when, and how it may be appropriate to limit life-sustaining medical therapy. Further, parents whose infants suffer severe neurologic damage may seek recourse in the form of a medical malpractice lawsuit. This study uses several hypothetical cases to highlight important ethical and legal considerations in the care of infants with HIE.

Sandra E. Juul and Thomas R. Wood

Historically, neonatal neuroscience boasted a robust and successful preclinical pipeline for therapeutic interventions, in particular for the treatment of hypoxic-ischemic encephalopathy (HIE). However, since the successful translation of therapeutic hypothermia (TH), several high-profile failures of promising adjunctive therapies, in addition to the lack of benefit of TH in lower resource settings, have brought to light critical issues in that same pipeline. Using recent data from clinical trials of erythropoietin as an example, the authors highlight several key challenges facing preclinical neonatal neuroscience for HIE therapeutic development and propose key areas where model development and collaboration across the field in general can ensure ongoing success in treatment development for HIE worldwide.

PROGRAM OBJECTIVE
The goal of *Clinics in Perinatology* is to keep practicing perinatologists, neonatologists, obstetricians, practicing physicians and residents up to date with current clinical practice in perinatology by providing timely articles reviewing the state of the art in patient care.

TARGET AUDIENCE
Perinatologists, neonatologists, obstetricians, practicing physicians, residents and healthcare professionals who provide patient care utilizing findings from *Clinics in Perinatology*.

LEARNING OBJECTIVES
Upon completion of this activity, participants will be able to:
1. Recognize perinatal brain injury is multifactorial.
2. Discuss established therapies to improve neurodevelopment outcomes after hypoxic-ischemic encephalopathy (HIE).
3. Review EEG as an objective biomarker for hypoxic-ischemic encephalopathy (HIE), assisting in the assessment of HIE severity, treatment guidance, seizure detection, and outcome prediction.

ACCREDITATION
The Elsevier Office of Continuing Medical Education (EOCME) is accredited by the Accreditation Council for Continuing Medical Education (ACCME) to provide continuing medical education for physicians.

The EOCME designates this journal-based CME activity for a maximum of 15 *AMA PRA Category 1 Credit*(s)™. Physicians should claim only the credit commensurate with the extent of their participation in the activity.

All other health care professionals requesting continuing education credit for this enduring material will be issued a certificate of participation.

DISCLOSURE OF CONFLICTS OF INTEREST
The EOCME assesses conflict of interest with its instructors, faculty, planners, and other individuals who are in a position to control the content of CME activities. All relevant conflicts of interest that are identified are thoroughly vetted by EOCME for fair balance, scientific objectivity, and patient care recommendations. EOCME is committed to providing its learners with CME activities that promote improvements or quality in healthcare and not a specific proprietary business or a commercial interest.

The planning committee, staff, authors, and editors listed below have identified no financial relationships or relationships to products or devices they or their spouse/life partner have with commercial interest related to the content of this CME activity:
Afaf Ahmed, MBBS; Tayyba Anwar, MD; Nada Badawi, PhD; Nadia Badawi, AM; Alice C. Baker, MD, MPH; John Barks, MD, PhD; Nitesh Barthwal; Lynn Bitar, MD, MSc; Stephanie M. Boyd, MBBS(Hons), BS (Med), MPHTM, FRACP; Aoife Branagan, MSc; Constance Burgod, MRes, PhD; Lina F. Chalak, MD, MSCS; Alexa K. Craig, MD; Joanne O. Davidson, PhD; Linda S. de Vries, MD, PhD; Simerdeep K. Dhillon, PhD; Steven M. Donn, MD, FAAP, FAARC; Roger G. Faix, MD; Jonathan M. Fanaroff, MD, JD; Reema Garegrat, MD, DNB, MRCPCH; Hannah C. Glass, MDCM, MAS; Shona C. Goldsmith, PhD, BPhty(Hons); Pierre Gressens, MD, PhD; Alistair J. Gunn, MBChB, PhD; Kerry Holland; Rod W. Hunt, PhD, FRACP, FRCP(UK); Simone L. Huntingford, BComm/BSc, MBBS, FRACP; Terrie Inder, MBChB, MD; Lucky Jain, MD, MBA; Sandra E. Juul, MD, PhD; Wendy C. King, PhD; Abbot R. Laptook, MD; Monica Lemmon, MD; Michelle Littlejohn; Michelle Machie, MD; Sarah J. McIntyre, PhD, MPS, BAppSc(OT) Hons; Mark R. Mercurio, MD, MA; Eleanor J. Molloy, PhD; Sara Munoz-Blanco, MD; Pallavi Muraleedharan, MHA, PhD; Karin B. Nelson, MD; John M. O'Toole, PhD; Betsy Pilon; Jacopo Proietti, MD; Mark S. Scher, MD; Seetha Shankaran, MD; Renée A. Shellhaas, MD, MS; Jonathan L. Slaughter, MD, MPH; Barbara Stonestreet, MD; Jeyanthi Surendrakumar; Sudhin Thayyil, MD, FRCPCH, PhD; Regina L. Triplett, MD, MS; Stephen R. Wisniewski, PhD; Thomas R. Wood, BM BCh, PhD

The planning committee, staff, authors, and editors listed below have identified financial relationships or relationships to products or devices they or their spouse/life partner have with commercial interest related to the content of this CME activity:
Geraldine B. Boylan, PhD: *Consultant*: Nihon Kohden; Ownership Interest: Kephala Ltd, CergenX Ltd

Deirdre M. Murray, MD, PhD: *Ownership Interest*: Liltoda Ltd

UNAPPROVED/OFF-LABEL USE DISCLOSURE

The EOCME requires CME faculty to disclose to the participants:

1. When products or procedures being discussed are off-label, unlabelled, experimental, and/or investigational (not US Food and Drug Administration [FDA] approved); and
2. Any limitations on the information presented, such as data that are preliminary or that represent ongoing research, interim analyses, and/or unsupported opinions. Faculty may discuss information about pharmaceutical agents that is outside of FDA-approved labelling. This information is intended solely for CME and is not intended to promote off-label use of these medications. If you have any questions, contact the medical affairs department of the manufacturer for the most recent prescribing information.

TO ENROLL

To enroll in the *Clinics in Perinatology* Continuing Medical Education program, call customer service at 1-800-654-2452 or sign up online at http://www.theclinics.com/home/cme. The CME program is available to subscribers for an additional annual fee of USD 254.00.

METHOD OF PARTICIPATION

In order to claim credit, participants must complete the following:

1. Complete enrolment as indicated above.
2. Read the activity.
3. Complete the CME Test and Evaluation. Participants must achieve a score of 70% on the test. All CME Tests and Evaluations must be completed online.

CME INQUIRIES/SPECIAL NEEDS

For all CME inquiries or special needs, please contact elsevierCME@elsevier.com.

CLINICS IN PERINATOLOGY

SERIES OF RELATED INTEREST

Obstetrics and Gynecology Clinics of North America
https://www.obgyn.theclinics.com

THE CLINICS ARE AVAILABLE ONLINE!
Access your subscription at:
www.theclinics.com

Foreword

Perinatal Asphyxia: Moving a Mountain

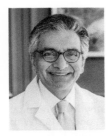

Lucky Jain, MD, MBA
Consulting Editor

Perinatal asphyxia continues to be a major cause of morbidity and mortality worldwide.[1,2] It is estimated that nearly 1 to 2 million babies across the globe die of birth asphyxia or suffer from its disabling consequences.[1] That number rivals nearly half of all births in the United States in any given year! The needle on this troubling statistic has largely stayed stuck, despite the many advances in maternal-fetal and neonatal care, which have transformed the survival of preterm babies after birth and have had a similar positive impact on outcome of babies with birth anomalies. In fact, recent studies show a paradoxical rise in perinatal hypoxic ischemic encephalopathy, albeit in limited cohorts (**Fig. 1**).[2]

Part of the problem lies in the complex nature of the problem with overlapping causes that are often hard to diagnose. The interplay between multiple causes of fetal compromise includes placental malperfusion, toxemia of pregnancy, and intrauterine hypoxia. Regardless of the cause, the consequences are all too familiar and can be devastating.

As Dr Chalak and the many esteemed authors in this issue of the *Clinics in Perinatology* point out, we need to start with standardization of definitions and terminology. There is hope that newer approaches, such as artificial intelligence and machine learning, will lead to earlier and more accurate appreciation of fetal jeopardy. A deeper look into the reproductive and pregnancy exposome may also yield new information about the maternal-placental-fetal interactions that are critical to a good outcome.

I want to congratulate Dr Chalak for assembling a true state-of-the-art offering on this subject. As always, I am grateful to the authors for their valuable contributions and to my publishing partners at Elsevier (Kerry Holland and Nitesh Barthwal) for their help in bringing this valuable resource to you. It may be hard to move the mountain of

Clin Perinatol 51 (2024) xix–xx
https://doi.org/10.1016/j.clp.2024.06.002
0095-5108/24/© 2024 Published by Elsevier Inc.

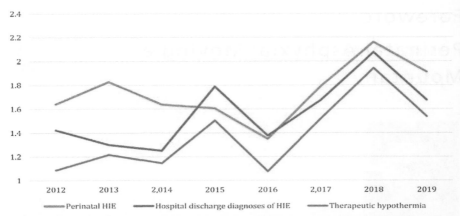

Fig. 1. Population incidence of perinatal hypoxic ischemic encephalopathy (HIE), hospital discharge diagnosis of HIE, and therapeutic hypothermia between 2012 and 2019. (With permission from Cornet M-C, Kuzniewicz M, Scheffler A, Forquer H, Hamilton E, Newman TB, Wu YW. Perinatal hypoxic ischemic encephalopathy: Incidence over time within a modern US birth cohort. Pediatr Neurol 2023 Dec:149:145-150. (Page 148).)

perinatal asphyxia, but we can surely begin by moving the "needle" in the right direction!

Lucky Jain, MD, MBA
Department of Pediatrics
Emory University School of Medicine
Children's Healthcare of Atlanta
2015 Uppergate Drive Northeast
Atlanta, GA 30322, USA

E-mail address:
ljain@emory.edu

REFERENCES

1. Jain L. Birth asphyxia and the inextricable intersection of fetal and neonatal physiology. Clin Perinatol 2016;43:xv–xvii.
2. Cornet M-C, Kuzniewicz M, Scheffler A, et al. Perinatal hypoxic ischemic encephalopathy: Incidence over time within a modern US birth cohort. Pediatr Neurol 2023;149:145–50.

Preface

Moving the Needle in Perinatal Asphyxia

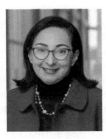

Lina F. Chalak, MD, MSCS
Editor

The last decade has witnessed remarkable strides in understanding, diagnosing, and managing perinatal asphyxia—a condition deemed nonmodifiable and managed solely with supportive care when I started my career in this topic over twenty-five years ago. I was fortunate to participate in the early translational preclinical studies among esteemed colleagues to establish mechanisms of neuroprotection with therapeutic hypothermia. This preclinical work translated into the first clinical hypothermia trials establishing a standard of care throughout the world in high-income countries for infants with moderate to severe hypoxic-ischemic encephalopathy.

This special issue of *Clinics in Perinatology* aims to illuminate the key developments and reflect on whether, collectively, we have succeeded in significantly altering the trajectory of perinatal asphyxia outcomes by delving into the advancements, breakthroughs, and challenges encountered in our collective endeavor to "move the needle" in perinatal asphyxia.

EARLY DETECTION AND DIAGNOSIS

One pivotal area of progress is the early detection and diagnosis of perinatal asphyxia. Improved understanding of antenatal and intrapartum risk factors, coupled with the widespread adoption of advanced imaging technologies and biomarker assessments, has enhanced our ability to identify at-risk pregnancies and intervene proactively. This special issue explores the impact of these advancements on reducing the incidence of perinatal asphyxia and improving outcomes. Finally, the launch of Cooling Effectivness Trial prospective Investigation of Mild Encephalopathy (COOL PRIME), a comparative effectiveness trial of mild hypoxic ischemic encephalopathy (HIE), offers to address the current conundrum of care after a decade of work to validate an early definition of mild HIE.

Clin Perinatol 51 (2024) xxi–xxiii
https://doi.org/10.1016/j.clp.2024.06.001
0095-5108/24/© 2024 Published by Elsevier Inc.

perinatology.theclinics.com

NEUROPROTECTIVE MODALITIES

The quest for effective neuroprotective strategies and treatment modalities has been a focal point of research and clinical trials in perinatal asphyxia. This decade focuses on new neuroprotective trials evaluating the expansion of treatment to other vulnerable unstudied populations and combination of added interventions. Three hypothermia trials since the first were sponsored by The Neonatal Research Network of the Eunice Kennedy Shriver National Institute of Child Health and Human Development in order to evaluate possible optimization of treatment (1) with deeper and longer cooling and (2) to determine if the eligibility window could be expanded to infants identified beyond the first 6 hours after birth, and (3) to the late preterm born at 33 0/7 to 35 6/7 weeks' gestational age. Safety is an important aspect of extending hypothermia or any neuroprotective therapy to new populations, including low- and middle-income countries. Similarly, trials funded by NINDS have demonstrated the lack of efficacy of erythropoietin injections in the term and preterm newborns at risk for asphyxia. The lessons learned from the negative trials and from translational models are discussed. This special issue explores the outcomes of these landmark studies and trials that have sought to minimize brain damage and improve the neurodevelopmental trajectories of infants affected by perinatal asphyxia.

While celebrating progress, it is equally important to acknowledge the persistent challenges and uncharted territories in perinatal asphyxia research and clinical practice. We address what barriers still impede access to care for developing countries with unmet needs.

Finally, it has been indeed a true privilege to have the world experts in neonatal asphyxia lend their knowledge and experience to create the state-of-the-art issue, and I am most grateful for their contributions. This special issue serves as a comprehensive exploration of the multifaceted journey we have undertaken in the last decade to alter the trajectory of perinatal asphyxia. Through insightful research contributions, we reflect on the past decade and envision a future where perinatal asphyxia is significantly mitigated, ensuring a healthier start for every newborn.

DEDICATION

I dedicate this issue to the memories of Dr Maria Papavoulous and Dr Tae Chung, whom we lost this year. Their contributions, though, are forever part of moving the needle in perinatal asphyxia. My personal gratitude to Abbot Laptook, Jeffrey Perlman, and Donna Ferriero, who set exacting standards for my career with their own trajectories, as well as to all my colleagues partnering in COOLPRIME for the amazing esprit de corps. This special issue is also dedicated to my colleagues in neonatal neurology, as collaborative teamwork has been a shared trait in our field.

DISCLOSURES

None.

FUNDING

Dr Lina F. Chalak is funded by NIH Grant 5R01NS102617, Patient-Centered Outcomes Research Institute® (PCORI®) Award. The views, statements, opinions presented in this work are solely the responsibility of the author(s) and do not necessarily represent the views of the PCORI®.

Lina F. Chalak, MD, MSCS
Neonatal–Perinatal Medicine
Fetal and Neonatal Neurological Intensive Care Unit/Fellowship Program
Department of Pediatrics
University of Texas Southwestern Medical School
5323 Harry Hines Boulevard
Dallas, TX 75390-9063, USA

E-mail address:
Lina.Chalak@utsouthwestern.edu

Causes and Terminology in Neonatal Encephalopathy

What is in a Name? Neonatal Encephalopathy, Hypoxic-ischemic Encephalopathy or Perinatal Asphyxia

Aoife Branagan, MB, MSc[a,b,c,d], Eleanor J. Molloy, MB, PhD[a,b,c,d,e,f,g,*], Nadia Badawi, MB, PhD[h,i,j], Karin B. Nelson, MD[k]

KEYWORDS

- Neonatal encephalopathy • Hypoxic ischemic encephalopathy • Perinatal asphyxia
- Brain injury

KEY POINTS

- Clinical research indicates that with modern obstetrics only a minority of neonatal encephalopathy (NE) is related to perinatal deprivation of oxygen, still less to oxygen deprivation only.
- Studies of genetics/genomics, metabolic disease, and the placenta are proving informative in identifying pathogenic pathways and etiologic subgroups in NE.
- Uniformity of definitions, agreement on study inclusions and exclusions, and a core set of descriptors of outcome would increase the comparability of datasets across studies of NE.

[a] Discipline of Paediatrics, Trinity College Dublin, The University of Dublin, Dublin, Ireland; [b] Trinity Translational Medicine Institute (TTMI), St James Hospital & Trinity Research in Childhood Centre (TRiCC), Dublin, Ireland; [c] Department of Paediatrics, The Coombe Hospital, 32 Kickham Road, Inchicore, Dublin 8, Dublin D08W2T0, Ireland; [d] Health Research Board Neonatal Encephalopathy PhD Training Network (NEPTuNE), Ireland; [e] Department of Neonatology, Children's Health Ireland, Dublin, Ireland; [f] Neurodisability, Children's Health Ireland (CHI) at Tallaght, Dublin, Ireland; [g] Department of Paediatrics, Trinity Centre for Health Sciences, Tallaght University Hospital, Dublin 24, Ireland; [h] Cerebral Palsy Alliance Research Institute, Specialty of Child & Adolescent Health, Sydney Medical School; [i] Faculty of Medicine & Health, Department of Paediatrics, The University of Sydney, PO Box 171, Allambie Heights, Sydney, New South Wales 2100, Australia; [j] Grace Centre for Newborn Intensive Care, Sydney Children's Hospital Network, The University of Sydney, Westmead, New South Wales, Australia; [k] National Institutes of Health, National Institute of Neurological Diseases and Stroke, 050 Military Road NEW, Apt 815, Washington, DC 20015, USA
* Corresponding author. Department of Paediatrics, Trinity Centre for Health Sciences, Tallaght University Hospital, Dublin 24, Ireland.
E-mail address: Eleanor.molloy@tcd.ie

Clin Perinatol 51 (2024) 521–534
https://doi.org/10.1016/j.clp.2024.04.015
0095-5108/24/© 2024 Elsevier Inc. All rights are reserved, including those for text and data mining, AI training, and similar technologies.
perinatology.theclinics.com

INTRODUCTION

Experimental and clinical observations make it clear that severe and prolonged deprivation of oxygen in the fetus/neonate can lead to injury to the brain and to increased mortality and neurologic morbidity. Neonatal encephalopathy (NE), hypoxic-ischemic encephalopathy (HIE), and perinatal asphyxia are terms used in clinical practice and medical literature to describe this brain injury. However, many non-asphyxial factors can cause or contribute to NE. It is now widely agreed that HIE is the subset of NE that is due to birth asphyxia, either as a sole etiology or, more commonly, as a contributing factor. Yet the terms NE and HIE continue to be used with differing meanings or interchangeably, causing confusion for clinicians, researchers, and families.

Why has it been so difficult achieve clarity about terms describing neurologic depression in the human infant? A newborn has a limited range of ways to manifest illness, and these are chiefly nonspecific, so that identifying the causal pathway in each infant requires thoughtful investigation. The chief treatment for NE is therapeutic hypothermia, which is most effective if begun early[1] so decisions about treatment must take place in a brief period and a hectic setting, with an ill infant and an immediately post-partum mother. Most births of term infants with encephalopathy take place at outlying hospitals and facilities, and records of family history, pregnancy, and birth are often sparse. There are pressing needs to obtain informed parental consents for treatment and transport (including placenta, and genetic studies particularly if the infant is *in extremis*). Thus, there is an immediate need for a descriptive working diagnosis based on rapid clinical assessment. Later, there is need for a final diagnosis that incorporates information derived from later-performed diagnostic procedures, review of records, and initial follow-up.

The authors propose that NE is the initial working diagnosis, to be followed by NE due to X cause, as investigation reveals (**Fig. 1**). *If HIE is a final diagnosis, that means NE due to HIE, when other conditions have been excluded.*

NE has been defined by the American College of Obstetricians and Gynecologists/ American Academy of Pediatrics (ACOG-AAP) as a "clinical syndrome of disturbed neurologic function in the first week after birth in an infant born at or beyond 35 weeks of gestation, manifested by an abnormal level of consciousness or seizures, often accompanied by difficulty with initiating and maintaining respiration and depression of tone and reflexes."[2] NE is a leading cause of neonatal death and disability in term and near-term infants, affecting 1.2 million infants globally per year. Up to 96% of those affected by NE are born in low-to-middle income countries,[3] where there are few effective neuroprotective strategies.[4,5] NE is a descriptive diagnosis. An early diagnosis of NE does not imply a specific or known etiology and as discussed later in this article, a variety of pathobiological states can present with these findings. A specific etiologic diagnosis is highly desirable because of implications for treatment, prognosis, and family planning. The more thorough the diagnostic process, the more likely it is that an underlying contributing or determinative pathology is identified.[6]

HIE is a subgroup of NE. The occurrence of a "sentinel event" around the time of birth, such as a cord accident or uterine rupture, suggest HIE, but many neonates with NE have not experienced abnormal birth events. Low Apgar scores and acidosis are consistent with HIE but are themselves consequences of prior processes and do not establish the nature of the initiating process. Genetic vulnerabilities may differ.[7] ACOG-AAP recommend that HIE be used as a final diagnosis only when diagnostic studies have been completed. Sometimes, despite best efforts during the neonatal period, the diagnosis may not be made until many years later or following the birth of another sibling with a similar presentation.

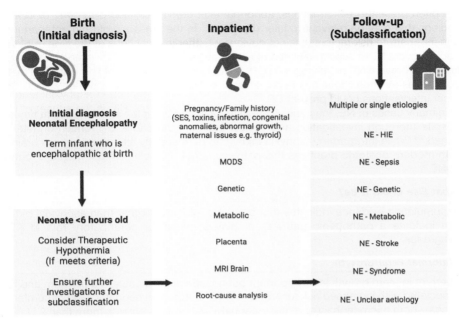

Fig. 1. Neonatal encephalopathy: Moving from an initial diagnosis to a subclassification. At birth a term infant who has signs of encephalopathy should be diagnosed as having NE. Following initial resuscitation and where indicated, therapeutic hypothermia commenced, further thorough investigations are required to subclassify the etiologic diagnosis.

The relevance of experimental models of birth asphyxia to human NE/HIE cannot be assumed. In animal models, the fetus/infant is usually the product of an uncomplicated pregnancy and birth, and the dose and duration of hypoxia ischemia are controlled, so the term HIE can be used precisely. In contrast, events in human neonates are often complex, with a range of prenatal complications whose impact on outcome is difficult to establish. Abnormal births often follow abnormal pregnancies. It is likely that much HIE is a culmination of a cascade of events.[8,9]

How Much of Neonatal Encephalopathy is Hypoxic-ischemic Encephalopathy?

In the few controlled studies of NE in defined populations in modern obstetric settings, most infants with NE have not experienced asphyxial birth, and especially not asphyxia *only*.[8–10] Risk factors are often multiple and may interact. A prospective population-based study reported an acute intrapartum event in 4% of 164 term infants with moderate or severe NE, while 69% had only antenatal risk factors and 24% had a mixture of antenatal and intrapartum risks.[8] The medical histories of asphyxiated neonates are often complicated and are not uniformly recorded. For example, one of the main risk factors for HIE is placental abruption. Early defects in the development of deep placental vascularization may play an important role in abruption and influence its severity.[11] Abruption has its own set of risk factors, including maternal autoimmune disease or cocaine use which are not always recorded.[12]

Cerebral palsy (CP) is a highly feared outcome in infants with NE and is often attributed to asphyxial birth, sometimes on slender evidence. Features of asphyxial birth were present more often in children with a later diagnosis of CP than in controls, but the difference in those frequencies was not large.[13–16] Furthermore, non-asphyxial conditions are often present—malformations, abnormal fetal growth, clotting disorders, or other findings that may be relevant to later disability.[17] In the presence of both antepartum and intrapartum risk factors, it is not obvious whether interventions at the time of birth could prevent NE or subsequent neurologic disability. Few intrapartum interventions are known to prevent NE or later spastic CP. A Cochrane review did not find evidence that continuous electronic fetal monitoring in labor or treatment of severe pre-eclampsia or other interventions could prevent CP.[18]

In many cases of NE, the cause is multifactorial and complex in origin, and at times despite thorough investigation and clinical acumen, the cause will remain undetermined.[10] While intrapartum asphyxia injury can permanently alter the newborn brain, with modern obstetric practices this pathway is not the sole or most frequent route to NE.

What Else Could It Be?

Accumulating evidence indicates that a number of factors other than asphyxial birth can indicate a pathogenic pathway or play a causal or contributory role in NE subgroups.[19,20]

Abnormal Fetal Growth

Aberrant in utero growth is an important but nonspecific indicator of a problem and is associated with increased risk for NE[8] and CP.[21,22] Unusual neonatal head circumferences—both microcephaly and macrocephaly, with measurements more than 2 standard deviations above or below norms for gestational age and gender—are risk factors for abnormal neurologic outcome.[21,22] Normal head size at birth followed by deceleration of head growth over the next months, with crossing of grid lines, is consistent with brain-destructive perinatal disorders or progressive disease. As with head size, both excessive and insufficient fetal growth are associated with increased risk.[21,22] Poor fetal growth in a child with one or more major malformations is associated with especially high risk of later neurologic abnormality. Environmental toxins, including the ubiquitous PFASs, have joined the lengthy list of exposures that can impair fetal growth.[23]

Birth Defects

Major congenital malformations are strongly associated with risk of NE.[24] Birth defects are also strongly associated with poor fetal growth; a combination that is present in many infants survivors of NE who develop CP.[14] In a large population-based study, co-existence of aberrant fetal growth and malformations was much more common than asphyxial birth in infants with later-recognized CP.[14] Improved imaging should enable earlier diagnosis of malformations in growth-restricted infants and thus identify heightened CP risk.

In infants with congenital heart defects, adverse neurologic outcomes may relate to acute postnatal events, including diagnostic and therapeutic interventions, but cardiac and brain malformations may coexist before any intervention.[25,26]

Placenta

The placenta is a temporary but critical organ, with unique genes and processes. Successful placental development is critical for survival and optimal development of the fetus. Maternal stressors may impact on placental gene expression, perhaps affecting DNA methylation, cell cycle regulation, and epigenetic pathways.[27]

Even gross examination of the placenta and cord, conducted routinely by trained medical personnel, can be informative: in a population-based study, gross placental infarcts were 8 times more frequent in children with later-identified spastic CP and were concentrated in survivors of NE.[28]

Babies with NE commonly have abnormal placentas, whether or not their births were considered asphyxial.[29-32] Recent reports, many using the Amsterdam consensus criteria,[33] have divided placental findings into maternal vascular malperfusion, fetal vascular malperfusion (FVM; including umbilical cord lesions), acute chorioamnionitis, and chronic villitis, or combinations of these lesions.[34] FVM, characterized by reduced or absent perfusion of the fetal villous parenchyma, may be of special relevance to NE.[32,35-37] FVM may also be associated with fetal growth restriction and with later neurologic and development disorders.[38] FVM is thought to originate before the final 48 hours preceding birth and was observed 3 to 4 times more often in infants with NE than controls.[8,39] FVM was often associated with abnormal electronic fetal monitoring patterns in labor and, therefore with emergency caesarean section, a sequence suggestive of birth asphyxia, but the placental changes and poor fetal growth predate the onset of labor.

Evidence of placental inflammation is more frequently observed in the placentas of term infants with NE than in controls (see the later discussion in this article). Placental infection can mimic birth asphyxia, perhaps via interference with and prolongation of labor, and possibly through effects on fetal movements that contribute to normal labor. Placental inflammation occurs with differing frequency in differing populations and may, along with other correlates of infection, be more frequent with poverty.

Informed examination of the placenta is an important part of the workup of a baby with NE. Once slides have been made, these can be circulated electronically for expert interpretation.

Genetic/Genomic

An increasing number of studies have documented the relevance of genetic factors in NE. In a large cohort in China, Yang and colleagues observed that 11.7% of 366 neonates with NE had pathogenic or probably pathogenic variants on whole exome sequencing; an additional 2.7% had variants of unknown significance. Genes related to NE were observed in nearly half with NE and seizures.[40] Other investigators focused on NE in the absence of recognized asphyxia, finding genetic abnormalities in 36%.[41,42] Another Chinese study examined 133 neonates with NE, of whom 68 had HIE as judged by sentinel birth events or Apgar score 7 or less. Around 29% had positive results on next-generation sequencing.[43] These investigators concluded that genetic diseases were not rare even in neonates with NE who had hypoxic births. Genetic factors may modify the vulnerability of the fetus to injurious antepartum and intrapartum events.[7,44]

Infants with seizures and/or hypotonia are especially likely to yield genetic abnormalities. Tonic seizures were often associated with sodium channel gene defects, suggesting that sodium channel-blocking medications warrant trial.[45] In cultures with high rates of consanguinity, genetic studies are of special importance. Dried blood spots routinely collected in the newborn period can be examined by whole-genome sequencing and yield a genetic diagnosis.[46]

About 1 in 4 infants who survive NE have later diagnoses of CP, and about a third of CP in term infants is genetic in origin.[47] Genes associated with hereditary spastic diplegia, clotting disorders, vascular disease, inflammation, and other pathogenetic mechanisms have been observed with relative frequency in CP, leading to better understanding of pathogenesis,[48] and have sometimes influenced clinical management.[49] Because of its utility in family counseling and prognosis and possible therapeutic implications, "comprehensive and early genomic testing is a crucial component of the routine diagnostic work-up in people with CP."[50]

Infection

Infection is a commonly described cause of brain injury, manifested as intracranial infections such as meningitis or congenital infections. In animal models of neonatal brain injury endotoxin-sensitisation in addition to hypoxia-ischemia cause a synergistic effect with exacerbation of brain injury.[51–53] Human neonates with infection are less responsive to therapeutic hypothermia and infection has been well described in the etiology of NE.[54] CP and NE are strongly associated with chorioamnionitis.[55,56] Spastic and quadriplegic CP are associated with the combination of HIE and infection.[57] Children with CP and a maternal history of infection more frequently had NE, with lower Apgar scores, more need for intubation and inotropes, and more seizures.[57]

Inflammation is associated with abnormal neurologic outcomes and abnormal neuroimaging in infants with NE. Inflammatory cytokines such as IL-6 can predict outcome.[58,59] Infants with NE had chorioamnionitis in 40% of cases, with 11% having a sentinel event.[60] In the large Vermont Oxford network, there was associated antenatal inflammation in 24% of NE.[61] Interpretation of the sepsis evaluation in neonates undergoing therapeutic hypothermia is difficult, as cooling delays the rise in CRP and may cause decreased leukocyte and neutrophil counts.[62] Attempts to optimize pathogen recognition have demonstrated success in LMICs with doubling of the recognition of microbes with polymerase chain reaction (PCR) use.[63]

Group B Streptococcus (GBS), *Escherichia coli*, Listeria monocytogenes, and congenital syphilis can present with NE. Tann and colleagues found higher mortality in infants with both NE and GBS infection.[64] The neuroprotective effect of TH in an animal model was dependent on the pathogen and was more protective in gram-positive versus gram-negative infections. Culture yielded 3.6%, increasing to 8.95% with PCR; more infants with NE had pathogenic bacteria than controls.[63] Herpes simplex enters the differential diagnosis of early neonatal seizures even when the mother is asymptomatic.[65] Although parechovirus/enterovirus, rotavirus, and chikungunya virus are usually postnatally acquired, chikungunya virus can present as NE in half of cases.[66] Parvovirus may be implicated if there is severe anemia at birth.[66] Cytomegalovirus and Zika virus are associated with brain injury but more commonly manifest after the early newborn period and infrequently present with NE alone.[66] COVID 19 has also been associated with neurologic injury and neurodevelopmental delay in a subset of affected infants. Song and colleagues reported an increase in admissions for HIE assessing during the pandemic.[67]

Infection is in general more frequent in impoverished than in more prosperous settings. A systematic review of the association of outcome of NE with and without perinatal infection found many relevant studies, but few were without serious risk of bias. Further studies of high quality are needed for confident assessment of the role of infection in adverse outcome of NE.[68]

Metabolic

Many metabolic disorders manifest in the newborn period with suboptimal nutrition, abnormal neuroimaging, and hypoglycemia.[69,70] Latzer and colleagues found 256 inherited metabolic disorders associated with a variety of epilepsies; often presenting in the neonatal period.[71] As 20% were deemed drug treatable, it is important to recognize these etiologies.

Urea cycle defects, amino acid, and organic acid disorders can present in the first hours or days with toxic metabolite accumulation in the central nervous system, manifesting as persistent metabolic acidosis, hyperlactemia, intractable hypoglycemia, cardiorespiratory compromise, and organomegaly.[72,73] Detailed metabolic workup and family history are useful in the diagnosis.

Perinatal Stroke

Stroke in the perinatal period is estimated to occur in about 1 per 1100 term live-births,[74] and is thus more common in newborns than at any other time until old age. Strokes are mostly arterial ischemic in nature, and commonly present with seizures, which lead to neuroimaging and thus diagnosis. In many cases a diagnosis is made after the newborn period when hemiparesis is recognized. About half of children with perinatal stroke experience long-term disability, with hemiparesis and seizure disorders, but disability is not severe in the majority.[75]

The placenta has been suspected as a source of embolic material in perinatal stroke, but the onset of seizures is most common a day or two after birth, so the placenta has often been discarded by the time seizures occur. In a review of studies that could compare placentas of neonates with and without NE or seizures, FVM was significantly more common in those with NE and/or seizures.[37] Heritable hematologic risk factors are often sought and sometimes found in neonatal strokes but except in cultures in which consanguinity is common, perinatal stroke is rarely observed in more than one child in a sibship.

Toxins

Modern life is increasingly complicated by exposure to potential toxins in food, water, and air. Phthalates and "forever chemicals" such as per- and polyfluoroalkyl substances are virtually ubiquitous and found in many human tissues including placentas and breast milk. These agents affect endocrine, inflammatory, metabolic, and other functions. Impact upon human birthweight and head size has been documented.[76–79] Combinatorial effects are likely. A full assessment of the influence of these and other toxins such as lead and mercury, on the placenta and developing brain await further examination.

Social and Economic Factors

NE is more frequent in neonates born to families of low socioeconomic status, according to population-based controlled studies.[8,80,81] Neonatal seizures were four times more common in poor communities.[82] Importantly, the effectiveness of hypothermia and adjuvants in the therapy of depressed neonates appears to differ in economically depressed as compared with wealthier nations.

Studies of the risk factors for NE and HIE classically focus on factors known in the delivery room and seldom report social circumstances, although neonatal *mortality* is clearly influenced by level of care of the locus of birth and measures of socioeconomic status. Economic status, in turn, is related to parental health, height, and weight, frequency and nature of infections, diet, level of care at delivery, and cultural factors including consanguinity. Studies of risk factors for NE and HIE that include the social environment and its correlates are needed.

Future Research on NE

Neonatal units capable of identifying and treating NE and pursuing differential diagnosis should be established and funded. These should agree on terminology and employ similar inclusion and exclusion criteria, procedures for evaluation and follow-up and standardized approach to neuroimaging. Placentas should receive gross description, sampling, and selective storage. Placental examination by a perinatal pathologist should be routine, and a spot of blood collected on filter paper (as in neonatal metabolic testing) retained for future genetic and biochemical microanalyses.

TERMINOLOGY

As recent research increases our understanding of the biology underlying NE and the often-complex pathways by which NE arises, there is a need to reexamine the vocabulary we use to discuss neurologic depression in term and near-term infants, and its subgroups. Uniform terminology is needed to harmonize data collection and interpretation, to focus research, and to communicate contemporary understanding to families and later to patients. It is difficult to assess the contribution of asphyxial birth to NE because the common markers of asphyxia—abnormal level of consciousness with low Apgar scores and acidosis—are results of their own causes as well as contributors, if untreated, to further injury. The advent of therapeutic hypothermia has enabled neonatologists to limit injury in these ill neonates. The role of asphyxial birth alone has been over-estimated, and underlying genetic, metabolic, infectious, placenta-related or yet-unknown factors often determine outcome.

Work has recently been completed on a Delphi process to identify a core set of outcomes for treatment trials of NE, to increase comparability of results.[83] A major factor influencing outcome is etiology: chicken pox and smallpox have different outcomes, however treated. Uniform specification and definition of eligibility criteria are needed using information available at the time of study inclusion is decided. Secondary analyses should include descriptors of the population and its medical and sociologic features. Special efforts are warranted to characterize study subjects in low-middle income countries, where NE is most frequent, with fewest known options for treatment, and where paucity of resources may hinder investigation and management.

The DEFINE group is working toward consensus definition that will facilitate research and communication among clinicians and with families. We propose the term NE as an early working-diagnosis, guiding use of therapeutic hypothermia and other immediate interventions, to be supplemented by a diagnosis of NE due to HIE or to other factors, as a final diagnosis once workup is complete.

SUMMARY

There has been an understandable impetus to describe babies with NE as having HIE since the advent of therapeutic hypothermia has finally given neonatologists a tool to help those seriously unwell term babies. However, even when it appears that a baby has an acute hypoxia-ischemia-related encephalopathy with low Apgar scores, a low cord pH, and therapeutic hypothermia is commenced, there is still an imperative to search for other factors that underlie or contribute to the illness. The more thorough the investigation, the more likely it is that relevant contributory factors are identified, which may open up additional treatment opportunities. Using common terminology and definitions will support this etiological search and has many advantages for harmonizing data collection and research internationally.

Best Practices

What is the current best practice for management and identification of etiology of NE?

- Infants with signs suggestive of NE should be evaluated immediately for evidence of hypoxia-ischemia.
- If acute hypoxia-ischemia is the suspected cause of a moderate/severe encephalopathy, therapeutic hypothermia should be commenced within 6 hours of birth to maximize the neuroprotective benefit of treatment.

What changes in current practice are likely to improve outcomes?

- A diagnosis of NE should be provided initially with consideration to treatment with therapeutic hypothermia, a more specific diagnosis of NE due to HIE, or NE due to another or multiple etiologies identified once investigations are complete.
- For neonates requiring neoental intensive care unit (NICU) admission for NE, placenta to laboratory, and a blood spot on filter paper stored for possible later genetic/genomic assessment and biochemical microanalyses.
- . Consider fetal growth, malformations, family history, and socioeconomic setting in the workup of child with NE.

Major recommendations:

- Standardization of terminology and definitions for neonatal brain disorders and their outcomes
- Consensus guidelines on investigations of etiology for use in clinical practice and research, suggesting both minimal and optimal levels for units of differing capabilities.
- Studies of diagnostic yield of specific investigations in workup of children who experienced NE, preferably from population-based samples.

DISCLOSURE

The authors have nothing to disclose.

FUNDING

Eleanor Molloy and Aoife Branagan are supported by funding from the Health Research Board, Ireland via funding of the NEPTUNE PhD program, project number 207928, award number 15278.

REFERENCES

1. Jacobs SE, Berg M, Hunt R, et al. Cooling for newborns with hypoxic ischaemic encephalopathy. Cochrane Database Syst Rev 2013;2013(1):Cd003311.
2. Executive summary: neonatal encephalopathy and neurologic outcome, second edition. Report of the American College of Obstetricians and Gynecologists' task force on neonatal encephalopathy. Obstet Gynecol 2014;123(4):896–901.
3. Lee AC, Kozuki N, Blencowe H, et al. Intrapartum-related neonatal encephalopathy incidence and impairment at regional and global levels for 2010 with trends from 1990. Pediatr Res 2013;74(Suppl 1):50–72.
4. Thayyil S, Pant S, Montaldo P, et al. Hypothermia for moderate or severe neonatal encephalopathy in low-income and middle-income countries (HELIX): a randomised controlled trial in India, Sri Lanka, and Bangladesh. Lancet Global Health 2021;9(9):e1273–85.
5. Krishnan V, Kumar V, Shankaran S, et al. Rise and fall of therapeutic hypothermia in low-resource settings: lessons from the HELIX Trial. Indian J Pediatr 2021. https://doi.org/10.1007/s12098-021-03861-y.
6. McIntyre S, Badawi N, Blair E, et al. Does aetiology of neonatal encephalopathy and hypoxic-ischaemic encephalopathy influence the outcome of treatment? Dev Med Child Neurol 2015;57(Suppl 3):2–7.
7. Woodward KE, Murthy P, Mineyko A, et al. Identifying genetic susceptibility in neonates with hypoxic-ischemic encephalopathy: a retrospective case series. J Child Neurol 2023;38(1–2):16–24.

8. Badawi N, Kurinczuk JJ, Keogh JM, et al. Antepartum risk factors for newborn encephalopathy: the Western Australian case-control study. Br Med J 1998; 317(7172):1549–53.

9. Badawi N, Kurinczuk JJ, Keogh JM, et al. Intrapartum risk factors for newborn encephalopathy: the Western Australian case-control study. Br Med J 1998; 317(7172):1554–8.

10. McIntyre S, Nelson KB, Mulkey SB, et al. Neonatal encephalopathy: focus on epidemiology and underexplored aspects of etiology. Semin Fetal Neonatal Med 2021;26(4):101265.

11. Jenabi E, Salimi Z, Ayubi E, et al. The environmental risk factors prior to conception associated with placental abruption: an umbrella review. Syst Rev 2022; 11(1):55.

12. Brandt JS, Ananth CV. Placental abruption at near-term and term gestations: pathophysiology, epidemiology, diagnosis, and management. Am J Obstet Gynecol 2023;228(5s):S1313–s1329.

13. Nelson KB, Ellenberg JH. Antecedents of cerebral palsy. Multivariate analysis of risk. N Engl J Med 1986;315(2):81–6.

14. McIntyre S, Blair E, Badawi N, et al. Antecedents of cerebral palsy and perinatal death in term and late preterm singletons. Obstet Gynecol 2013;122(4):869–77.

15. McIntyre S, Badawi N, Brown C, et al. Population case-control study of cerebral palsy: neonatal predictors for low-risk term singletons. Pediatrics 2011;127(3): e667–73.

16. Galea C, McIntyre S, Smithers-Sheedy H, et al. Cerebral palsy trends in Australia (1995-2009): a population-based observational study. Dev Med Child Neurol 2019;61(2):186–93.

17. Nelson KB, Grether JK. Selection of neonates for neuroprotective therapies: one set of criteria applied to a population. Arch Pediatr Adolesc Med 1999;153(4): 393–8.

18. Shepherd E, Salam RA, Middleton P, et al. Antenatal and intrapartum interventions for preventing cerebral palsy: an overview of Cochrane systematic reviews. Cochrane Database Syst Rev 2017;8(8):Cd012077.

19. Russ JB, Simmons R, Glass HC. Neonatal encephalopathy: beyond hypoxic-ischemic encephalopathy. NeoReviews 2021;22(3):e148–62.

20. Sandoval Karamian AG, Mercimek-Andrews S, Mohammad K, et al. Neonatal encephalopathy: etiologies other than hypoxic-ischemic encephalopathy. Semin Fetal Neonatal Med 2021;26(5):101272.

21. Blair EM, Nelson KB. Fetal growth restriction and risk of cerebral palsy in singletons born after at least 35 weeks' gestation. Am J Obstet Gynecol 2015;212(4): 520.e1–7.

22. Streja E, Miller JE, Wu C, et al. Disproportionate fetal growth and the risk for congenital cerebral palsy in singleton births. PLoS One 2015;10(5):e0126743.

23. Gundacker C, Audouze K, Widhalm R, et al. Reduced birth weight and exposure to per- and polyfluoroalkyl substances: a review of possible underlying mechanisms using the AOP-HelpFinder. Toxics 2022;10(11).

24. Felix JF, Badawi N, Kurinczuk JJ, et al. Birth defects in children with newborn encephalopathy. Dev Med Child Neurol 2000;42(12):803–8.

25. Waller DK, Keddie AM, Canfield MA, et al. Do infants with major congenital anomalies have an excess of macrosomia? Teratology 2001;64(6):311–7.

26. Vega Puyal L, Llurba E, Ferrer Q, et al. Neurodevelopmental outcomes in congenital heart disease: usefulness of biomarkers of brain injury. An Pediatr 2024; 100(1):13–24.

27. Gheorghe CP, Goyal R, Mittal A, et al. Gene expression in the placenta: maternal stress and epigenetic responses. Int J Dev Biol 2010;54(2–3):507–23.
28. Blair E, de Groot J, Nelson KB. Placental infarction identified by macroscopic examination and risk of cerebral palsy in infants at 35 weeks of gestational age and over. Am J Obstet Gynecol 2011;205(2):124.e1–7.
29. Chalak L, Redline RW, Goodman AM, et al. Acute and chronic placental abnormalities in a multicenter cohort of newborn infants with hypoxic-ischemic encephalopathy. J Pediatr 2021;237:190–6.
30. Lachapelle J, Chen M, Oskoui M, et al. Placental pathology in asphyxiated newborns treated with therapeutic hypothermia. J Neonatal Perinat Med 2015. https://doi.org/10.3233/npm-15814068.
31. Fox A, Doyle E, Geary M, et al. Placental pathology and neonatal encephalopathy. Int J Gynaecol Obstet 2023;160(1):22–7.
32. Kim CF, Carreon CK, James KE, et al. Gross and histologic placental abnormalities associated with neonatal hypoxic-ischemic encephalopathy. Pediatr Dev Pathol 2023. https://doi.org/10.1177/10935266231195166. 10935266231195166.
33. Khong TY, Mooney EE, Ariel I, et al. Sampling and definitions of placental lesions: amsterdam placental workshop group consensus statement. Arch Pathol Lab Med 2016;140(7):698–713.
34. Penn AA, Wintermark P, Chalak LF, et al. Placental contribution to neonatal encephalopathy. Semin Fetal Neonatal Med 2021;26(4):101276.
35. McDonald DG, Kelehan P, McMenamin JB, et al. Placental fetal thrombotic vasculopathy is associated with neonatal encephalopathy. Hum Pathol 2004;35(7):875–80.
36. Vik T, Redline R, Nelson KB, et al. The placenta in neonatal encephalopathy: a case-control study. J Pediatr 2018;202:77–85.e3.
37. Spinillo A, Dominoni M, Mas FD, et al. Placental fetal vascular malperfusion, neonatal neurologic morbidity, and infant neurodevelopmental outcomes: a systematic review and meta-analysis. Am J Obstet Gynecol 2023;229(6):632–40.e2.
38. Gardella B, Dominoni M, Caporali C, et al. Placental features of fetal vascular malperfusion and infant neurodevelopmental outcomes at 2 years of age in severe fetal growth restriction. Am J Obstet Gynecol 2021;225(4):413.e1–11.
39. Loverro MT, Di Naro E, Nicolardi V, et al. Pregnancy complications, correlation with placental pathology and neonatal outcomes. Front Clin Diabetes Healthc 2021;2:807192.
40. Yang L, Chen X, Liu X, et al. Clinical features and underlying genetic causes in neonatal encephalopathy: a large cohort study. Clin Genet 2020;98(4):365–73.
41. Lenahan A, Mietzsch U, Wood TR, et al. Characteristics, genetic testing, and diagnoses of infants with neonatal encephalopathy not due to hypoxic ischemic encephalopathy: a cohort study. J Pediatr 2023;260:113533.
42. Bruun TUJ, DesRoches CL, Wilson D, et al. Prospective cohort study for identification of underlying genetic causes in neonatal encephalopathy using whole-exome sequencing. Genet Med 2018;20(5):486–94.
43. Xiao TT, Yang L, Wu BB, et al. [Genotype and phenotype analysis of neonates with neonatal encephalopathy complicated with perinatal hypoxic event]. Zhonghua Er Ke Za Zhi 2021;59(4):280–5.
44. Balada R, Tebé C, León M, et al. Enquiring beneath the surface: can a gene expression assay shed light into the heterogeneity among newborns with neonatal encephalopathy? Pediatr Res 2020;88(3):451–8.

45. Cornet MC, Morabito V, Lederer D, et al. Neonatal presentation of genetic epilepsies: early differentiation from acute provoked seizures. Epilepsia 2021; 62(8):1907–20.

46. Owen MJ, Lenberg J, Feigenbaum A, et al. Postmortem whole-genome sequencing on a dried blood spot identifies a novel homozygous SUOX variant causing isolated sulfite oxidase deficiency. Cold Spring Harb Mol Case Stud 2021;7(3).

47. Evans MI, Britt DW, Devoe LD. Etiology and ontogeny of cerebral palsy: implications for practice and research. Reprod Sci 2023.

48. Xu Y, Li Y, Richard SA, et al. Genetic pathways in cerebral palsy: a review of the implications for precision diagnosis and understanding disease mechanisms. Neural Regen Res 2024;19(7):1499–508.

49. van Eyk CL, Webber DL, Minoche AE, et al. Yield of clinically reportable genetic variants in unselected cerebral palsy by whole genome sequencing. NPJ Genom Med 2021;6(1):74.

50. van Eyk CL, Fahey MC, Gecz J. Redefining cerebral palsies as a diverse group of neurodevelopmental disorders with genetic aetiology. Nat Rev Neurol 2023;19(9): 542–55.

51. Mallard C, Wang X. Infection-induced vulnerability of perinatal brain injury. Neurol Res Int 2012;2012:102153.

52. Nelson KB, Leviton A. How much of neonatal encephalopathy is due to birth asphyxia? Am J Dis Child 1991;145(11):1325–31.

53. Aslam S, Strickland T, Molloy EJ. Neonatal encephalopathy: need for recognition of multiple etiologies for optimal management. Front Pediatr 2019;7:142.

54. Martinello KA, Meehan C, Avdic-Belltheus A, et al. Acute LPS sensitization and continuous infusion exacerbates hypoxic brain injury in a piglet model of neonatal encephalopathy. Sci Rep 2019;9(1):10184.

55. Nelson KB, Willoughby RE. Infection, inflammation and the risk of cerebral palsy. Curr Opin Neurol 2000;13(2):133–9.

56. Willoughby RE Jr, Nelson KB. Chorioamnionitis and brain injury. Clin Perinatol 2002;29(4):603–21.

57. Nelson KB, Grether JK. Potentially asphyxiating conditions and spastic cerebral palsy in infants of normal birth weight. Am J Obstet Gynecol 1998; 179(2):507–13.

58. Shalak LF, Laptook AR, Jafri HS, et al. Clinical chorioamnionitis, elevated cytokines, and brain injury in term infants. Pediatrics 2002;110(4):673–80.

59. O'Hare FM, Watson RW, O'Neill A, et al. Serial cytokine alterations and abnormal neuroimaging in newborn infants with encephalopathy. Acta Paediatr 2017; 106(4):561–7.

60. Parker SJ, Kuzniewicz M, Niki H, et al. Antenatal and intrapartum risk factors for hypoxic-ischemic encephalopathy in a US birth cohort. J Pediatr 2018;203: 163–9.

61. Nelson KB, Bingham P, Edwards EM, et al. Antecedents of neonatal encephalopathy in the Vermont Oxford network encephalopathy registry. Pediatrics 2012; 130(5):878–86.

62. Chakkarapani E, Davis J, Thoresen M. Therapeutic hypothermia delays the C-reactive protein response and suppresses white blood cell and platelet count in infants with neonatal encephalopathy. Arch Dis Child Fetal Neonatal Ed 2014; 99(6):F458–63.

63. Tann CJ, Nkurunziza P, Nakakeeto M, et al. Prevalence of bloodstream pathogens is higher in neonatal encephalopathy cases vs. controls using a novel panel of real-time PCR assays. PLoS One 2014;9(5):e97259.

64. Tann CJ, Martinello KA, Sadoo S, et al. Neonatal encephalopathy with group b streptococcal disease worldwide: systematic review, investigator group datasets, and meta-analysis. Clin Infect Dis 2017;65(suppl_2):S173–s189.

65. Akhtar LN, Szpara ML. Viral genetic diversity and its potential contributions to the development and progression of neonatal herpes simplex virus (HSV) disease. Curr Clin Microbiol Rep 2019;6(4):249–56.

66. de Vries LS. Viral infections and the neonatal brain. Semin Pediatr Neurol 2019; 32:100769.

67. Song D, Narasimhan SR, Huang A, et al. Increased newborn NICU admission for evaluation of hypoxic-ischemic encephalopathy during COVID-19 pandemic in a public hospital. Front Pediatr 2023;11:1206137.

68. Andersen M, Pedersen MV, Andelius TCK, et al. Neurological outcome following newborn encephalopathy with and without perinatal infection: a systematic review. Front Pediatr 2021;9:787804.

69. Tan ES. Inborn errors of metabolism presenting as neonatal encephalopathy: practical tips for clinicians. Ann Acad Med Singapore 2008;37(12 Suppl): 94–103.

70. Molloy EJ, El-Dib M, Juul SE, et al. Neuroprotective therapies in the NICU in term infants: present and future. Pediatr Res 2023;93(7):1819–27.

71. Latzer IT, Blau N, Ferreira CR, et al. Clinical and biochemical footprints of inherited metabolic diseases. XV. Epilepsies. Mol Genet Metabol 2023;140(3): 107690.

72. O'Dea M, Sweetman D, Bonifacio SL, et al. Management of multi organ dysfunction in neonatal encephalopathy. Front Pediatr 2020;8:239.

73. Saudubray JM, Garcia-Cazorla À. Inborn errors of metabolism overview: pathophysiology, manifestations, evaluation, and management. Pediatr Clin North Am 2018;65(2):179–208.

74. Roy B, Webb A, Walker K, et al. Risk factors for perinatal stroke in term infants: a case-control study in Australia. J Paediatr Child Health 2023;59(4):673–9.

75. Giraud A, Dinomais M, Garel P, et al. Perinatal inflammation exposure and developmental outcomes 7 years after neonatal arterial ischaemic stroke. Dev Med Child Neurol 2023;65(8):1073–80.

76. Gui SY, Chen YN, Wu KJ, et al. Association between exposure to per- and polyfluoroalkyl substances and birth outcomes: a systematic review and meta-analysis. Front Public Health 2022;10:855348.

77. Liu B, Lu X, Jiang A, et al. Influence of maternal endocrine disrupting chemicals exposure on adverse pregnancy outcomes: a systematic review and meta-analysis. Ecotoxicol Environ Saf 2024;270:115851.

78. Trasande L, Nelson ME, Alshawabkeh A, et al. Prenatal phthalate exposure and adverse birth outcomes in the USA: a prospective analysis of births and estimates of attributable burden and costs. Lancet Planet Health 2024; 8(2):e74–85.

79. Siddique S, Chaudhry MN, Ahmad SR, et al. Ecological and human health hazards; integrated risk assessment of organochlorine pesticides (OCPs) from the Chenab River, Pakistan. Sci Total Environ 2023;882:163504.

80. Blume HK, Loch CM, Li CI. Neonatal encephalopathy and socioeconomic status: population-based case-control study. Arch Pediatr Adolesc Med 2007;161(7): 663–8.

81. Battin M, Sadler L, Masson V, et al. Neonatal encephalopathy in New Zealand: demographics and clinical outcome. J Paediatr Child Health 2016; 52(6):632–6.
82. Tanous O, Haj-Yahya KT, Ershead A, et al. Communal poverty is a significant risk factor for neonatal seizures. Neuropediatrics 2023;54(5):322–7.
83. Quirke FA, Ariff S, Battin MR, et al. COHESION: a core outcome set for the treatment of neonatal encephalopathy. Pediatr Res 2023. https://doi.org/10.1038/s41390-023-02938-y.

Neonatal Encephalopathy is a Complex Phenotype Representing Reproductive and Pregnancy Exposome Effects on the Maternal-Placental-Fetal Triad

Mark S. Scher, MD

KEYWORDS

- Maternal-placental-fetal triad • Neonatal encephalopathy
- Hypoxic-ischemic encephalopathy • Placental disease
- Gene-environment interactions • Neural exposome • Social determinants of health

KEY POINTS

- Consider timing and etiologies affecting maternal-placental-fetal triad disease pathways when evaluating neonatal encephalopathy.
- Reproductive, pregnancy, and placental exposomes influence the fetal neural exposome through toxic stressor interplay.
- Future biosignatures will detect maladaptive gene-environment interactions before conception through 2 years of life to improve neurotherapeutic interventions.
- Equitable healthcare delivery strengthens a brain capital strategy that prolongs survival with an improved quality of life.

INTRODUCTION

A 2-step diagnostic strategy promotes person-centric evaluations[1,2] of neonatal encephalopathy (NE): (1) recognize phenotypes over time to identify diseases affecting each woman, maternal-placental-fetal triad (MPF) triad, and neonate that impair the fetal brain; and (2) correlate etiopathogenesis during each developmental interval contributing to phenotypes. Serial evaluations re-assess diagnoses to accurately identify timing and etiologies associated with NE. This neonatal minority is comparatively at

Division of Pediatric Neurology, Department of Pediatrics, Fetal/Neonatal Neurology Program, Case Western Reserve University School of Medicine, Rainbow Babies and Children's Hospital/MacDonald Hospital for Women, University Hospitals Cleveland Medical Center, 22315 Canterbury Lane, Shaker Heights, OH 44122, USA
E-mail address: Mark.s.scher@gmail.com

Clin Perinatol 51 (2024) 535–550
https://doi.org/10.1016/j.clp.2024.04.001
0095-5108/24/© 2024 Elsevier Inc. All rights reserved.
perinatology.theclinics.com

greater risk than the "silent majority" for neurologic sequelae presenting before 2 years of age.[3]

Preconception and pregnancy perspectives strengthen evaluations during first 1000 days to distinguish functional neurodiversity from permanent brain disorders and offer effective interventions and prognosis. Eighty percent of brain connectivity occurs during this first critical/sensitive period of developmental neuroplasticity, followed by adolescence and reproductive senescence. Fetal and neonatal neurology (FNN) practice advances diagnostic and therapeutic approaches using developmental origins of health and disease (DoHaD) principles that consider reproductive and pregnancy health. Benefits and risks will be better predicted during each and successive generations. Social determinants of health (SDH) integrated into a brain capital strategy reduce health disparities toward equitable healthcare for all women to improve outcomes for their children.[4]

THE EXPOSOME CONCEPT APPLIED TO FETAL NEONATAL NEUROLOGY

NE represents one of the "great neonatal neurologic syndromes" (GNNS) often associated with seizures and stroke.[1] Diagnostic complexity regarding timing and etiology of the GNNS resemble the "great obstetric syndromes", referring to placental maldevelopment that impairs the MPF triad with adverse outcomes.[5] GNNS also represent trimester-specific vulnerabilities or diseases of the MPF triad with associated fetal brain injuries. Peripartum and neonatal diseases initiate or worsen damage. Maternal levels of care provide limited surveillance without recognizing many disease pathways. No single or combination of biomarkers accurately predicts the onset or worsening of injuries expressed as NE. Multiple etiologies include hypoxia-ischemia (HI) with variable clinical expressions. Future diagnostic strategies will expand neurotherapeutic options before and after birth.

The exposome is an epidemiologic concept referring to the totality of stressors with positive or negative influences.[6] The neural exposome specifically refers to the brain's responses from endogenous and exogenous toxic stressor interplay (TSI) (**Fig. 1**A).[7] Diagnosis and prognosis improve by considering a functional exposome specific to critical or sensitive periods of neuroplasticity. Deep-state learning using population health prediction models improve person-centric healthcare (**Fig. 1**B).[8]

This article stresses reproductive and pregnancy exposome effects on the MPF triad that impair the fetal neural exposome with NE expression. Antepartum brain vulnerabilities or injuries often combine with peripartum and neonatal events. Childhood diseases with adverse childhood experiences[9] further impair brain health with life-long consequences.

THE REPRODUCTIVE EXPOSOME

Women are vulnerable to life-long exposome effects during their reproductive years (**Fig. 2**)[10]. The periconceptional period introduces risks during 1 or multiple pregnancies, enhanced with unplanned pregnancies particularly during adolescence.[11,12] TSI threatens the MPF triad throughout each pregnancy, affected by a social exposome that enhances vulnerabilities from health disparities, which further reduces outcomes.[13]

Hypertension, diabetes, obesity, and mental health disorders exemplify complex MPF triad diseases associated with TSI that impair reproductive health starting during childhood before each pregnancy. Pollutants combined with SDH represent complex exogenous toxic stressor exposures then interact with a woman's biological system to produce preclinical or active fetal brain diseases.

A

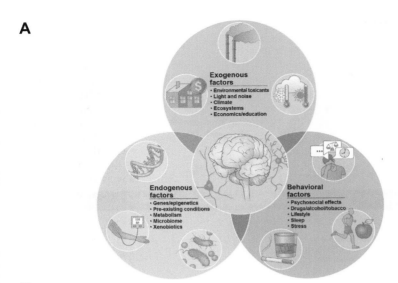

B

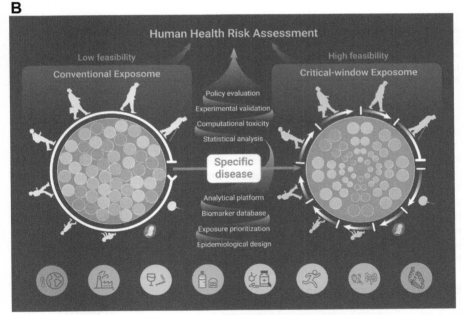

Fig. 1. (*A*) The neural exposome is depicted as overlapping influences among multiple endogenous and exogenous toxic stressors.[7] Endogenous factors encompass multisystemic diseases including mental health disorders and behavioral factors, as well as social determinants of health (SDH) with lifestyle choices. The examples cite represent a more extensive list of factors.(*B*) The functional exposome prioritizes person-centric exposome factors identified across the developmental-aging continuum from conception to old age. This approach improves feasibility by applying time-dependent windows to better assess human health risk (note the organized color order represent specific person identification). Critical-sensitive periods of neuroplasticity across the lifespan correlate specific phenotypes with disease pathways. Exogenous and endogenous toxic stressor interplay (TSI) use meta-analysis to prioritize the usage of large data sets from population health metrics to identify person-centric

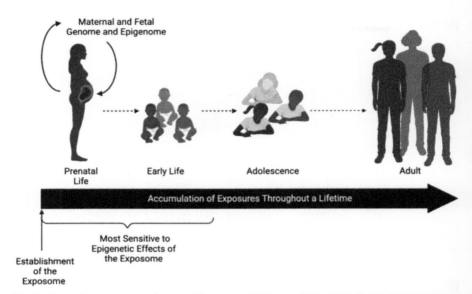

Fig. 2. The epigenome remains sensitive to environmental insults. Epigenetic patterns are established before conception and sustained during rapid tissue development during pregnancy and early postnatal life. These environmental perturbations to epigenetic programming can serve as biomarkers of past exposures and predictors of future diseases later in life and across generations. Additional exposures during childhood, adolescence, and adulthood may impart further epigenetic alterations. (Created with BioRender.com.)

Etiopathogenetic mechanisms affect reproductive health through inflammatory, oxidative, and HI disease pathways with adversities to the MPF triad. Periconception and first trimester testing provide detection of pregnancy-related diseases that impair a dynamic fetal neural exposome. Multispecialty consultations enhance fetal surveillance with time-sensitive interventions through shared clinical decisions with women.

Parental or de novo allelic alterations produce genetic abnormalities in the conceptus, enhanced by MPF triad diseases. Whole exome sequencing and high through-put next-generation genomic technologies suggest genetic risks despite negative karyotypic and microarray screens.[13,14] Epigenetic biomarkers such as the methylome will offer biologic age assessments of diseases.[15] Post-translational biosignatures represent altered gene-environment (G x E) interactions with fetal brain health risks, influencing subsequent pregnancies through epigenetic memory.[16]

THE PREGNANCY EXPOSOME

MPF triad effects to the fetal neural exposome guide FNN diagnoses throughout pregnancy applied to NE evaluations. No specific biomarkers optimally assess all factors

factors more accurately. Appropriate epidemiologic designs, followed by exposure prioritization, biomarker databases, analytical platforms, statistical analyses, computational toxicity estimations, experimental validation, and health policy applications must be standardized for a specific country or region. (Mingliang Fang, et al., Exposome in human health: Utopia or wonderland?, The Innovation, 2 (4), 2021, 100172, https://doi.org/10.1016/j.xinn.2021.100172.)

influencing the pregnancy exposome. Maternal levels of care offer limited surveillance[17] without detecting most fetal brain disorders.

Environmental science education improves maternal health care delivery by identifying TSI that compromises pregnancies.[18] Environmental threats throughout the Global South (ie, countries in the regions of Latin America, Africa, Asia, and Oceania), as well as high-income country medical deserts[19] reduce healthcare delivery given inadequate resources. Research methodologies are underpowered by small sample sizes, exclusion of vulnerable populations, and biased choices of study variables. Interdisciplinary FNN training helps close this information gap by integrating knowledge of TSI effects on the MPF triad with NE. Studies designed with SDH factors provide person-centric applications before and during each pregnancy.[20]

Physiologic adaptations during pregnancy preserve MPF triad health[21] while adverse biological-chemical TSI interactions impair inter-connected biological systems. Hypertensive, metabolic, mental health, and autoimmune-inflammatory disease states exemplify conditions that worsen during each pregnancy to threaten maternal-fetal dyad health with fetal neural exposome impairments. Maternal body fluid, placental, and cord blood biomarkers can assess maternal and fetal micro-environments,[20] representing a broad range of biological-chemical interactions that contribute to maternal diseases.[22] Few biomarkers, however, correlate TSI specifically with fetal brain risks. Pregnancy exposome investigations will offer greater recognition of fetal brain disorders associated with NE. Examples highlight pregnancy exposome effects on the fetal neural exposome.

Hypertensive Disorders

Hypertensive disorders of pregnancy affect 5% to 8% of the world's female population.[23] One study assessed non-targeted placental samples suggesting future omics-based systems biology investigations linking the woman's biological systems with with TSI with pregnancy induced hypertension (PIH) expression: (1) mechanisms link gene signatures and human metabolites with physiologic effects, (2) specific xenobiotic risks are identified, and (3) combined xenobiotic exposures (primary vs secondary; intentional vs unplanned) affect different individuals.[24] Reported maternal levels of phthalates, perfluoroalkyl acids, and endocrine disruptors suggest correlations with placental maldevelopment, combining genomic and epigenome placental analyses of understudied chemicals to PIH.[25]

Gestational Diabetes Mellitus and Diabesity

Nutritional diseases combined with environmental pollutant exposures combine to express gestational diabetes mellitus (GDM). Obesity increases metabolic risks for GDM and co-morbid diseases. Identifying risk factors improve understanding of disease pathways. Reducing TSI effects[26] lessen glucose intolerance and GDM disease consequences. Placental vasculopathies associated with GDM, gestational diabesity and PIH will be discussed in the placental exposome section.

Autoimmune Disorders

The woman's immune system physiologically adjusts to the semi-allogenic fetus to preserve health. Pro- and anti-inflammatory states are balanced to optimize uterine remodeling, fetal growth, and maturation, with immune homeostasis that protects the MPF triad.[27] Non-infectious autoimmune phenotypes represent diverse maternal inflammatory diseases that impair immune interactions and contribute to childhood brain disorders. A machine learning study evaluated immune fingerprints, representing a lifetime exposome using prenatal disease prediction. The maternal immune activation

(MIA) process discussed in the placental exposome section highlights immunologic dysfunction with sequelae based on DoHaD principles.[28,29]

Maternal-Fetal Infectious or Inflammatory Responses

Many communicable diseases produce inflammatory placental responses,[30] represented by chronic villitis of unknown etiology, chronic deciduitis-chorionitis, eosinophilic T-cell vasculitis, and chronic histiocytic intervillositis. Acute or subacute chorioamnionitis or funisitis contribute to peripartum preterm and full-term complications with NE. Two disease pathways impact the fetal immune system[31]: (1) upregulation of host immune responses with excessive release of harmful cytokine species in the placenta, cord, and fetal brain; and (2) human leukocyte antigens (HLA) transcript perturbation increases risks of fetal semi-allogenic graft rejection with miscarriage or fetal diseases. Neurologic sequelae result from any one of the disease pathways.[32] Xenobiotics impair placental functions, increasing morbidities from infections exacerbated by health disparities. Public health attention is needed to identify and appropriately treat women with congenital and acute infectious illnesses.

Mental Health Disorders and Substance Exposure

Prenatal corticosteroid and adrenergic hormone surges from maternal hypothalamic-pituitary-adrenal axis dysfunction occur with mental health disorders. Recreational or prescribed controlled substances increase adverse effects. While cannabidiol is currently a popular choice for recreational and medicinal benefits, neurotoxicity occurs with combined use of alcohol, tobacco, amphetamines, and opiates. Prescribed central nervous system-active psychoactive and antiepileptic medications also contribute to similar toxic neuronal effects.[2]

Harmful Effects from Treatment Interventions

Prenatal to postnatal inflammatory, oxidative stress, and asphyxia disease pathways injure the MPF triad and neonate with treatments for maternal diseases. Antibiotic administration for maternal infections alters fetal gut microbiota. Impaired fetal neuronal development through exaggerated systemic inflammatory disease pathways alters angiogenesis and neurogenesis within the fetal blood-brain barrier.[33] Preterm neonates incur postnatal brain injuries with systemic diseases such as necrotizing enterocolitis and sepsis.[34]

Xenobiotic Exposures with Climate Change

Excessive organophosphate pesticides are common agricultural residues that contribute to fetal neurologic diseases with postnatal disease expression,[35] exaggerated by global climate change. Upregulated pro-inflammatory cytokines alter gene expressions with non-infectious inflammatory responses, worsened by xenobiotic-induced climate changes. Childhood exposures worsen brain injuries across the lifespan.

Social Determinants of Health

Maternal populations with healthcare disparities are more vulnerable to xenobiotics. Food and economic insecurity amplify MPF triad disease effects particularly for persons of color,[36] contributing to impaired fetal brain development. A public health exposome study correlated factors pregnancy-related mortality with health behaviors, social determinants, and environmental exposures. Proximal, intermediate and distal risks[37] from TSI also apply to maternal and fetal morbidities that influence NE. Resilience or vulnerability regarding these risks influence mother's childcare with childhood brain disorders. A model-of-care framework describes a life-course approach inclusive of preconception, pregnancy, and postpartum healthcare. This social-ecological model identifies individual, interpersonal, institutional, community, and policy targets that promote positive woman-child dyad health interventions, supported by her partner and family[38] **(Fig. 3)**.

THE PLACENTAL EXPOSOME

Placental exposome effects impair MPF triad health.[2] Time-dependent placental disease pathways influence NE. Perinatal pathology applied to developmental neuropathologic effects[39] improve NE evaluations contributing to childhood sequelae.

TSI impairs placental energy-substrate delivery, waste removal, and growth factor production and transport.[40] Following suboptimal oocyte implantation and embryonic pre-functional placental maldevelopment contribute to fetal brain anomalies or destructive lesions, depending on trimester effects to the MPF triad. Dysgenesis occurs during the first half of pregnancy while destructive fetal brain lesions occur during the latter half of pregnancy. HI, oxidative stress, and inflammation represent 3 disease pathways that contribute to adverse placental exposome effects on neuronal populations and connections. G x E interactions influence susceptibility to pregnancy-related diseases through defective fetal brain-placental axis communication, worsened by TSI.[41] Representative placental lesions exemplify etiopathogenesis.[42] Placental-brain imaging modalities using fMRI combined with exomic or high through-put genetic testing offer future diagnostic opportunities.[43]

Epigenetic molecular biomarkers link complex placental mechanisms from TSI to the MPF triad with unfavorable outcomes. Developmental programming of chronic disease helps explain evolving brain disorders through reproductive senescence.

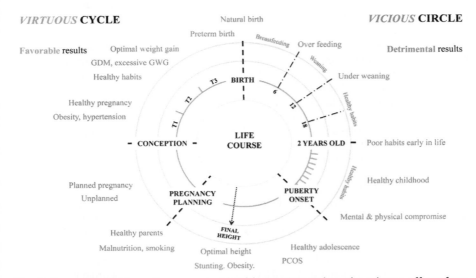

Fig. 3. Favorable ("virtuous"-green color) health practices reduce the adverse effects from unfavorable ("vicious"- red color) health practices across the lifespan beginning with reproductive followed by pregnancy health. GDM, gestational diabetes mellitus; GWG, gestational weight gain; PCOS, polycystic ovarian syndrome; T1, first trimester; T2, second trimester; T3, third trimester. (Yap, F., Loy, S.L., Ku, C.W. et al. A Golden Thread approach to transforming Maternal and Child Health in Singapore. BMC Pregnancy Childbirth 22, 561 (2022). https://doi.org/10.1186/s12884-022-04893-8.)

Placental dysfunction mediated by xenobiotic-altered transporters affects metabolizing enzymes with biological-chemical interactions specific to the person.[2]

Maternal Immune Activation

MIA initiates after blastocyte implantation 2 to 8 days following fertilization. Immune intolerance results from suboptimal attachment between the embryos as the semi-allogenic graft to the mother as the host. Impaired precursor trophoblastic cell development induces inflammatory disease pathways with miscarriage or system-specific health risks to the surviving embryo. Defective microglial precursors migrate from the secondary yolk sac, impairing progenitor neuronal pathways within the neural plate.[44] The functional hemochorial placenta replacing the yolk sac after gestational week 10 to 12 continues to impair precursor neuronal and glial cell populations within transient brain structures. Dysgenesis continues during the second half of pregnancy within the subplate zone and early cortical plate, combined with destructive lesions that disrupt the 6-layered cerebral cortex. Villous dysmaturity, chronic villitis, and vasculopathies correlate with anomalous and destructive brain lesions. Childhood autistic spectrum disorder, cerebral palsy, epilepsy, as well as later life neurodegenerative and stroke syndromes are phenotypes correlated with MIA-induced fetal brain maldevelopment.[45] Conventional MRI often detect only nonspecific markers such as gliosis and atrophy. Future fetal neuroimaging structural-functional assessments using fMRI and volumetric information will improve detection.[43]

MIA-associated inflammatory, oxidative, and hypoxic mechanisms reprogram fetal brain and immune systems with TSI.[28] Microglia, the peripheral immune system, and colonization of gut microbiota are altered through epigenetic disease pathways influencing fetal brain maldevelopment. Inflammatory and non-inflammatory factors induce release of pathogen-associated molecular patterns and damage-associated molecular patterns within the MPF triad. Toll-like receptors on maternal peripheral innate immune and placental cells are activated by these patterns, mediated by gestational-age specific cytokine species. Abnormal immune mediators alter passive placental transport and active metabolic, neuroendocrine, and stress signaling pathways. Abnormal epigenetic memory within fetal microglia and immune cells worsens throughout pregnancy.[28] Endogenous maternal diseases and stressors with xenobiotic exposures worsen fetal brain lesions. A postnatal double-hit initiated by placental disease enhance abnormal systemic-brain immune pathway interactions during critical periods of neuroplasticity throughout the lifespan. Abnormal peripheral inflammatory signals from TSI activate abnormal brain immune cells, with chronic inflammatory alterations noted within aging brain and peripheral systems.

Ischemic Placental Syndrome

Ischemic placental syndrome (IPS) involves TSI with defective angiogenesis. Shallow spiral artery remodeling results from precursor trophoblastic cellular maldevelopment,[46] reducing placental flow. Decidual thrombotic lesions on the maternal surface or avascular chorionic villi with thrombi on the fetal surface are representative placental lesions worsening MPF triad diseases associated with gestational diabetes or PIH.[47] Fetal growth restriction (FGR) can be associated with fetal brain injury, even with subtle FGR calculated by the ponderal index.[48]

First trimester umbilical cord lesions increase adverse TSI effects from IPS. Narrowed cord vascular diameters reduce placental blood flow. Two embryonic stalks connect the yolk sac to the embryo; the vitelline duct loses function and the umbilical duct form mature structures.[49] Marginal or velamentous umbilical cord insertions, true knots, and excessive coiling indices result after anomalous first-trimester cord.

Oxygen, glucose, and growth factor delivery and waste removal reduction contribute to fetal brain lesions.[2]

Fetal Inflammatory Response

Fetal inflammatory response (FIR) represents a third placental disease mechanism associated with TSI, representing 1 of 4 histopathologic lesions correlating with neurologic sequelae.[50] "FIR type 1" represents an acute immune response.[31] Activated monocytes, macrophages, and neutrophils correlate with placental disease before and during parturition with 2 disease pathways: (1) inflammatory mediator-induced asphyxia results after reduced blood vessel caliber size and contractility responsivity with vasoconstriction of placenta orcord and fetal brain microvasculature; and (2) inflammatory mediator cytosolic injury within mitochondria and nuclear damage of genetic material result in cell death or dysfunction.[32] TSI affects FIR[51] worsening dysregulation of epithelial cell and macrophage immune responses with disruption of the cervicovaginal barrier.[51]

"FIR type 2"[31] involves chronic HLA transcript perturbations, threatening fetal semiallograft rejection during the first half of pregnancy. Chronic villitis[52] can be associated with FIR type 2, contributing to later FIR type 1 disease pathways.

THE NEONATAL EXPOSOME

Peripartum events before delivery are associated with NE. Adverse reproductive and pregnancy exposome effects potentially impair the MPF triad during fetal-to-neonatal transition. Antepartum and intrapartum surveillance tests offer limited guidance to adjust obstetric strategies that improve outcomes without accurately identifying timing or etiology associated with NE. Diagnostic challenges often combine remote and acute effects on the MPF triad expressed by the neonatal exposome.

Sentinel Events Close to Delivery

Abruptio placenta, cord prolapse, and uterine rupture represent acute and unpredictable challenges to neonatal neurocritical care, often combined with antepartum vulnerabilities or injuries associated with NE.[1] Fetal brain injuries may precede intrapartum events: (1) primary or secondary uterine ruptures are pre-conception anomalous or destructive myometrial lesions. Adenomyosis and scarring represent chronic uterine lesions with peripartum fetal stress from uterine rupture[53]; (2) cord prolapse usually associated with abnormally long cords, may also be accompanied by abnormal placental bed insertion with reduced placental blood flow. Abnormal nuchal cord coiling, entanglement, true knots, and hypoplastic umbilical tissue development occur with either short or long cords often have first trimester occurrence, contributing to chronic HI from reduced placental blood flow blood flow closer to delivery[49]; and (3) abruptio placenta correlates with abnormal first trimester placental maldevelopment.[46] Shallow spiral artery placental penetration correlates with vasculopathies contributing to antepartum HI. Unexpected membrane separation during parturition later results in acute blood loss with peripartum HI.

Non-Sentinel Events

Resuscitative interventions for children with NE are more often not associated with sentinel events. Reliance on intrapartum fetal surveillance has limited specificity and sensitivity. Fetal heart rate patterns, fetal blood oximetry, and intrauterine pressures help choose delivery options. Physiologic changes suggesting fetal distress occur more often during the second stage of labor, representing complex disease pathways without the ability to predict pre-existing MPF triad diseases. Current tests lack precision to identify the child with NE at increased risk for acute or chronic brain injury.

A robust physiologic reflex preferentially protects fetal brain, heart, and adrenal gland. This peripheral chemoreflex (PCR) is activated by the baroreflex often associated with fetal hypoxia.[54] Aerobic to anaerobic conversion of glucose metabolism releases 3 rather than 18 ATP molecules in the form of lactate and pyruvate without oxidative phosphorylation. PCR can be activated before or during parturition to preserve life and health. The low incidence of NE affecting 1 to 3/1000 of full-term newborns suggests PCR is an effective neuroprotective mechanism, given only a small percentage of symptomatic neonates benefit less or have no protection with resultant sequelae.[55]

Neonatal EncephalopathyPresentations Evolve Through Discharge

Descriptive criteria define 3 stages of NE[56] based on reduced arousal with altered muscle tone, often associated with dysautonomia, seizures, and multiorgan system dysfunction with metabolic acidosis. Survivors more often express motor sequelae commonly referred to as cerebral palsy,[3] often accompanied by co-morbidities regarding cognition, language, and social adaptive skills. Vision and hearing deficits, epilepsy, and mental health disorders may also be expressed.

Published guidelines recommend therapeutic hypothermia (THT) to treat more severe stages of NE,[57] assuming less than 4 hours to 6 hours of intrapartum HI. Lower mortality risks and less severe sequalae may result with limited predictive value. Considerable heterogeneity exists regarding etiology and timing of disease pathways[58] during intensive care evaluations after THT. Controversies remain regarding treatment of "mild' forms of NE,[59] as unnecessary or ineffective given timing and etiologies associated with MPF triad disease pathways.

Mimicry of HIE requires serial assessments as additional diagnostic information is ascertained.[2] Serial examination, multi-organ analyses, electroencephalography (EEG), multimodal neuroimaging, placenta-cord pathology, and genetic assessments improve prognostic accuracy without necessarily elucidating timing and etiologies. Survivors may clinically improve or resolve phenotypic abnormalities but remain at risk for sequelae. Significant neuroimaging or EEG pattern abnormalities offer stronger predictive value, usually associated with children who remain neurologically abnormal after discharge when delayed milestones and associated co-morbidities present.

THE PEDIATRIC EXPOSOME

The minority with NE more likely requires pediatric follow-up, coordinating primary pediatric care, early intervention programs, and pediatric subspecialty services. Developmental and paroxysmal disorders are principal reasons for outpatient or hospital orintensive care evaluations, often coincident with communicable and noncommunicable adverse events that may contribute to brain injury.

Several of healthy children more often present with similar phenotypes compared with the symptomatic neonatal minority. Paucity of accurate information based on maternal reportage or prenatal testing impedes recognition of impaired reproductive and pregnancy exposomes affecting the fetal neural exposome. Re-evaluations consider complex G x E disease pathways affecting the pediatric exposome using targeted diagnostic studies.[60]

Equitable Diagnostic and Therapeutic Advances "Move the Needle"

Restructuring reproductive and pregnancy healthcare will help identify more women and their partners who conceive children at risk for neurologic sequelae. Only a small percentage presents with NE, often following a healthy prenatal medical course. Equitable health care delivery must consider SDH when providing medical services. Population health policies rely on available resources specific to high-income versus low-moderate income countries. Medical deserts within any community introduce health disparities with negative outcomes,[19] including pregnant women.[61] More successful population health goals can be achieved with advances that benefit all women and children, independent of race-ethnicity, social-economic class, gender identity, or geographic isolation.

Three research agendas exemplify improved detection and intervention strategies that can "move the needle" to improve brain health, integrating equitable healthcare strategies for each mother-child dyad. Deep-state learning platforms will more successfully identify factors to reduce adverse maternal and fetal outcomes associated with NE[62].

1. Untargeted and targeting "omics" testing use genomic, proteomic, metabolomic, and transcriptomic biosignatures for reproductive health and pregnancy planning. Screening during preassigned intervals during pregnancy[17] may be supplemented by more frequent encounters when MPF triad diseases are identified, elucidating trimester, and region-specific effects on fetal brain. "Omics" technologies are applied after identifying NE to assess GNNS, often in the context of multisystem diseases (eg, congenital heart disease and sepsis) that contribute to brain injuries. These biosignatures later identify children during the first 2 years of age when childhood diseases present in the outpatient or hospital setting. This "omics" technology builds on whole exome sequencing and high through-put genomic association studies to better identify mitotic and posttranslational G x E effects on the neural exposome.

2. Volumetric and quantitative MRI imaging assess the placenta-brain axis relative to MPF triad health at preassigned intervals during pregnancy,[43] visualizing brain structures starting during the early second trimester, with postnatal brain neuroimaging comparisons.

3. Tissue-specific exosome biosignatures evaluate systemic-specific cellular bi-products associated with disease pathways. Different exosomes, classified by size and function, potentially detect MPF triad diseases by targeting neuronal or placental cell populations affected by TSI, and deliver pharmaceuticals to block or mitigate disease pathway effects that impair the brain-placenta axis[63](**Fig. 4**). These placental and neuronal bio-signatures can be associated with primary, secondary, and tertiary stages of neurodegeneration[64] (**Fig. 5**). Preventive, rescue, or reparative treatments can be chosen based on prenatal or postnatal timing and etiologies associated with disease pathways.

Genomic, proteomic, metabolomic, or transcriptomic biomarkers will be designed to treat disease pathways, based on regulatory genetic processes.[65] Neuroprotective strategies will be chosen based on biosignatures during pre-clinical stages of disease, as well as with abnormal phenotypes such as NE.

INVESTING IN A BRAIN CAPITAL STRATEGY

A life-course brain capital strategy promotes the science of social-to-biological transitions[2] when evaluating NE in the context of effects on the fetal neural exposome from reproductive and pregnancy exposomes. Brain research, innovation, regulatory, and funding systems require interdisciplinary FNN principles and practice to improve an understanding of normal and abnormal brain maturation and aging across each and

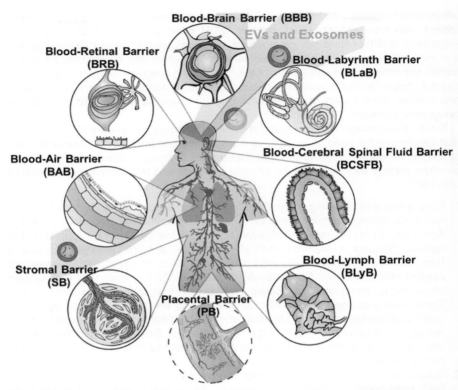

Fig. 4. Essential biological barriers are penetrated by exosomes that regulate cellular functions and drug delivery.[63]

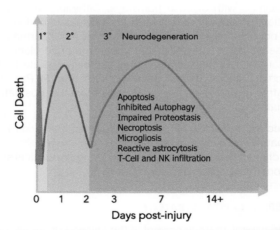

Fig. 5. Stages of neurodegeneration represent disease pathways identified with hypoxia-ischemia (HI) represent multiple mechanisms with primary, secondary, and tertiary stages of injury. (Levison, S. W., Rocha-Ferreira, E., Kim, B. H., Hagberg, H., Fleiss, B., Gressens, P., & Dobrowolski, R. (2022). Mechanisms of tertiary neurodegeneration after neonatal hypoxic-ischemic brain damage. Pediatric Medicine, 5, 28. https://doi.org/10.21037/pm-20-104.)

successive lifespans. Applying a fetal neural exposome concept to clinical practice better identifies functional neurodiversity or permanent sequelae to offer more accurate interventions and prognosis.

DISCLOSURE

There are no commercial or financial conflicts and no funding sources to disclose.

Best practices

- Integrate reproductive and pregnancy bio-social health risks to the maternal-placental-fetal triad when evaluating neonatal encephalopathy.
- Reassess with serial evaluations timing and etiologies contributing to the expression of neonatal encephalopathy.
- Apply the exposome concept to an understanding of a dynamic fetal neural exposome influenced by reproductive and pregnancy factors contributing to neonatal encephalopathy.
- Investigate for gene-environment interactions throughout childhood that best explain neurologic phenotypes of neurodiversity or disease.

REFERENCES

1. Scher MS. "The first thousand days"define a fetal/neonatal neurology program. Front. Pediatr 2021;9:1–28.
2. Scher MS. Interdisciplinary fetal-neonatal neurology training applies neural exposome perspectives to neurology principles and practice. Front Neurol 2023;14.
3. Yang M, Eide S, Tam EW, et al. Worsening of cerebral palsy following neonatal encephalopathy: a meta-analysis. Adv Neurol 2023;2:1719.
4. Scher MS. The neural exposome influences the preterm fetal-to-neonatal connectome. Pediatr Res 2023. https://doi.org/10.1038/s41390-023-02804-x.
5. Brosens I, Pijnenborg R, Vercruysse L, et al. The "great Obstetrical Syndromes" are associated with disorders of deep placentation. Am J Obstet Gynecol 2011; 204:193–201.
6. Wild CP. Complementing the genome with an "exposome": the outstanding challenge of environmental exposure measurement in molecular epidemiology. Cancer Epidemiol Biomarkers Prev 2005;14:1847–50.
7. Tamiz AP, Koroshetz WJ, Dhruv NT, et al. A focus on the neural exposome. Neuron 2022;110:1286–9.
8. Fang M, Hu L, Chen D, et al. Exposome in human health: utopia or wonderland? Innovation 2021;2.
9. Mamun A, Biswas T, Scott J, et al. Adverse childhood experiences, the risk of pregnancy complications and adverse pregnancy outcomes: a systematic review and meta-analysis. BMJ Open 2023;13.
10. Colwell ML, Townsel C, Petroff RL, et al. Epigenetics and the exposome: DNA methylation as a proxy for health impacts of prenatal environmental exposures. Exposome 2023;3.
11. Kiely M, El-Mohandes AAE, Gantz MG, et al. Understanding the association of biomedical, psychosocial and behavioral risks with adverse pregnancy outcomes among African-Americans in Washington, DC. Matern Child Health J 2011;15(Suppl 1).

12. Diabelková J, Rimárová K, Dorko E, et al. Adolescent pregnancy outcomes and risk factors. Int J Environ Res Publ Health 2023;20.

13. Deguen S, Amuzu M, Simoncic V, et al. Exposome and social vulnerability: an overview of the literature review. Int J Environ Res Publ Health 2022;19.

14. Chen M, Guan Y, Huang R, et al. Associations between the maternal exposome and metabolome during pregnancy. Environ Health Perspect 2022;130.

15. de Prado-Bert P, Ruiz-Arenas C, Vives-Usano M, et al. The early-life exposome and epigenetic age acceleration in children. Environ Int 2021;155.

16. Ambeskovic M, Roseboom TJ, Metz GAS. Transgenerational effects of early environmental insults on aging and disease incidence. Neurosci Biobehav Rev 2020; 117:297–316.

17. Menard MK, Menard MK, Kilpatrick S, et al. Levels of maternal care. Am J Obstet Gynecol 2015;212:259–71.

18. Dranitsaris G, Johnston M, Poirier S, et al. Are health care providers who work with cancer drugs at an increased risk for toxic events? A systematic review and meta-analysis of the literature. J Oncol Pharm Pract 2005;11:69–78.

19. Hguyen A., Van Meijgaard E., Kim S., et al., Mapping healthcare deserts. 2021. The GoodRx Research Team. goodrx.com, from the National Council for Prescription Drug Programs, Inc. (NCPDP), January 2021-December 2021, data QPharmnacy Database v3.1.

20. Zhang P, Carlsten C, Chaleckis R, et al. Defining the scope of exposome studies and research needs from a multidisciplinary perspective. Environ Sci Technol Lett 2021;8:839–52.

21. Napso T, Yong HEJ, Lopez-Tello J, et al. The role of placental hormones in mediating maternal adaptations to support pregnancy and lactation. Front Physiol 2018;9.

22. Wright ML, Starkweather AR, York TP. Mechanisms of the maternal exposome and implications for health outcomes. Adv Nurs Sci 2016;39:E17–30.

23. Than NG, Romero R, Tarca AL, et al. Integrated systems biology approach identifies novel maternal and placental pathways of preeclampsia. Front Immunol 2018;9.

24. Chao A, Grossman J, Carberry C, et al. Integrative exposomic, transcriptomic, epigenomic analyses of human placental samples links understudied chemicals to preeclampsia. Environ Int 2022;167.

25. Wu M, Yan F, Liu Q, et al. Effects of xenobiotic compounds on preeclampsia and potential mechanisms. Toxics 2023;11.

26. Rudge MVC, Alves FCB, Hallur RLS, et al. Consequences of the exposome to gestational diabetes mellitus. Biochim Biophys Acta Gen Subj 2023;1867.

27. Ronsmans S, Sørig Hougaard K, Nawrot TS, et al. The EXIMIOUS project-Mapping exposure-induced immune effects: connecting the exposome and the immunome. Environ Epidemiol 2022;6:E193.

28. Han VX, Patel S, Jones HF, et al. Maternal immune activation and neuroinflammation in human neurodevelopmental disorders. Nat Rev Neurol 2021;17:564–79.

29. Goldstein JA, Norris SA, Aronoff DM. DOHaD at the intersection of maternal immune activation and maternal metabolic stress: a scoping review. Journal of Developmental Origins of Health and Disease 2017;8:273–83.

30. Goldstein JA, Gallagher K, Beck C, et al. Maternal-fetal inflammation in the placenta and the developmental origins of health and disease. Front Immunol 2020;11.

31. Para R, Romero R, Miller D, et al. The distinct immune nature of the fetal inflammatory response syndrome type I and type II. ImmunoHorizons 2021;5:735–51.

32. Scher MS. Neurologic outcome after fetal inflammatory response syndrome: trimester-specific considerations. Semin Fetal Neonatal Med 2020;25:101137.

33. Tam SJ, Watts RJ. Connecting vascular and nervous system development: angiogenesis and the blood-brain barrier. Annu Rev Neurosci 2010;33:379–408.

34. Klerk DH, van Avezaath LK, Loeffen EAH, et al. Fetal–neonatal exposure to antibiotics and NEC development: a systematic review and meta-analysis. Front Pediatr 2023;10.

35. Naughton SX, Terry AV. Neurotoxicity in acute and repeated organophosphate exposure. Toxicology 2018;408:101–12.

36. Vineis P, Barouki R. The exposome as the science of social-to-biological transitions. Environ Int 2022;165.

37. Harville EW, Kruse AN, Zhao Q. The impact of early-life exposures on women's reproductive health in adulthood. Curr. Epidemiol. Reports 2021;8:175–89.

38. Yap F, Loy SL, Ku CW, et al. A golden thread approach to transforming maternal and child health in Singapore. BMC Pregnancy Childbirth 2022;22.

39. Fox A, Doyle E, Geary M, et al. Placental pathology and neonatal encephalopathy. Int J Gynecol Obstet 2023;160:22–7.

40. Hodyl NA, Aboustate N, Bianco-Miotto T, et al. Child neurodevelopmental outcomes following preterm and term birth: what can the placenta tell us? Placenta 2017;57:79–86.

41. Rosenfeld CS. Transcriptomics and other omics approaches to investigate effects of xenobiotics on the placenta. Front Cell Dev Biol 2021;9.

42. Redline RW, Roberts DJ, Parast MM, et al. Placental pathology is necessary to understand common pregnancy complications and achieve an improved taxonomy of obstetrical disease. Am J Obstet Gynecol 2023;228:187–202.

43. De Asis-Cruz J, Andescavage N, Limperopoulos C. Adverse prenatal exposures and fetal brain development: insights from advanced fetal magnetic resonance imaging. Biol. Psychiatry Cogn. Neurosci. Neuroimaging 2021. https://doi.org/10.1016/j.bpsc.2021.11.009.

44. Cuadros MA, Sepulveda MR, Martin-Oliva D, et al. Microglia and microglia-like cells: similar but different. Front Cell Neurosci 2022;16.

45. Meyer U. Neurodevelopmental resilience and susceptibility to maternal immune activation. Trends Neurosci 2019;42:793–806.

46. Brosens I, Puttemans P, Benagiano G. Placental bed research: I. The placental bed: from spiral arteries remodeling to the great obstetrical syndromes. Am J Obstet Gynecol 2019;221:437–56.

47. Romero R, Jung E, Chaiworapongsa T, et al. Toward a new taxonomy of obstetrical disease: improved performance of maternal blood biomarkers for the great obstetrical syndromes when classified according to placental pathology. Am J Obstet Gynecol 2022;227:615, e1-e25.

48. Landmann E, Reiss I, Misselwitz B, et al. Ponderal index for discrimination between symmetric and asymmetric growth restriction: percentiles for neonates from 30 weeks to 43 weeks of gestation. J Matern Neonatal Med 2006;19:157–60.

49. Vrabie SC, Novac L, Manolea MM, et al. In: Abnormalities of the umbilical cord, In: Congenital anomalies - from the embryo to the neonate. UK: InTech; 2018. https://doi.org/10.5772/intechopen.72666.

50. Khong TY, Mooney EE, Ariel I, et al. Sampling and definitions of placental lesions: amsterdam placental workshop group consensus statement. Arch Pathol Lab Med 2016;140:698–713.

51. Kindschuh WF, Baldini F, Liu MC, et al. Preterm birth is associated with xenobiotics and predicted by the vaginal metabolome. Nat Microbiol 2023;8:246–59.

52. Ernst LM, Bockoven C, Freedman A, et al. Chronic villitis of unknown etiology: investigations into viral pathogenesis. Placenta 2021;107:24–30.
53. Rees C, van Vliet H, Siebers A, et al. The ADENO study: ADenomyosis and its effect on neonatal and obstetric outcomes: a retrospective population-based study. Am J Obstet Gynecol 2022. https://doi.org/10.1016/j.ajog.2022.12.013.
54. Lear CA, Wassink G, Westgate JA, et al. The peripheral chemoreflex: indefatigable guardian of fetal physiological adaptation to labour. J Physiol 2018;596: 5611–23.
55. American College of Obstetricians and Gynecologists' Task Force on Neonatal Encephalopathy. Neonatal encephalopathy and neurologic outcome, second edition. 2014, reaffrimed. Obstet Gynecol 2019;123:896–901.
56. Sarnat HB, Flores-Sarnat L, Fajardo C, et al. Sarnat grading scale for neonatal encephalopathy after 45 years: an update proposal. Pediatr Neurol 2020;113:75–9.
57. Jacobs SE, Berg M, Hunt R, et al. Cooling for newborns with hypoxic ischaemic encephalopathy. Cochrane Database Syst Rev 2013;2013.
58. Molloy EJ, El-Dib M, Juul SE, et al. Neuroprotective therapies in the NICU in term infants: present and future. Pediatr Res 2022. https://doi.org/10.1038/s41390-022-02295-2.
59. Chalak L. New horizons in mild hypoxic-ischemic encephalopathy: a standardized algorithm to move past conundrum of care. Clin Perinatol 2022;49:279–94.
60. Scher MS. Gene-environment interactions during the first thousand days influence childhood neurological diagnosis. Semin Pediatr Neurol 2022;100970. https://doi.org/10.1016/j.spen.2022.100970.
61. Brigance C, Lucas R, Jones E, et al. Nowhere to go: maternity care deserts across the U.S. (Report No. 3). March of Dimes 2022;1–36.
62. Mennickent D, Rodríguez A, Opazo MC, et al. Machine learning applied in maternal and fetal health: a narrative review focused on pregnancy diseases and complications. Front Endocrinol 2023;14:1130139.
63. Elliott RO, He M. Unlocking the power of exosomes for crossing biological barriers in drug delivery. Pharmaceutics 2021;13:1–20.
64. Levison SW, Rocha-Ferreira E, Kim BH, et al. Mechanisms of tertiary neurodegeneration after neonatal hypoxic-ischemic brain damage. Pediatric Medicine 2022;5.
65. Loebrich S, Nedivi E. The function of activity-regulated genes in the nervous system. Physiol Rev 2009;89:1079–103.

Uncovering the Role of Inflammation with Asphyxia in the Newborn

Simerdeep K. Dhillon, PhD[a], Pierre Gressens, MD, PhD[b],
John Barks, MD, PhD[c], Alistair J. Gunn, MBChB, PhD[a],*

KEYWORDS

- Hypoxia-ischemia • Inflammation • Anti-inflammatory treatments

KEY POINTS

- Acute and chronic inflammation triggered after hypoxia-ischemia (HI) is a critical mediator of secondary cell loss and subsequent injury and repair during the tertiary phase.
- HI can co-occur with perinatal inflammation or infection, and modulation of the immune responses to HI by pre-existing inflammation can be associated with either exacerbation or attenuation of neural injury.
- There is mixed clinical and preclinical evidence for the reduced efficacy of therapeutic hypothermia in the presence of perinatal infection/inflammation.
- Recent preclinical data suggest that targeting acute inflammatory processes after HI may be a viable strategy for treating inflammation-sensitized HI.

INTRODUCTION

Hypoxia-ischemia (HI) before or at birth is the single most common cause of perinatal brain injury in term infants, affecting approximately 1.5 to 3/1000 live births annually in high-income countries, leading to approximately 1 million neonatal deaths and life-long disabilities in survivors around the world.[1] Exposure to HI is also a significant contributor to the multifactorial etiology of preterm brain damage. A large cohort study reported that rates of hypoxic-ischemic encephalopathy (HIE) in preterm infants were significantly higher than at term, with moderate–severe HIE in 37.3/1000 preterm-born infants.[2]

Other etiologies associated with neonatal encephalopathy include perinatal infections, placental pathologies, and maternal comorbidities.[3] The amniotic cavity is maintained sterile in a healthy pregnancy. Pathogens can invade the amniotic cavity via

[a] Department of Physiology, The University of Auckland, 85 Park Road, Grafton, Auckland 1023, New Zealand; [b] Université Paris Cité, NeuroDiderot, Inserm, F-75019 Paris, France; [c] Department of Pediatrics and Communicable Diseases, The University of Michigan, 2018 MLB, Ann Arbor, MI 48109, USA
* Corresponding author.
E-mail address: aj.gunn@auckland.ac.nz

Clin Perinatol 51 (2024) 551–564
https://doi.org/10.1016/j.clp.2024.04.012
0095-5108/24/© 2024 Elsevier Inc. All rights reserved.
perinatology.theclinics.com

placental transfer from maternal blood or ascend from the lower genital tract, causing intra-amniotic infection and fetal inflammation and infection.[4] Intrauterine inflammation can also be induced in the absence of microbes by endogenous molecules associated with cellular stress and damage.[5] Intra-amniotic infection or inflammation induces an inflammatory response in the fetal tissues in direct contact with amniotic fluid and subsequently can lead to a robust systemic and cerebral inflammatory response and associated brain injury.[6]

Retrospective cohort studies have reported inflammatory placental pathology and fetal inflammation in approximately 43% of term-born infants, in the absence of evidence for sentinel events. Moreover, histologic funisitis was an independent risk factor for neonatal encephalopathy.[7] Histologic chorioamnionitis is reported in nearly 95% of preterm births at 21 to 24 weeks of gestation and in about 10% of deliveries at 33 to 36 weeks and is associated with an increased risk of MRI abnormalities at term equivalent age and delayed brain maturation.[8,9] Babies can also be exposed to infectious microorganisms during birth or postnatally. Early-onset sepsis occurs within 72 hours after birth and is associated with microorganisms acquired in utero or during birth; its incidence is reported as 0.56 to 0.79 per 1000 live births in term-born infants and 13.5 per 1000 in very preterm infants.[10,11] In turn, neonatal sepsis is associated with an increased risk of developing brain injury and adverse neurodevelopmental outcomes.[12]

Importantly, these inflammatory insults can also occur in combination with HI and have a cumulative contribution to the pathogenesis of perinatal brain injury. For example, compared with the population, a higher incidence of early neonatal infections is reported in term infants with HIE.[13] Chorioamnionitis and fetal vasculitis are also commonly observed in term infants with perinatal asphyxia.[3] In a subset of the high-dose erythropoietin for asphyxia and encephalopathy trial participants, nearly 40% (124 of 321) had evidence of histologic chorioamnionitis.[14] These placental pathologies are associated with acute electroencephalographic (EEG) abnormalities, injury severity on MRI, and adverse neurodevelopmental outcomes in term infants treated with therapeutic hypothermia.[15,16]

To change outcomes, we need to improve our understanding of the pathogenesis of perinatal brain injury and the complex interactions between different etiologies. Inflammation is the common mediator of neural injury for multiple perinatal insults.[17] This review discusses the role of acute and chronic inflammation in mediating neural injury after HI, modification of neuro-inflammatory responses with a combination of HI and inflammatory insults and potential interventions.

Acute Inflammatory Response After Hypoxia-Ischemia

HI events trigger a cascade of inflammatory processes, which play a crucial role in the evolution of injury over weeks. Reperfusion after HI is typically associated with transient recovery of mitochondrial function and cerebral metabolism during the latent phase. Despite no reduction in cerebral perfusion, this transient recovery can be followed by secondary deterioration of oxidative metabolism from 6 to 8 hours and ultimately bulk cell loss.[18] The acute pro-inflammatory processes during the latent phase have been shown to contribute to the progression of secondary deterioration and cell loss (**Fig. 1**).

Microglia are the resident immune-responsive cells. They are involved in immune surveillance, synaptic pruning, neuronal hemostasis, and establishing network connectivity in the developing brain.[19] Exposure of the microglial pattern recognition receptors to damage-associated molecules released after HI, leads to diffuse microglia activation.[20] "Activated" microglia undergo morphologic and functional

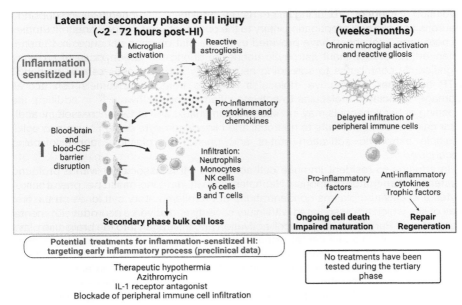

Fig. 1. Flow diagram showing inflammatory processes during the latent, secondary, and tertiary phases of HI injury, modulation of early inflammatory processes with pre-existing inflammatory challenge and potential neuroprotective treatments for inflammation-sensitized HI. Created with BioRender.com

changes, including upregulation of toll-like receptors expression, initiation of phagocytosis, and increased production of effector molecules like reactive oxygen species and inflammatory cytokines, and these inflammatory mediators can directly activate extrinsic cell death pathways.[19] It is important to appreciate that microglial activation is complex and encompasses multiple states; thus, this term should be considered to be short-hand for a highly polymorphic reality.[21]

Intense microglial activation and upregulation of pro-inflammatory cytokines like tumor necrosis factor (TNF), interleukin (IL)-1β and IL-6 have been observed as early as 2 to 3 hours after HI in preclinical studies.[22] The degree of acute neuro-inflammatory response was associated with neuronal loss within 24 hours after HI, and attenuation of the excessive early neuro-inflammation is neuroprotective.[22] In contrast, in neonatal mice, complete depletion of microglia significantly exacerbated brain injury at 3 days after HI, highlighting an endogenous neuroprotective role of acute microglial activation.[23] Consequently, the field has tended to focus on the functional categorization of microglia into M1 (activated: pro-inflammatory) and M2 (anti-inflammatory) phenotypes after HI and targeting induction of M2 phenotype for neuroprotection.[19] However, it is now recognized that such phenotypic classification may overly simplify the complexity of dynamic changes in microglia that are intricately associated with their local environment changes.[21] Understanding the temporal pattern of diverse microglial transcriptional changes after neonatal HI will aid the development of treatment strategies.

Astrocytes are important in maintaining homeostasis and a stable environment for normal neuronal function. Astrocytes respond to HI with morphologic changes such as hypertrophy of the cell body and processes, increased intermediate filaments, and changes in gene and protein expression.[24] Astrocytes can contribute to the evolution of injury by producing inflammatory cytokines, disrupting trophic support to neurons and glia and propagating injury to the previously undamaged areas.[25] Studies in near-term fetal sheep have provided evidence that opening of connexin 43 hemichannel (the predominant astrocytic connexin) during the latent phase of recovery significantly contributes to spreading neural injury and increases seizure burden.[26] ATP and other neuroactive molecules released from hemichannels can act as damage-associated molecules to activate inflammatory pathways.[25] In addition, the opening of hemichannels may increase calcium influx, and in turn increased intracellular calcium can contribute to neuronal and oligodendrocyte death.[25] Like microglia, multiple astrocytic activation states and phenotypic plasticity are also being recognized.[27]

In addition to resident immune cell activation, HI is associated with a profound systemic inflammatory response. Neonates with HIE have increased peripheral leukocytes and elevated plasma concentrations of proinflammatory cytokines on the first day of life, which are associated with injury severity and adverse neurodevelopmental outcomes.[28] Peripheral immune cell activation and infiltration into the brain also plays a significant role in acute neural damage after HI. Recruitment of peripheral immune cells into the brain is facilitated by chemokine upregulation and transient disruption and increased permeability of the blood–brain barrier after HI[29]; in addition, alterations of the blood–cerebrospinal fluid barrier may facilitate immune cell infiltration.[30]

Studies in neonatal rodents have examined the temporal profile of peripheral immune cell recruitment into the brain after HI. In P9 mice, circulating neutrophils in the blood increased 12 hours post-HI, followed by infiltration into the brain, with cerebral neutrophil counts peaking at 24 hours, and then declining by 72 hours post-HI.[31] Similarly, other preclinical studies have shown waves of cerebral infiltration of peripheral monocytes, gamma-delta-T cells, natural killer cells, and peripheral B and T cells after neonatal HI.[32,33] More importantly, early depletion of peripheral immune cells in different models was consistently neuroprotective.[31,32] These data denote that acute peripheral immune cell infiltration contributes to the secondary phase of damage after HI. However, the precise time course of expression of different cells and their role in injury evolution needs further investigation. Peripheral immune cells can exacerbate neuro-inflammatory response by promoting glial activation, formation of neutrophil extracellular traps, and increased production of reactive oxygen species and pro-inflammatory cytokines.[34]

Tertiary Phase: Chronic Inflammation

The secondary phase of cell death lasts approximately 72 hours after severe HI. It resolves into a tertiary phase involving both ongoing cell death and repair and reorganization.[18] Serial imaging studies in term neonates with HIE have reported that subtle abnormalities in the regional signal intensity seen in the first few days after birth become more apparent by the end of the first week, and an MRI scan after 1 month can show gross changes such as volume loss, cysts, gliosis, and impaired myelination.[35] Similarly, preclinical studies have shown delayed evolution of injury over weeks after HI.[36] There is limited understanding of the mechanisms of this delayed evolution of injury, but there is evidence to support the role of chronic neuroinflammation.

In preterm fetal sheep exposed to severe HI, diffuse white matter loss and maturational arrest at 3 to 7 days post-HI evolve into severe cystic injury and white matter atrophy over 2 to 3 weeks.[37] The development of these cystic lesions in fetal sheep was preceded by intense local microgliosis. Treatment with a TNF inhibitor during the tertiary phase attenuated cystic white matter damage and improved neurorepair, supporting the concept that inflammation is a key mediator of the delayed evolution of injury.[38] Region-dependent, biphasic microglial activation over 2 weeks after

HI was also observed in neonatal mice.[33] In term-equivalent fetal sheep, neuronal loss, white matter damage, development of lesions, and EEG dysfunction at 7 days after 30 minutes cerebral ischemia were associated with persistent microgliosis and astrogliosis and upregulation for pro-inflammatory microglia.[39] Altered microenvironment with chronic microglial activation and reactive gliosis in the tertiary phase also contributes to impaired maturational processes, leading to microstructural abnormalities.[40]

Beneficial Effects of Microglia

Along with detrimental effects, microglia activation may also play a role in tissue remodeling and neurorepair. Based on activation of specific cell surface receptors, microglia phagocytose cellular debris and provide neurotrophic support for the surviving cells by releasing growth factors.[41] In response to chronic stress in mice, IL-4 signaling-driven hippocampal microglia triggered neurogenesis mediated by brain-derived growth factor.[42] Studies in mouse models of spinal cord injury have shown that exosomes from the M2 subtype of microglia can modulate astrocyte activation and promote axonal regrowth.[43] Microglia can also aid in myelin regeneration, and in part, this reparative microglial response is mediated by infiltering peripheral immune cells.[44]

Peripheral immune cell infiltration during the tertiary phase corresponds with the period of initiation of repair and regeneration. For example, there is a biphasic pattern of myeloid cell recruitment into the neonatal mouse brain after HI, with a second peak 1 week post-HI.[45] Similarly, peripheral adaptive immune cells (T lymphocytes) were recruited into the brain at 1 and 2 weeks, and CD69-expressing B lymphocytes were upregulated in the damaged brain up to 3 months post-HI in neonatal mice.[33] The relative contribution of immune cell to protection and repair after HI in the immature brain needs extensive further research.

Sustained Inflammation in Infants with Neonatal Encephalopathy

Consistent with the preclinical data for persistent inflammation after HI, there is mounting evidence from recent clinical trials that alterations in inflammatory response persist well beyond the early postnatal period in both preterm and term infants with neonatal encephalopathy. Term neonates with HIE treated with therapeutic hypothermia were reported to have higher plasma concentrations of TNF, IL-2, IL-8, and IL-6 at school age than age-matched controls.[46] Prospective cohort studies in term infants with neonatal encephalopathy showed altered cytokine levels in whole blood samples in response to endotoxin exposure during the first 4 days of life, including lower production of pro-inflammatory mediators IL-8, IL-2, IL-6, TNF, granulocyte–macrophage colony-stimulating factor than healthy controls.[47] The difference in baseline and endotoxin-stimulated TNF production was associated with injury severity on MRI. Hypo-responsiveness to stimulation with gram-negative bacterial cell wall mimetics lipopolysaccharide (LPS) was also reported in children with cerebral palsy.[48] In contrast, preterm-born children with periventricular leukomalacia and cerebral palsy were reported to have increased plasma concentration of TNF-α and hyper-responsiveness to inflammatory stimulus at 7 years of age.[49] These findings highlight that the initial response to HI has the potential to either program the immune system for an aggravated response to a secondary inflammatory challenge or induce tolerance to it.

Complex Interaction Between Hypoxia-Ischemia and Inflammatory Insult

Given the high incidence of perinatal inflammation, babies are likely to be exposed to multiple injurious insults. Therefore, there is a need to consider whether pre-existing inflammation would modify the adaptation to HI and the severity of subsequent neural injury. In a small cohort study in preterm infants, Stark and colleagues showed that histologic chorioamnionitis was associated with increased cerebral oxygen consumption on the first day of life,[50] suggesting that pre-existing inflammation could potentially accelerate metabolic decompensation during HI and alter post-HI recovery. Similarly, in term neonates undergoing therapeutic hypothermia, the presence of histologic chorioamnionitis was associated with worsening of metabolic acidosis within the first 6 hours after birth,[51] implying that the combined insults can exacerbate the severity of HIE.

The additive effect of HI and inflammation is not unexpected. However, considerable preclinical evidence shows that depending on the order, severity, and time interval between the insults, inflammation can modulate the response to HI in a positive (tolerance) or negative (sensitization) manner.[52] For example, in preterm fetal sheep exposed to a chronic low dose of LPS (100–250 ng/day for 5 days), superimposed with bolus injections of 1 μg, there was significantly reduced white matter damage with HI at 4 hours after the last bolus of LPS.[53]

In contrast, sensitization is seen with the shorter or longer intervals between the insults. In P7 rats, exposure to LPS at 2 or 72 hours before HI also exacerbated neural injury.[54] Aggravation of neural injury was associated with altered immune responsiveness to HI, involving TLR4 and the recruitment of the MyD88 adaptor protein and increased NF-kβ signaling.[55] In P9 mice, exposure to LPS 14 hours before HI was associated with a greater acute rise in proinflammatory markers, microglia activation, and neutrophil infiltration compared to HI alone and resulted in progressive exacerbation of diffuse to cystic neural injury over 15 days post-HI.[56]

Sensitization has also been demonstrated in an excitotoxic model of perinatal brain damage. Excitotoxicity is a major mechanism leading to secondary neuronal cell death in neonatal HIE.[18] Intracerebral injection of ibotenate, an agonist of glutamatergic NMDA and metabotropic receptors, at P5 or P10 induces cortical neuronal cell death, mimicking cell death observed in HIE and related animal models.[57,58] Pre-treating the mouse pups (P1-P5) with systemic administration of pro-inflammatory cytokines (IL-1beta, IL-6, or TNF-alpha) significantly exacerbated the excitotoxic neuronal cell death through recruitment of reactive microglia and de-sensitization of glutamate receptors via GRK2 inhibition.[59] Similarly, pre-treatment with a Th2 cytokine (IL-9) in mouse pups exacerbated ibotenate-induced neuronal cell death through mast cell recruitment and histamine release.[60,61]

The increased infiltration of peripheral immune cells also contributes to ongoing neural damage. For example, monocytes infiltrating the brain after inflammation-sensitized HI in neonatal mice transformed into pathologic microglia, which persisted for months after the insult.[62] In rats exposed to a combination of LPS and HI in utero on embryonic day 18, the peripheral blood mononuclear cells were hyper-reactive and had a robust proinflammatory response to LPS stimulation until adulthood.[63] These data suggest a potential increase in long-term vulnerability to subsequent inflammatory challenges. Importantly, altered inflammatory profile could modulate the protective effect of neurotherapeutics.

Efficacy of Therapeutic Hypothermia for Inflammation-Sensitized Hypoxia-Ischemia

Therapeutic hypothermia is now standard care for term neonates with moderate-to-severe HIE in high-income countries. Despite significantly reducing death and disability, therapeutic hypothermia is only partially neuroprotective, with a number needed to treat of 7 ([95% CI 5–10], 8 studies, 1344 infants).[64] Further, a recent large randomized controlled trial has raised concerns that therapeutic hypothermia did not improve outcomes in low- and middle-income settings.[65] The reason why some infants do not benefit from therapeutic hypothermia is not entirely understood. However, it is postulated that hypothermia treatment might not be effective for neonates with inflammation-sensitized HI injury.[4]

Small studies have reported that in neonates with HIE treated with therapeutic hypothermia, placental abnormalities, including histologic chorioamnionitis, were independently associated with brain injury severity and adverse neurodevelopmental outcomes.[15,66] These findings suggest that therapeutic hypothermia might be less effective in neonates with prior exposure to perinatal inflammation. By contrast, other studies reported no association between placental pathology and MRI findings and neurodevelopmental outcomes after hypothermia treatment.[67,68] Similarly, neonates with sepsis being treated with hypothermia had greater requirements for intensive care support, but they did not have higher mortality.[69] However, the impact on neurodevelopmental outcomes is unknown. Studies with large sample sizes and better-quality evidence are still needed to address the concerns about the effectiveness of therapeutic hypothermia in neonates sensitized with prior infection/inflammation.

Evidence from preclinical studies also supports these concerns. In P7 rats exposed to systemic LPS injection followed by HI after a 4 h delay, LPS sensitization significantly increased brain area loss, apoptosis, microgliosis, and astrogliosis compared with vehicle-HI controls, and treatment with hypothermia did not ameliorate these effects.[70] In contrast, studies in P7 rats using gram-positive bacterial mimetics to induce inflammatory sensitization 8 hours before HI reported that hypothermia was highly neuroprotective,[71] suggesting that hypothermia can still be effective in the presence of gram-positive bacterial infections. Recently, 2 studies have examined hypothermic neuroprotection for LPS-sensitized HI in newborn piglets (human term-equivalent).[72,73] Both these studies reported that hypothermia did not improve acute EEG recovery, MR spectroscopy parameters, and cell survival. These studies used short, sub-optimal durations of therapeutic hypothermia (14–24 hours) and thus there is a need for large animal translational studies using clinical protocols of hypothermia.

Antibiotic Treatment for Perinatal Infections

The efficacy of broad-spectrum antibiotics for managing perinatal infections has been examined for preterm or pre-labor rupture of membranes at term, intra-amniotic infections, and neonatal sepsis.[74] There is no convincing evidence for maternal and neonatal benefit with antibiotic use for prelabor rupture of membranes at term.[75] Indeed, prophylactic antibiotic treatment for preterm rupture of membranes appears to be associated with increased neonatal mortality (Relative Risk 1.57) although there may have been reduced maternal infection.[76] In a randomized control trial in women presenting with spontaneous preterm labor (n = 4221), maternal administration of erythromycin for preterm labor with intact membranes was associated with increased risk of functional impairments and cerebral palsy among the children at 7 years of age.[77] Large randomized control trials are needed to assess the benefits and risks associated with antibiotic regimens for treating early-onset neonatal sepsis. Prolonged use of antibiotics can be associated with antibiotic resistance and longer-term adverse outcomes such as necrotizing enterocolitis and brain injury, especially in preterm neonates without proven infection.[74] Further, in infants undergoing therapeutic hypothermia, the pharmacodynamics of antibiotics may also be modulated by cooling,[78] suggesting the need for careful assessment of dosage and potential adverse effects in infants with perinatal infection and HIE.

Preclinical Studies of Anti-Inflammatory Therapies for Inflammation-Sensitized Hypoxia-Ischemia

In preclinical studies, targeting acute inflammatory processes after inflammation-sensitized HI may confer neuroprotection.[79] For example, in P7 rats exposed to systemic LPS injection and HI after a 4 h delay, intranasally administered of NF-kβ inhibitor (Tat-NBD peptide) at 10 minutes post-insult, reduced atrophy of cortex, striatum, and hippocampus at 1 week post-HI.[55] Similarly, early blockade of peripheral immune cell trafficking into the brain early after LPS–HI using agents such as chemokine receptor antagonist for monocyte blockade, fingolimod for lymphocyte blockade significantly reduces brain tissue loss and improved cognitive function in neonatal rodents.[62,80]

Recent studies have focused on examining the neuroprotective potential of clinically available anti-inflammatory drugs. In P7 rats exposed to gram-negative or gram-positive bacterial mimetics (using LPS or Pam3CysSerLys4) sensitized HI, treatment with 5 doses (22.5 mg/kg, intraperitoneal [i.p.]) of azithromycin starting 2 hours post-HI was associated with improvement in intact tissue volume and sensorimotor function at P35.[81] Similarly, in P4 mice with *Staphylococcus epidermidis*-potentiated HI, i.p. injection of antibiotic vancomycin given 2 minutes after the insult was associated with reduced cortical, deep gray matter and white matter loss at 9 days post-HI.[82]

Recombinant erythropoietin has potent anti-inflammatory properties, and there is preclinical evidence that potentially it could be used to reprogram microglia toward beneficial functions.[83] However, in P17 ferret kits, repeated doses of erythropoietin at 0, 24, 48 hours and 7 days after inflammation-sensitized HI provided no significant neuroprotection.[84] Clinically, high-dose erythropoietin given from 24 hours after birth to 32 weeks postmenstrual age did not improve neurodevelopmental outcomes in extremely preterm infants, suggesting that it is not an effective strategy.[85]

SUMMARY

Inflammation is critical in mediating both secondary and tertiary phase injury and neuro-repair processes after HI. Inflammatory challenges associated with perinatal infections can commonly co-occur with HI. Preclinical studies show exacerbation of neural damage after HI in the presence of pre-existing inflammation and that therapeutic hypothermia may be ineffective for the neural injury associated with a combination of inflammation and HI. However, this needs further investigation in translational large animal studies with optimal duration of hypothermia, as there is no conclusive clinical evidence for the lack or reduced efficacy of neuroprotection with therapeutic hypothermia in neonates with sepsis or chorioamnionitis. Immunomodulatory and anti-inflammatory agents have shown promising neuroprotective effects for inflammation-sensitized HI in neonatal rodents. These studies were limited by the relatively early start time of treatments. Future studies are needed to assess whether these treatments will still be beneficial if started with a clinically realistic delay after the insult and if they will have an additive neuroprotective effect with therapeutic hypothermia.

Best Practices

The current practice for HIE with pre-existing inflammation

- There is considerable speculation in the field that hypothermia treatment might not be effective for neonates sensitized with prior infection/inflammation.

Major recommendations

- Large animal translational studies using clinical protocols of hypothermia and clinical studies with large sample sizes and better-quality evidence are needed to resolve the concerns about the effectiveness of therapeutic hypothermia for inflammation-sensitized HI injury and to test novel add-on therapies.

Bibliographic Source(s)

Mir IN, Johnson-Welch SF, Nelson DB, Brown LS, Rosenfeld CR, Chalak LF. Placental pathology is associated with severity of neonatal encephalopathy and adverse developmental outcomes following hypothermia. Am J Obstet Gynecol. 2015;213(6):849 e1-7.

Wintermark P, Boyd T, Gregas MC, Labrecque M, Hansen A. Placental pathology in asphyxiated newborns meeting the criteria for therapeutic hypothermia. Am J Obstet Gynecol. 2010;203(6):579 e1-9.

Gonzalez FF, Voldal E, Comstock BA, Mayock DE, Goodman AM, Cornet MC, et al. Placental Histologic Abnormalities and 2-Year Outcomes in Neonatal Hypoxic-Ischemic Encephalopathy. Neonatology. 2023;120(6):760-7.

Kovatis KZ, Mackley A, Antunes M, Holmes PJ, Daugherty RJ, Paul D. Relationship Between Placental Weight and Placental Pathology With MRI Findings in Mild to Moderate Hypoxic Ischemic Encephalopathy. Cureus. 2022;14(5):e24854.

Falck M, Osredkar D, Maes E, Flatebo T, Wood TR, Sabir H, et al. Hypothermic Neuronal Rescue from Infection-Sensitised Hypoxic-Ischaemic Brain Injury Is Pathogen Dependent. Developmental neuroscience. 2017;39(1–4):238-47.

Andersen M, Andersen HB, Andelius TCK, Hansen LH, Pinnerup R, Bjerre M, et al. No neuroprotective effect of therapeutic hypothermia following lipopolysaccharide-sensitized hypoxia-ischemia: a newborn piglet study. Frontiers in pediatrics. 2023;11:1,268,237.

Martinello KA, Meehan C, Avdic-Belltheus A, Lingam I, Mutshiya T, Yang Q, et al. Hypothermia is not therapeutic in a neonatal piglet model of inflammation-sensitized hypoxia-ischemia. Pediatr Res. 2022;91(6):1416-27.

DISCLOSURE

The authors have nothing to disclose.

FUNDING

The authors' research discussed in this paper was supported by the Health Research Council of New Zealand (grant numbers: 17/601 and 22/559), the Auckland Medical Research Foundation (Grant number 1123012) and CureKids (Grant number 3631). PG is supported by grants from Inserm, Université Paris Cité, Horizon 2020 Framework Program of the European Union (grant agreement no. 874721/PREMSTEM), ANR, ERANET-NEURON (VasOX), Fondation Princesse Grace de Monaco, and an additional grant from "Investissement d'Avenir -ANR-11-INBS-0011-" NeurATRIS.

REFERENCES

1. Ahearne CE, Boylan GB, Murray DM. Short and long term prognosis in perinatal asphyxia: an update. World J Clin Pediatr 2016;5(1):67–74.
2. Manuck TA, Rice MM, Bailit JL, et al. Preterm neonatal morbidity and mortality by gestational age: a contemporary cohort. Am J Obstet Gynecol 2016;215(1):103 e1–14.

3. Fox A, Doyle E, Geary M, et al. Placental pathology and neonatal encephalopathy. Int J Gynaecol Obstet 2023;160(1):22–7.

4. Andersen M, Pedersen MV, Andelius TCK, et al. Neurological outcome following newborn encephalopathy with and without perinatal infection: a systematic review. Front Pediatr 2021;9:787804.

5. Abbah J, Vacher CM, Goldstein EZ, et al. Oxidative stress-induced damage to the developing Hippocampus is mediated by GSK3beta. J Neurosci 2022; 42(24):4812–27.

6. Kemp MW, Molloy TJ, Usuda H, et al. Outside-in? Acute fetal systemic inflammation in very preterm chronically catheterized sheep fetuses is not driven by cells in the fetal blood. Am J Obstet Gynecol 2016;214(2):281 e1–10.

7. Novak CM, Eke AC, Ozen M, et al. Risk factors for neonatal hypoxic-ischemic encephalopathy in the absence of sentinel events. Am J Perinatol 2019;36(1):27–33.

8. Kim CJ, Romero R, Chaemsaithong P, et al. Acute chorioamnionitis and funisitis: definition, pathologic features, and clinical significance. Am J Obstet Gynecol 2015;213(4 Suppl):S29–52.

9. Jain VG, Willis KA, Jobe A, et al. Chorioamnionitis and neonatal outcomes. Pediatr Res 2022;91(2):289–96.

10. Cailes B, Kortsalioudaki C, Buttery J, et al. Epidemiology of UK neonatal infections: the neonIN infection surveillance network. Arch Dis Child Fetal Neonatal Ed 2018;103(6):F547–53.

11. Flannery DD, Edwards EM, Puopolo KM, et al. Early-onset sepsis among very preterm infants. Pediatrics 2021;148(4).

12. Smilga AS, Garfinkle J, Ng P, et al. Neonatal infection in children with cerebral palsy: a registry-based cohort study. Pediatr Neurol 2018;80:77–83.

13. Rao R, Lee KS, Zaniletti I, et al. Antimicrobial therapy utilization in neonates with hypoxic-ischemic encephalopathy (HIE): a report from the Children's Hospital Neonatal Database (CHND). J Perinatol 2020;40(1):70–8.

14. Chalak L, Redline RW, Goodman AM, et al. Acute and chronic placental abnormalities in a multicenter cohort of newborn infants with hypoxic-ischemic encephalopathy. J Pediatr 2021;237:190–6.

15. Mir IN, Johnson-Welch SF, Nelson DB, et al. Placental pathology is associated with severity of neonatal encephalopathy and adverse developmental outcomes following hypothermia. Am J Obstet Gynecol 2015;213(6):849 e1–7.

16. Stone AC, Strickland KC, Tanaka DT, et al. The association of placental pathology and neurodevelopmental outcomes in patients with neonatal encephalopathy. Pediatr Res 2023;94(5):1696–706.

17. Hagberg H, Mallard C, Ferriero DM, et al. The role of inflammation in perinatal brain injury. Nat Rev Neurol 2015;11(4):192–208.

18. Davidson JO, Gonzalez F, Gressens P, et al. Update on mechanisms of the pathophysiology of neonatal encephalopathy. Semin Fetal Neonatal Med 2021;26(5): 101267.

19. Fleiss B, Van Steenwinckel J, Bokobza C, et al. Microglia-mediated neurodegeneration in perinatal brain injuries. Biomolecules 2021;11(1).

20. Quan H, Zhang R. Microglia dynamic response and phenotype heterogeneity in neural regeneration following hypoxic-ischemic brain injury. Front Immunol 2023; 14:1320271.

21. Paolicelli RC, Sierra A, Stevens B, et al. Microglia states and nomenclature: a field at its crossroads. Neuron 2022;110(21):3458–83.

22. Teo EJ, Chand KK, Miller SM, et al. Early evolution of glial morphology and inflammatory cytokines following hypoxic-ischemic injury in the newborn piglet brain. Sci Rep 2023;13(1):282.
23. Tsuji S, Di Martino E, Mukai T, et al. Aggravated brain injury after neonatal hypoxic ischemia in microglia-depleted mice. J Neuroinflammation 2020;17(1):111.
24. Mallard C, Davidson JO, Tan S, et al. Astrocytes and microglia in acute cerebral injury underlying cerebral palsy associated with preterm birth. Pediatr Res 2014; 75(1–2):234–40.
25. Zhou KQ, Green CR, Bennet L, et al. The role of connexin and pannexin channels in perinatal brain injury and inflammation. Front Physiol 2019;10:141.
26. Davidson JO, Green CR, Bennet L, et al. A key role for connexin hemichannels in spreading ischemic brain injury. Curr Drug Targets 2013;14(1):36–46.
27. Giovannoni F, Quintana FJ. The role of astrocytes in CNS inflammation. Trends Immunol 2020;41(9):805–19.
28. McGowan MM, O'Kane AC, Vezina G, et al. Serial plasma biomarkers of brain injury in infants with neonatal encephalopathy treated with therapeutic hypothermia. Pediatr Res 2021;90(6):1228–34.
29. Mallard C, Ek CJ, Vexler ZS. The myth of the immature barrier systems in the developing brain: role in perinatal brain injury. J Physiol 2018;596(23):5655–64.
30. Mottahedin A, Blondel S, Ek J, et al. N-acetylcysteine inhibits bacterial lipopeptide-mediated neutrophil transmigration through the choroid plexus in the developing brain. Acta neuropathologica communications 2020;8(1):4.
31. Mülling K, Fischer AJ, Siakaeva E, et al. Neutrophil dynamics, plasticity and function in acute neurodegeneration following neonatal hypoxia-ischemia. Brain Behav Immun 2021;92:234–44.
32. Albertsson AM, Zhang X, Vontell R, et al. γδ T cells contribute to injury in the developing brain. Am J Pathol 2018;188(3):757–67.
33. Winerdal M, Winerdal ME, Kinn J, et al. Long lasting local and systemic inflammation after cerebral hypoxic ischemia in newborn mice. PLoS One 2012;7(5): e36422.
34. Herz J, Bendix I, Felderhoff-Muser U. Peripheral immune cells and perinatal brain injury: a double-edged sword? Pediatr Res 2022;91(2):392–403.
35. Parmentier CEJ, de Vries LS, Groenendaal F. Magnetic resonance imaging in (Near-) Term infants with hypoxic-ischemic encephalopathy. Diagnostics 2022;12(3).
36. Geddes R, Vannucci RC, Vannucci SJ. Delayed cerebral atrophy following moderate hypoxia-ischemia in the immature rat. Dev Neurosci 2001;23(3):180–5.
37. Lear BA, Lear CA, Davidson JO, et al. Tertiary cystic white matter injury as a potential phenomenon after hypoxia-ischaemia in preterm f sheep. Brain Commun 2021;3(2):fcab024.
38. Lear CA, Lear BA, Davidson JO, et al. Tumour necrosis factor blockade after asphyxia in foetal sheep ameliorates cystic white matter injury. Brain 2023; 146(4):1453–66.
39. Zhou KQ, Bennet L, Wassink G, et al. Persistent cortical and white matter inflammation after therapeutic hypothermia for ischemia in near-term fetal sheep. J Neuroinflammation 2022;19(1):139.
40. Volpe JJ. Dysmaturation of premature brain: importance, cellular mechanisms, and potential interventions. Pediatr Neurol 2019;95:42–66.
41. Fisch U, Brégère C, Geier F, et al. Neonatal hypoxia-ischemia in rat elicits a region-specific neurotrophic response in SVZ microglia. J Neuroinflammation 2020;17(1):26.

42. Zhang J, Rong P, Zhang L, et al. IL4-driven microglia modulate stress resilience through BDNF-dependent neurogenesis. Sci Adv 2021;7(12).

43. Zhang J, Hu D, Li L, et al. M2 microglia-derived exosomes promote spinal cord injury recovery in mice by alleviating A1 astrocyte activation. Mol Neurobiol 2024. https://doi.org/10.1007/s12035-024-04026-6.

44. Shi L, Sun Z, Su W, et al. Treg cell-derived osteopontin promotes microglia-mediated white matter repair after ischemic stroke. Immunity 2021;54(7):1527–15242 e8.

45. Smith PLP, Mottahedin A, Svedin P, et al. Peripheral myeloid cells contribute to brain injury in male neonatal mice. J Neuroinflammation 2018;15(1):301.

46. Zareen Z, Strickland T, Eneaney VM, et al. Cytokine dysregulation persists in childhood post Neonatal Encephalopathy. BMC Neurol 2020;20(1):115.

47. O'Dea MI, Kelly LA, McKenna E, et al. Altered cytokine endotoxin responses in neonatal encephalopathy predict MRI outcomes. Front Pediat 2021;9:734540.

48. Zareen Z, Strickland T, Fallah L, et al. Cytokine dysregulation in children with cerebral palsy. Dev Med Child Neurol 2021;63(4):407–12.

49. Lin CY, Chang YC, Wang ST, et al. Altered inflammatory responses in preterm children with cerebral palsy. Ann Neurol 2010;68(2):204–12.

50. Stark MJ, Hodyl NA, Belegar VK, et al. Intrauterine inflammation, cerebral oxygen consumption and susceptibility to early brain injury in very preterm newborns. Arch Dis Child Fetal Neonatal Ed 2016;101(2):F137–42.

51. Johnson CT, Burd I, Raghunathan R, et al. Perinatal inflammation/infection and its association with correction of metabolic acidosis in hypoxic-ischemic encephalopathy. J Perinatol 2016;36(6):448–52.

52. Dhillon SK, Lear CA, Galinsky R, et al. The fetus at the tipping point: modifying the outcome of fetal asphyxia. J Physiol 2018;596(23):5571–92.

53. van den Heuij LG, Mathai S, Davidson JO, et al. Synergistic white matter protection with acute-on-chronic endotoxin and subsequent asphyxia in preterm fetal sheep. J Neuroinflammation 2014;11(1):89.

54. Eklind S, Mallard C, Arvidsson P, et al. Lipopolysaccharide induces both a primary and a secondary phase of sensitization in the developing rat brain. Pediatr Res 2005;58(1):112–6.

55. Yang D, Sun YY, Lin X, et al. Intranasal delivery of cell-penetrating anti-NF-κB peptides (Tat-NBD) alleviates infection-sensitized hypoxic-ischemic brain injury. Exp Neurol 2013;247:447–55.

56. Bonestroo HJ, Heijnen CJ, Groenendaal F, et al. Development of cerebral gray and white matter injury and cerebral inflammation over time after inflammatory perinatal asphyxia. Dev Neurosci 2015;37(1):78–94.

57. Marret S, Mukendi R, Gadisseux JF, et al. Effect of ibotenate on brain development: an excitotoxic mouse model of microgyria and posthypoxic-like lesions. JNEN (J Neuropathol Exp Neurol) 1995;54(3):358–70.

58. Dommergues MA, Patkai J, Renauld JC, et al. Proinflammatory cytokines and interleukin-9 exacerbate excitotoxic lesions of the newborn murine neopallium. Ann Neurol 2000;47(1):54–63.

59. Degos V, Peineau S, Nijboer C, et al. G protein-coupled receptor kinase 2 and group I metabotropic glutamate receptors mediate inflammation-induced sensitization to excitotoxic neurodegeneration. Ann Neurol 2013;73(5):667–78.

60. Patkai J, Mesples B, Dommergues MA, et al. Deleterious effects of IL-9-activated mast cells and neuroprotection by antihistamine drugs in the developing mouse brain. Pediatr Res 2001;50(2):222–30.

61. Mesplès B, Fontaine RH, Lelièvre V, et al. Neuronal TGF-beta1 mediates IL-9/mast cell interaction and exacerbates excitotoxicity in newborn mice. Neurobiol Dis 2005;18(1):193–205.
62. Chen HR, Chen CW, Kuo YM, et al. Monocytes promote acute neuroinflammation and become pathological microglia in neonatal hypoxic-ischemic brain injury. Theranostics 2022;12(2):512–29.
63. Kitase Y, Chin EM, Ramachandra S, et al. Sustained peripheral immune hyper-reactivity (SPIHR): an enduring biomarker of altered inflammatory responses in adult rats after perinatal brain injury. J Neuroinflammation 2021;18(1):242.
64. Jacobs SE, Berg M, Hunt R, et al. Cooling for newborns with hypoxic ischaemic encephalopathy. Cochrane Database Syst Rev 2013;2013(1):CD003311.
65. Thayyil S, Pant S, Montaldo P, et al. Hypothermia for moderate or severe neonatal encephalopathy in low-income and middle-income countries (HELIX): a randomised controlled trial in India, Sri Lanka, and Bangladesh. Lancet Global Health 2021;9(9):e1273–85.
66. Wintermark P, Boyd T, Gregas MC, Labrecque M, Hansen A. Placental pathology in asphyxiated newborns meeting the criteria for therapeutic hypothermia. Am J Obstet Gynecol 2010;203(6):579 e1–9.
67. Gonzalez FF, Voldal E, Comstock BA, et al. Placental Histologic Abnormalities and 2-Year Outcomes in Neonatal Hypoxic-Ischemic Encephalopathy. Neonatology 2023;120(6):760–77.
68. Kovatis KZ, Mackley A, Antunes M, et al. Relationship between placental weight and placental pathology with MRI findings in mild to moderate hypoxic ischemic encephalopathy. Cureus 2022;14(5):e24854.
69. Sibbin K, Crawford TM, Stark M, et al. Therapeutic hypothermia for neonatal encephalopathy with sepsis: a retrospective cohort study. BMJ Paediat Open 2022;6(1).
70. Osredkar D, Sabir H, Falck M, et al. Hypothermia does not reverse cellular responses caused by lipopolysaccharide in neonatal hypoxic-ischaemic brain injury. Dev Neurosci 2015;37(4–5):390–7.
71. Falck M, Osredkar D, Maes E, et al. Hypothermic neuronal rescue from infection-sensitised hypoxic-ischaemic brain injury is pathogen dependent. Developmental Neuroscience 2017;39(1-4):238–47.
72. Andersen M, Andersen HB, Andelius TCK, et al. No neuroprotective effect of therapeutic hypothermia following lipopolysaccharide-sensitized hypoxia-ischemia: a newborn piglet study. Frontiers in pediatrics 2023;11:1268237.
73. Martinello KA, Meehan C, Avdic-Belltheus A, et al. Hypothermia is not therapeutic in a neonatal piglet model of inflammation-sensitized hypoxia-ischemia. Pediatr Res 2022;91(6):1416–27.
74. Shah NM, Charani E, Ming D, et al. Antimicrobial stewardship and targeted therapies in the changing landscape of maternal sepsis. J Int Med 2024;4(1):46–61.
75. Wojcieszek AM, Stock OM, Flenady V. Antibiotics for prelabour rupture of membranes at or near term. Cochrane Database Syst Rev 2014;2014(10):CD001807.
76. Flenady V, Hawley G, Stock OM, et al. Prophylactic antibiotics for inhibiting preterm labour with intact membranes. Cochrane Database Syst Rev 2013;12:CD000246.
77. Kenyon S, Pike K, Jones DR, et al. Childhood outcomes after prescription of antibiotics to pregnant women with spontaneous preterm labour: 7-year follow-up of the ORACLE II trial. Lancet 2008;372(9646):1319–27.

78. Matcha S, Raj EA, Mahadevan R, et al. Pharmacometric approach to assist dosage regimen design in neonates undergoing therapeutic hypothermia. Pediatr Res 2022;92(1):249–54.
79. Tetorou K, Sisa C, Iqbal A, et al. Current therapies for neonatal hypoxic-ischaemic and infection-sensitised hypoxic-ischaemic brain damage. Front Synaptic Neurosci 2021;13:709301.
80. Yang D, Sun YY, Bhaumik SK, et al. Blocking lymphocyte trafficking with FTY720 prevents inflammation-sensitized hypoxic-ischemic brain injury in newborns. J Neurosci 2014;34(49):16467–81.
81. Barks JDE, Liu Y, Dopp IA, et al. Azithromycin reduces inflammation-amplified hypoxic-ischemic brain injury in neonatal rats. Pediatr Res 2022;92(2):415–23.
82. Lai JCY, Svedin P, Ek CJ, et al. Vancomycin is protective in a neonatal mouse model of Staphylococcus epidermidis-potentiated hypoxic-ischemic brain injury. Antimicrob Agents Chemother 2020;64(3).
83. Fumagalli M, Lombardi M, Gressens P, et al. How to reprogram microglia toward beneficial functions. Glia 2018;66(12):2531–49.
84. Corry KA, White OR, Shearlock AE, et al. Evaluating neuroprotective effects of uridine, erythropoietin, and therapeutic hypothermia in a ferret model of inflammation-sensitized hypoxic-ischemic encephalopathy. Int J Mol Sci 2021;22(18).
85. Juul SE, Comstock BA, Wadhawan R, et al. A randomized trial of erythropoietin for neuroprotection in preterm infants. N Engl J Med 2020;382(3):233–43.

Reverse Therapy
Impact of Hyperthermia and Rewarming on Newborn Outcomes

Lina F. Chalak, MD, MSCS[a],*, Joanne O. Davidson, PhD[b,c],
Alistair J. Gunn, MBChB, PhD[d]

KEYWORDS

- Therapeutic hypothermia • Hypoxic-ischemic encephalopathy • Pyrexia
- Rewarming • Animal models

KEY POINTS

- Preclinical and clinicals trials suggest hyperthermia after asphyxia represents a double-hit insult and is associated with worse outcomes.
- Avoidance of hyperthermia is strongly recommended.
- Reversal of therapy with rewarming should be monitored with EEG to detect sublinical seizures.

EVIDENCE FROM PRECLINICAL MODELS

Therapeutic hypothermia is now well established to improve neurodevelopmental outcomes after hypoxic-ischemic encephalopathy (HIE). Although the overall principles of treatment are well established, there is little strong evidence to guide many smaller clinical questions. It is well established that hyperthermia of even 1 °C to 2 °C during hypoxia-ischemia (HI) worsens damage, and promotes pan-necrosis in both adult animals[1,2] and postnatal day (P) 7 rats.[3,4] The impact of hyperthermia after reperfusion from HI is much more complex. This article will address the effects of HI and increased temperature on the neurovascular unit in preclinical and clinical models.

The impact of changes in temperature after HI is best understood in relation to the evolution of injury. Optimally, hypothermia should be started as soon as possible in the early recovery ('latent') phase, when oxidative metabolism has partially or fully

[a] Department of Pediatrics, Neonatal-Perinatal Medicine, University of Texas Southwestern Medical School, 5323 Harry Hines Boulevard, Dallas, TX 75390-9063, USA; [b] Department of Physiology, University of Auckland, Private Bag 92019, Auckland 1023, New Zealand; [c] Department of Paediatrics, University of Auckland, Private Bag 92019, Auckland 1023, New Zealand; [d] Department of Physiology, Faculty of Medical and Health Sciences, University of Auckland, Private Bag 92019, Auckland 1142, New Zealand
* Corresponding author.
E-mail address: lina.chalak@utsouthwestern.edu

Clin Perinatol 51 (2024) 565–572
https://doi.org/10.1016/j.clp.2024.04.002
perinatology.theclinics.com

recovered, and before the onset of delayed mitochondrial failure.[5] This phase typically lasts around 6 hours, and in moderate to severe HIE is followed by secondary deterioration with seizures, cytotoxic edema, and ultimately failure of mitochondrial oxidative metabolism. Hypothermia needs to be continued until the end of this phase, which lasts for approximately 72 hours. After this time, ongoing tertiary cell loss and remodeling may continue for weeks, months and years. However, there is now robust animal evidence that extended cooling to 120°C after HI does not further improve neuroprotection.[6]

The specific clinical question then is whether the speed of rewarming and hyperthermia from 72 h and later after HI, in the tertiary phase, affects outcomes. To the best of our knowledge there is no direct evidence. In adult rats, as little as 3 hours of moderate (2 °C–3 °C) hyperthermia, induced 24 hours after either global or brief focal ischemia in the adult rat, exacerbated histologic injury.[7,8] Further, adult rats exposed to transient global ischemia develop spontaneous hyperthermia, to 38.5°C or more from 21 hours to 63 hours after ischemia,[9] and preventing hyperthermia with an antipyretic between 12 hours and 72 hours substantially reduced neuronal loss after 7 days recovery. Interestingly, the protective effect of the antipyretic alone was greatly reduced after 2 months recovery,[10] such that combined moderate hypothermia, from 2 hours to 9 hours after HI, plus prevention of late hyperthermia was needed for long-term neuroprotection. Similarly, after hypothermic cardiac arrest in piglets, followed by rectal temperatures of 34 °C, 37 °C or 40 °C, respectively, for 24 hours, histologic and behavioral scores were significantly worse after hyperthermia than hypothermia,[11] with intermediate outcomes after normothermia.

The original randomized clinical trials of therapeutic hypothermia all aimed to rewarm neonates after hypothermia at a rate of 0.5°C per hour.[12,13] It is important to appreciate though that this reflected a very conservative approach in the absence of strong evidence. Many animal studies examined rewarming after suboptimal and short periods of hypothermia. For example, in adult gerbils, rapid rewarming over 30 minutes after 2 hours of hypothermia was associated with transient uncoupling of cerebral circulation and metabolism leading to increased extracellular glutamate and lactate levels.[14] Further, after traumatic brain injury in adult rats rapid rewarming over 15 minutes, after 1 hour of hypothermia, exacerbated traumatic axonal injury and impaired cerebrovascular responsiveness compared with rewarming over 90 minutes.[15] In neonatal piglets, after brief post-HI hypothermia for just 18 hours; rapid rewarming (4°C per hour) was associated with increased cortical apoptosis compared with slow rewarming (0.5°C per hour).[16] Potentially, this could reflect either a beneficial effect of slow rewarming, or confounding from the greater duration of mild hypothermia during slow compared with rapid rewarming.

In near-term fetal sheep, rapid and spontaneous rewarming over approximately 30 minutes, after a clinical protocol of 72 hours of head cooling, was associated with increased electrographic seizures in 5 by 9 animals in the ischemia-hypothermia group compared with 1 by 13 animals in the ischemia-normothermia group.[17] However, the absolute number of seizures was small and hypothermia was associated with better electroencephalography (EEG) recovery and neuronal survival compared with normothermia despite these transient EEG changes.[18]

In the same paradigm in near-term (0.85 gestation) fetal sheep, after 30 min of cerebral ischemia followed by normothermia, fetuses were randomized to 48 hours hypothermia with rapid rewarming over 1 hour, 48 hour hypothermia with slow rewarming over 24 hours, or 72 hours hypothermia with rapid rewarming.[19] After 48 hours of hypothermia, this very slow rewarming protocol was associated with improved recovery of EEG power compared with rapid rewarming (P<.05, **Fig. 1**), but was not different

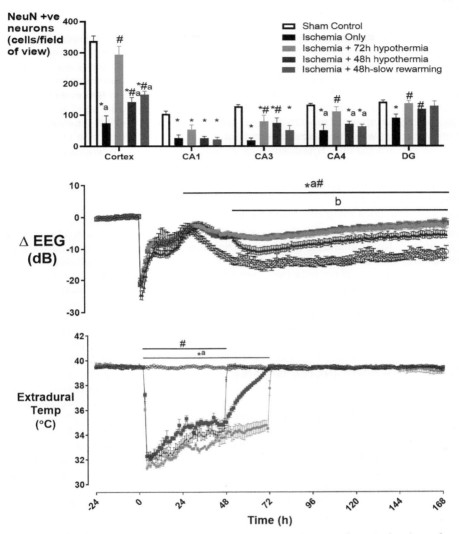

Fig. 1. Impact of slow rewarming after head cooling. Top: Neuronal survival 7 days after 30 minutes of global cerebral ischemia in the sham control (n = 9), ischemia-normothermia (n = 8), ischemia-48-h hypothermia (n = 8), ischemia-48-h hypothermia-slow-rewarming (n = 7) and ischemia-72-h hypothermia (n = 8) groups. Middle: Changes in electroencephalography (EEG) power before, during and after 30 min of global cerebral ischemia (time zero). Bottom: Change in extradural temperature before, during and after 30 min of global cerebral ischemia (time zero) in the near-term fetal sheep. Asterisk denotes P<.05 versus sham control, hash denotes P<.05 versus ischemia-normothermia, a denotes P<.05 versus ischemia-72-h hypothermia. Data are mean ± SEM.[19]

from rapid rewarming after 72 hours of hypothermia. After 7 days recovery, neuronal survival was partially improved by both fast and slow rewarming after 48 hours hypothermia, but was significantly less protective than 72 hours hypothermia in the cortex and carbon anhydrase 4 (P<.05). Further, although all hypothermia protocols similarly improved total numbers of oligodendrocytes and myelin basic protein area, only ischemia-72 hours hypothermia attenuated loss of mature oligodendrocytes.[20]

Microglia were suppressed by all hypothermia protocols; the greatest reduction was seen after ischemia-72 hours hypothermia; and an intermediate effect after ischemia-slow rewarming. Thus, in conclusion, although electrographic recovery was partially improved by slow rewarming over 24 hours following cerebral hypothermia for 48 hours compared with hypothermia for 48 hours plus rapid rewarming, optimal white and gray matter protection was seen with hypothermia for 72 hours with rapid rewarming, suggesting that speed of rewarming is just not very important, and that the overall duration of cooling was the critical determinant of outcomes. Studies of a clinical slow rewarming protocol after hypothermia for 72 hours are currently in progress.

CLINICAL OUTCOMES WITH HYPERTHERMIA FOLLOWING HYPOXIC-ISCHEMIC ENCEPHALOPATHY
Does Clinical Rewarming Affect the Extent of Neuroprotection?

All randomized controlled trials of hypothermia to date have rewarmed at a rate of 0.5°C per hour.[21] No randomized controlled trials have investigated the optimal rate of rewarming after therapeutic hypothermia for infants with HIE. The rewarming regimen was uniformly set in all neonatal hypothermia trials to increase the core body temperature by 0.5°C per hour until normothermia is achieved.[21] Rebound seizures during rewarming after 72 hours of hypothermia have been reported in clinical practice.[22-26]

The Systematic Monitoring of EEG in Asphyxiated Newborns during Rewarming after Hypothermia Therapy (SMaRT) study used continuous recording of raw EEG to assess the frequency of electrographic seizures before and during rewarming initiated at either 72 hours versus 120 hours during the National Institute of Child Health and Human Development (NICHD) optimizing cooling trial.[27] The study showed that 23% of infants had seizures during rewarming with increased risk of abnormal outcomes at 2 years, even after adjusting for baseline severity of encephalopathy (**Fig. 2**).

Compared with infants without seizures during rewarming, infants with these seizures were more likely to have abnormal background amplitude integrated electroencephalography and an incidence of basal ganglia-thalamic injury that was 2-fold higher than that of white matter injury.[27] Potentially, rewarming could re-activate inflammatory responses that have been suppressed during hypothermia. Alternatively, rewarming could lead to reversal of hypothermic suppression of oxidative stress and excitotoxin release.[28,29] There is no evidence though that rewarming at a slower rate would attenuate the increase in seizures noted with rewarming at 0.5°C per hour.

Physiologic Effects of Exposure to Hyperthermia

Infants exposed to maternal fever have a greater risk of birth depression, needing resuscitation, neonatal encephalopathy, and seizures.[30-34] In case–control studies maternal fever during labor was also associated with an increased risk of cerebral palsy (odds ratio 9.3, 95% confidence interval 2.7–31.0).[35] Presumptively, this association represents hyperthermia during HI itself.

The non-cooled control groups of the CoolCap study and the NICHD Neonatal Research Network whole body cooling trial demonstrated that among infants with HIE elevated infant temperatures are associated with worse outcomes between 18 hours and 22 months.[36,37] A surprising observation was the frequency of elevated esophageal temperatures during the 72 hour intervention. The mean esophageal temperature of all control infants over 72 hours was 37.2 plus minus 0.7 °C. After adjustment of co-variates, the odds of death or moderate orsevere disability was increased 4-fold for each 1 °C increase in the mean esophageal temperature and odds of death alone was associated with a 6.2-fold increase.[37] Similarly, non-cooled control infants

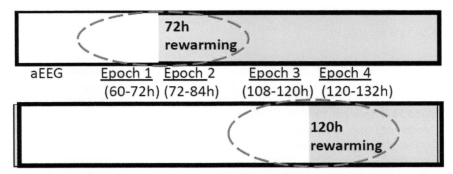

aEEG Data	Group Rewarming at 72 hrs (n=66)			Group Rewarming at 120 hrs (n=54)		
	Epoch 1	Epoch 2	P	Epoch 3	Epoch 4	P
Electrographic Seizure	9 (14%)	17 (27%)	0.007	5 (10%)	11 (21%)	0.03
Odds Ratio (95% C.I.) for having a seizure during later vs earlier epoch	2.7 (1.0, 7.5)		0.05	3.2 (0.9, 11.6)		0.07

Fig. 2. Seizures in the Systematic Monitoring of Electroencephalography (EEG) in Asphyxiated Newborns during Rewarming after Hypothermia Therapy (SMaRT) study.[27]

from the CoolCap trial who had 1 or more recorded temperature greater than or equal to 38 °C had a 3.2-higher odds of an unfavorable outcome (95% confidence interval 1.2–8.4).[36] At school age (6–7 years of age) there was a persisting association between elevated temperature and death or an intelligence quotient less than 70.[38]

The association between elevated temperature and adverse neurodevelopmental outcomes suggest that temperature may act as an independent variable for the observed outcomes but temperature dysregulation may also be a marker for brain injury severity. Critically, the evidence from analysis of the clinical trials applies to hyperthermia during the secondary phase after HI. These outcomes support the similar data in animals. Importantly, there is still a notable lack of evidence for the impact of late hyperthermia during the tertiary phase after rewarming therapeutic hypothermia. This will be an important topic for further research.

Best Practices

Current practice

- Rewarming is a stage of therapy reversal and should be titrated and monitored carefully.
- A core central temperature must be measured. Since axillary temperature is on average 0.5°C, one needs to correct by 0.5°C to avoid dangers associated with hyperthermia.[27]

DISCLOSURE

Nothing to disclose.

FUNDING

CHALAK R01 NS102617.

REFERENCES

1. Busto R, Dietrich WD, Globus MY, et al. Small differences in intraischemic brain temperature critically determine the extent of ischemic neuronal injury. J Cerebr Blood Flow Metabol 1987;7(6):729–38.
2. Dietrich WD, Busto R, Valdes I, et al. Effects of normothermic versus mild hyperthermic forebrain ischemia in rats. Stroke 1990;21(9):1318–25.
3. Tomimatsu T, Fukuda H, Endo M, et al. Effects of hypothermia on neonatal hypoxic-ischemic brain injury in the rat: phosphorylation of Akt, activation of caspase-3-like protease. Neurosci Lett 2001;312(1):21–4.
4. Mishima K, Ikeda T, Yoshikawa T, et al. Effects of hypothermia and hyperthermia on attentional and spatial learning deficits following neonatal hypoxia-ischemic insult in rats. Behav Brain Res 2004;151(1–2):209–17.
5. Wassink G, Davidson JO, Lear CA, et al. A working model for hypothermic neuroprotection. J Physiol 2018;596(23):5641–54.
6. Davidson JO, Wassink G, Yuill CA, et al. How long is too long for cerebral cooling after ischemia in fetal sheep? J Cerebr Blood Flow Metabol 2015;35(5):751–8.
7. Baena RC, Busto R, Dietrich WD, et al. Hyperthermia delayed by 24 hours aggravates neuronal damage in rat hippocampus following global ischemia. Neurology 1997;48(3):768–73.
8. Kim Y, Busto R, Dietrich WD, et al. Delayed postischemic hyperthermia in awake rats worsens the histopathological outcome of transient focal cerebral ischemia. Stroke 1996;27(12):2274–80.
9. Coimbra C, Boris-Moller F, Drake M, et al. Diminished neuronal damage in the rat brain by late treatment with the antipyretic drug dipyrone or cooling following cerebral ischemia. Acta Neuropathol 1996;92(5):447–53.
10. Coimbra C, Drake M, Boris-Moller F, et al. Long-lasting neuroprotective effect of postischemic hypothermia and treatment with an anti-inflammatory/antipyretic drug. Evidence for chronic encephalopathic processes following ischemia. Stroke 1996;27(9):1578–85.
11. Shum-Tim D, Nagashima M, Shinoka T, et al. Postischemic hyperthermia exacerbates neurologic injury after deep hypothermic circulatory arrest. J Thorac Cardiovasc Surg 1998;116(5):780–92.
12. Gluckman PD, Hanson MA. Developmental and epigenetic pathways to obesity: an evolutionary-developmental perspective. Int J Obes 2008;32(Suppl 7): S62–71.
13. Jacobs SE, Berg M, Hunt R, et al. Cooling for newborns with hypoxic ischaemic encephalopathy. Cochrane Database Syst Rev 2013;1:CD003311.
14. Nakamura T, Miyamoto O, Sumitani K, et al. Do rapid systemic changes of brain temperature have an influence on the brain? Acta Neurochir 2003;145(4):301–7.
15. Suehiro E, Povlishock JT. Exacerbation of traumatically induced axonal injury by rapid posthypothermic rewarming and attenuation of axonal change by cyclosporin A. J Neurosurg 2001;94(3):493–8.
16. Wang B, Armstrong JS, Reyes M, et al. White matter apoptosis is increased by delayed hypothermia and rewarming in a neonatal piglet model of hypoxic ischemic encephalopathy. Neuroscience 2016;316:296–310.

17. Gerrits LC, Battin MR, Bennet L, et al. Epileptiform activity during rewarming from moderate cerebral hypothermia in the near-term fetal sheep. Pediatr Res 2005; 57(3):342–6.

18. Gunn AJ, Gunn TR, de Haan HH, et al. Dramatic neuronal rescue with prolonged selective head cooling after ischemia in fetal lambs. J Clin Invest 1997;99(2): 248–56.

19. Davidson JO, Wassink G, Draghi V, et al. Limited benefit of slow rewarming after cerebral hypothermia for global cerebral ischemia in near-term fetal sheep. J Cerebr Blood Flow Metabol 2019;9(11):2246–57.

20. Draghi V, Wassink G, Zhou KQ, et al. Differential effects of slow rewarming after cerebral hypothermia on white matter recovery after global cerebral ischemia in near-term fetal sheep. Sci Rep 2019;9(1):10142.

21. Davies A, Wassink G, Bennet L, et al. Can we further optimize therapeutic hypothermia for hypoxic-ischemic encephalopathy? Neural Regen Res 2019;14(10): 1678–83.

22. Battin MR, Bennet L, Gunn AJ. Rebound seizures during rewarming. Pediatrics 2004;114(5):1369.

23. Azzopardi D, Brocklehurst P, Edwards D, et al. The TOBY Study. Whole body hypothermia for the treatment of perinatal asphyxial encephalopathy: a randomised controlled trial. BMC Pediatr 2008;8:17.

24. Yap V, Engel M, Takenouchi T, et al. Seizures are common in term infants undergoing head cooling. Pediatr Neurol 2009;41(5):327–31.

25. Shah DK, Wusthoff CJ, Clarke P, et al. Electrographic seizures are associated with brain injury in newborns undergoing therapeutic hypothermia. Arch Dis Child Fetal Neonatal Ed 2014;99(3):F219–24.

26. Kendall GS, Mathieson S, Meek J, et al. Recooling for rebound seizures after rewarming in neonatal encephalopathy. Pediatrics 2012;130(2):e451–5.

27. Chalak LF, Pappas A, Tan S, et al. Association between increased seizures during rewarming after hypothermia for neonatal hypoxic ischemic encephalopathy and abnormal neurodevelopmental outcomes at 2-Year Follow-up: a nested multisite cohort study. JAMA Neurol 2021;78(12):1484–93.

28. Hashimoto T, Yonetani M, Nakamura H. Selective brain hypothermia protects against hypoxic-ischemic injury in newborn rats by reducing hydroxyl radical production. Kobe J Med Sci 2003;49(3–4):83–91.

29. Nakashima K, Todd MM. Effects of hypothermia on the rate of excitatory amino acid release after ischemic depolarization. Stroke 1996;27(5):913–8.

30. Lieberman E, Lang J, Richardson DK, et al. Intrapartum maternal fever and neonatal outcome. Pediatrics 2000;105(1 Pt 1):8–13.

31. Lieberman E, Eichenwald E, Mathur G, et al. Intrapartum fever and unexplained seizures in term infants. Pediatrics 2000;106(5):983–8.

32. Impey L, Greenwood C, MacQuillan K, et al. Fever in labour and neonatal encephalopathy: a prospective cohort study. BJOG 2001;108(6):594–7.

33. Impey LW, Greenwood CE, Black RS, et al. The relationship between intrapartum maternal fever and neonatal acidosis as risk factors for neonatal encephalopathy. Am J Obstet Gynecol 2008;198(1):49 e1–e6.

34. Blume HK, Li CI, Loch CM, et al. Intrapartum fever and chorioamnionitis as risks for encephalopathy in term newborns: a case-control study. Dev Med Child Neurol 2008;50(1):19–24.

35. Grether JK, Nelson KB. Maternal infection and cerebral palsy in infants of normal birth weight. JAMA 1997;278(3):207–11.

36. Wyatt JS, Gluckman PD, Liu PY, et al. Determinants of outcomes after head cooling for neonatal encephalopathy. Pediatrics 2007;119(5):912–21.
37. Laptook A, Tyson J, Shankaran S, et al. Elevated temperature after hypoxic-ischemic encephalopathy: risk factor for adverse outcomes. Pediatrics 2008; 122(3):491–9.
38. Laptook AR, McDonald SA, Shankaran S, et al. Elevated temperature and 6- to 7-year outcome of neonatal encephalopathy. Ann Neurol 2013;73(4):520–8.

Treating Seizures and Improving Newborn Outcomes for Infants with Hypoxic-Ischemic Encephalopathy

Tayyba Anwar, MD[a], Regina L. Triplett, MD, MS[b],
Afaf Ahmed, MBBS[c], Hannah C. Glass, MDCM, MAS[d],
Renée A. Shellhaas, MD, MS[e],*

KEYWORDS

- Seizure • EEG • Phenobarbital • Neurocritical care • Epilepsy

KEY POINTS

- Continuous electroencephalographic monitoring is recommended for neonates with hypoxic-ischemic encephalopathy (HIE) to screen for seizures and evaluate evolution of the interictal background.
- Early recognition and effective treatment of seizures are key priorities for neonatal neuro-intensive care.
- First-line antiseizure medication remains phenobarbital while second line may include fosphenytoin, levetiracetam, or continuous infusions.
- Early discontinuation of antiseizure medication is safe in neonates with HIE following cessation of acute provoked seizures.

INTRODUCTION

Hypoxic-ischemic encephalopathy (HIE) is the most common cause of neonatal seizures.[1] Seizures in neonates with HIE peak in the first days after birth and are often subclinical.[1] Thus, these seizures are most accurately diagnosed by electroencephalography (EEG). Neonatal seizures are a medical emergency; early and effective

[a] Department of Neurology, Children's National Hospital, 111 Michigan Avenue Northwest, Washington, DC 20010, USA; [b] Department of Neurology, Washington University in St Louis, 1 Brookings Drive, Saint Louis, MO 63130, USA; [c] Division of Pediatric and Developmental Neurology, Department of Neurology, Washington University in St Louis, 1 Brookings Drive, Saint Louis, MO 63130, USA; [d] Department of Neurology, University of California San Francisco, 500 Parnassus Avenue, San Francisco, CA 94143, USA; [e] Department of Neurology, Washington University in St Louis, MSC 8091-29-12400, 660 South Euclid Avenue, Saint Louis, MO 63110, USA
* Corresponding author.
E-mail address: rshellhaas@wustl.edu

Clin Perinatol 51 (2024) 573–586
https://doi.org/10.1016/j.clp.2024.04.013

treatment to resolve seizures may lead to improved long-term neurodevelopmental outcomes. This study will outline the approach to timely evaluation and evidence-based treatment of HIE-associated seizures to improve outcomes in this population.

EVALUATION OF NEONATAL SEIZURES
Continuous Electroencephalographic Monitoring

Continuous electroencephalographic (cEEG) monitoring is the gold standard for seizure detection in neonates. The American Clinical Neurophysiology Society guideline recommends cEEG to detect seizures in high-risk populations such as newborns with HIE.[2] The EEG is used to detect electrographic seizures, confirm response to antiseizure medication (ASM), assess the interictal background to evaluate the degree of encephalopathy, and monitor the evolution of background changes over time. These data guide seizure treatment and inform discussions of prognosis for neonates with HIE.

Seizures and Status Epilepticus in Hypoxic-Ischemic Encephalopathy

About half of neonates with HIE who are treated with therapeutic hypothermia have EEG-confirmed seizures, and up to 20% have status epilepticus.[3–7] Among neonates with HIE who are not cooled, the risk of seizures is even higher.[8–10] Up to half of the seizures in HIE are clinically silent, and electroclinical uncoupling results in an even higher proportion of subclinical seizures after treatment with ASM.[3,11,12] Thus, evaluation and management of neonatal seizures are key aspects of neurocritical care for infants with HIE.

Predictors of Seizures in Neonates with Hypoxic-Ischemic Encephalopathy

Although the risk of acute provoked seizures is high among neonates with HIE, clinical characteristics (eg, gestational age, Apgar scores, and initial pH) do not reliably distinguish infants at highest risk.[3] While a suspected clinical seizure confers a risk for detecting seizures on EEG,[13,14] the initial EEG background pattern is, by far, the strongest predictor of seizures among neonates with HIE.[10,15] Among neonates with HIE treated with therapeutic hypothermia, excessive EEG background discontinuity or any severely abnormal background pattern (including burst suppression, depressed and undifferentiated, or inactive recording) is associated with an increased risk of acute provoked neonatal seizures.[3,6,13] The risk for acute seizures is independent of treatment with ASM prior to EEG initiation. Conversely, the risk of seizures is low when the initial EEG background is normal or mildly abnormal and has retained sleep–wake cycling.[5,13,16]

Timing of Seizures in Neonates with Hypoxic-Ischemic Encephalopathy

It is imperative that clinicians remain vigilant, with frequent assessment of the cEEG when the interictal background is moderately or severely abnormal, particularly in the first 24 hours, given the high risk of seizures. The median age at first seizure in HIE is ~4 to 20 hours after birth, and the maximum seizure burden is typically reached between 12 and 24 hours.[3,6,7,9] The timing of seizures is a manifestation of the secondary injury phase, when additional cell death occurs due to ongoing energy failure that results in increased excitotoxic neurotransmitter release, inflammation, and cytotoxic edema.[17]

With therapeutic hypothermia, the onset of seizures may be delayed and seizures may persist past the period of active cooling.[3,4,6,7] Therefore, many centers recommend cEEG monitoring throughout cooling and rewarming for all neonates treated with therapeutic hypothermia. Importantly, if seizures persist or worsen after active cooling, alternative diagnoses (eg, neonatal-onset epilepsy) must be considered.

NEURODEVELOPMENTAL OUTCOMES FOLLOWING HYPOXIC-ISCHEMIC ENCEPHALOPATHY-ASSOCIATED NEONATAL SEIZURES
Seizures and Brain Injury

Animal studies reveal that prolonged seizures in neonates induce or worsen brain injury via an increase in metabolic demands and formation of reactive oxygen species and inflammation that can cause tissue damage.[18,] This can lead to altered neuronal connectivity, receptor expression, and synaptic plasticity and, thereby, can result in long-lasting adverse effects on neurodevelopment.[18] In human neonates with HIE, seizure severity is associated with disruptions in brain metabolism as evidenced by an increase in lactate/choline ratio in the watershed areas and deep gray nuclei, as well as a decrease in the N-acetylaspartate/choline ratio in the watershed areas.[19] This effect is independent of the underlying structural patterns of brain injury seen on MRI for neonates with HIE.

More severe brain injury is also seen in neonates with higher seizure burden. Among 56 neonates with HIE who received therapeutic hypothermia and cEEG, 30% had confirmed seizures (30% of whom had status epilepticus and 40% had subclinical/EEG-only seizures).[20] Neonates with seizures were more likely to have a moderate–severe injury on brain MRI compared to those without (59% vs 26%), and all infants with status epilepticus had a moderate–severe injury.[21] Furthermore, the brain injury pattern was more often a cortical or near total injury among the neonates with seizures, providing critical evidence regarding the association between neonatal seizures and brain injury and suggesting a possible amplification of injury in the setting of high seizure burden.

Mortality

In neonates with HIE, high seizure burden and severe brain injury are significant risk factors for mortality.[1,22–24] In a prospective, multicenter study of 426 neonates with clinical and/or electrographic seizures of various etiologies, 17% died or were transferred to hospice care prior to discharge. Neonates with seizures due to HIE were at particularly high risk for death (21%–26%).[1,23] In the era of therapeutic hypothermia, deaths commonly follow the withdrawal of intensive care among neonates with severe HIE given their poor prognosis; half of these infants have seizures.[22] A high seizure burden ($\geq$7 total seizures) and status epilepticus are both independently associated with higher risk of death compared with a lower seizure burden (<7) or absence of status epilepticus.[1]

Cognitive and Motor Outcomes

Neonates with HIE and seizures are known to have high rates of long-term neurodisability (**Table 1**).[21,24–27] A prospective, multicenter study assessed the association of clinical neonatal seizures with the neurodevelopment of 77 term infants with HIE.[21] Cognitive and motor testing included a full scale IQ (FSIQ) using the Weschler scale of intelligence and the Gross Motor Function Classification System (GMFCS) (score $\geq$3 corresponding to a functional deficit and diagnosis of cerebral palsy) at 4 years of age. A composite seizure score ranging from 0 to 10 was assigned based on seizure frequency, timing of onset, ASMs, and EEG abnormalities. Severe seizures (cumulative seizure score $\geq$4) occurred in 14.3% of patients, mild-to-moderate seizures (cumulative seizure score 1–3) occurred in 18.2%, and no seizures were seen in the rest. Infants with severe seizures had more basal ganglia predominant injury on MRI while those with mild–moderate seizures had more watershed pattern of injury. After adjusting for degree of brain injury on MRI, there was a significant association between the

Table 1
Outcomes at 12–24 mo following neonatal seizures in hypoxic-ischemic encephalopathy

	McBride et al,[25] 2000	Glass et al,[21] 2009	Kharoshanykaya et al,[27] 2016	Basti et al,[28] 2020	Sewell et al,[29] 2023	Jagadish et al,[30] 2024
N	23	41	29	24	274	67
Normal (%)	44	–	17	77	66	46
Mortality (%)	30	39	24	–	5	–
Developmental delay (%)	56	61	62	11	34	54
Cerebral Palsy (%)	37	–	34	7	25	–
Epilepsy (%)	–	–	17	4	27	13

Adapted from Ref.[23]

presence and severity of seizures and developmental outcomes. Infants with severe seizures had a 30 point lower FSIQ (2 standard deviations) and infants with mild-to-moderate seizures had a 14 point lower FSIQ (1 standard deviation) compared with infants who had no seizures. The GMFCS scores were also significantly worse among neonates with seizures than those without.[21] In a second study, neonates with HIE and clinical seizures were assessed for outcomes including global developmental delay (significant delay in ≥2 domains) and cerebral palsy at age 2 years. Of these 62 neonates, 53% had global developmental delay and 45% had cerebral palsy.[26]

The causal effect of seizures on developmental outcome is supported by studies demonstrating a relationship between higher seizure burden and worse outcomes. This is particularly relevant for infants with HIE—who have a stronger correlation between seizure burden and worse Bayley III and Vineland II scores at the age of 17 to 31 months compared with infants with other acute provoked neonatal seizure etiologies.[31] An observational study on neonates with moderate–severe HIE assessed their neurodevelopmental outcomes at age 2 to 4 years.[27] Among the 47 neonates with HIE, 62% had cEEG-confirmed seizures. Seizures alone were not significantly associated with abnormal outcome; rather, seizure burden was more relevant. There was a 9 fold greater chance of an abnormal outcome with a total seizure burden greater than 40 minutes and an 8 fold greater chance of an abnormal outcome with maximal hourly seizure burden greater than 13 minutes per hour. This effect persisted after adjusting for HIE severity and treatment with therapeutic hypothermia.[27] In a subgroup of neonates with HIE, those with the highest cumulative duration of electrographic seizures had increased rates of death, microcephaly, and severe cerebral palsy.[25] Among neonates with status epilepticus, the total duration has been associated with worse scores on the Griffiths Mental Developmental Scale at the age of 18 months.[32]

Risk of Postneonatal Epilepsy

Following neonatal seizures in infants with HIE, 10% to 15% of survivors develop postneonatal epilepsy.[20,27,33] The provoked seizures subside, but recurrent unprovoked seizures (epilepsy) emerge after a quiescent period. Risk factors include neonatal seizures—especially status epilepticus—higher number of ASMs needed to control the seizures, severe encephalopathy, and/or severe injury on brain MRI.[20,33]

Prior to cooling, moderate–severe HIE was considered the most common symptomatic etiology of infantile epileptic spasms syndrome (IESS). Infants with HIE who do not receive therapeutic hypothermia are 6 times more likely to develop IESS by the age of 2 years than cooled infants.[34] In a prospective, multicenter study of the incidence and risk factors associated with the development of IESS among 204 survivors of acute symptomatic neonatal seizures, 12 (6%) developed IESS, of whom half had HIE.[35] Risk factors for IESS were stratified into a risk model and included (1) a severely abnormal EEG or 3 days or more with seizures recorded on EEG, (2) a deep gray or brainstem injury on MRI, and (3) an abnormal tone on discharge examination. IESS risk was 0% if none of these risk factors were present, 4% if 1 or 2 risk factors were present, and 57% if all 3 were present. Application of this risk model could aid parent counseling, tailored surveillance, and rapid diagnosis and treatment of IESS in high-risk infants.

Treating Electrographic Seizures

Neonatal seizures are defined by their EEG signatures—repetitive, evolving ictal rhythms with amplitude of 2 μV or greater, and duration of at least 10 seconds.[36] Electrographic only (or subclinical) seizures occur without obvious clinical manifestations and can only be detected by EEG.[37] Electroclinical seizures are confirmed on EEG and have associated clinical signs.[36]

Neonates with subclinical seizures have higher mortality rates than neonates with reported clinical seizures.[1] This may be, in part, due to the higher seizure burden encountered in those with subclinical seizures as they can be unrecognized for longer periods compared with clinical seizures. Neonates with subclinical seizures have MRI injury scores similar to those with electroclinical seizures—suggesting that subclinical and clinical seizures can be associated with similar degrees of brain injury.[20] Importantly, studies that include only neonates with clinically apparent seizures (without EEG confirmation) may inadvertently include infants whose paroxysmal events were not seizures.

Several randomized controlled trials (RCTs) have compared neonates with HIE who receive treatment of electrographic seizures versus treatment of only clinically apparent seizures. All of these studies excluded neonates with status epilepticus as the consensus among experts in the field is that such infants require aggressive treatment. In a multicenter RCT, 19 neonates with HIE were assigned to receive treatment of both amplitude-integrated EEG (aEEG)-diagnosed seizures and clinical seizures while 14 neonates were assigned to receive treatment of only clinically apparent seizures. The median duration of electrographic seizures (as quantified by aEEG) was longer in the clinical only treatment group (503 minutes) compared with the clinical plus aEEG-treated group (196 minutes), although the result did not reach statistical significance. Additionally, there was a trend toward more severe injury on MRI and longer seizure duration among neonates treated based only on clinical observation.[38]

In a similarly designed trial of 35 neonates with moderate–severe HIE and cEEG-confirmed seizures, 15 received treatment of electrographic *and* clinical seizures and 20 received treatment of only clinical seizures. In the cEEG group, there was a significantly shorter time to treatment after seizure onset, a decrease in the cumulative electrographic seizure burden, a decrease in the overall number of seizures, and lower MRI injury scores compared to the clinical treatment group.[39] Cognitive, language, and motor outcomes using Bayley Scales of Infant Development (BSID) were assessed at 18 to 24 months for all infants in the study (including the 26 without seizures). The neurodevelopmental outcomes between the 2 seizure treatment groups were not different, but when all babies (including those without seizures) were included, increased seizure burden was associated with worse scores across all domains on the BSID.

More recently, a larger (but still underpowered) trial randomized 86 neonates in each treatment arm (aEEG-guided vs clinical seizure treatment).[40] There was no difference in 2 year outcomes, including death or severe disability (ie, cerebral palsy, BSID scores 2 standard deviations below mean in any domain, blindness, or deafness) between the aEEG seizure treatment group and the clinical seizure treatment group. However, the authors acknowledge major study limitations. First, the study was underpowered due to early closure because of low recruitment and loss of clinical equipoise. Second, the study utilized aEEG, not cEEG, which affected the accuracy of seizure detection. Third, many babies were transferred from referring hospitals and were not monitored with aEEG until more than 12 hours after birth, which may have resulted in underdiagnosis of seizures and a delay of treatment in both groups. Although the quality of evidence for seizure treatment is limited, there is expert consensus to treat electrographic seizures as quickly as possible as a strategy to optimize neurodevelopmental outcome and minimize risk of postneonatal epilepsy.

MANAGEMENT OF ACUTE PROVOKED NEONATAL SEIZURES IN HYPOXIC-ISCHEMIC ENCEPHALOPATHY
Evidence for Current Guidelines

First-line and second-line medications for seizures in hypoxic-ischemic encephalopathy

By reducing brain injury, therapeutic hypothermia is a valuable advancement that decreases seizure burden in treated infants.[8,41] Therapeutic hypothermia is standard of care in neonates with moderate-to-severe HIE; however, up to 50% of treated infants continue to have seizures.[6,7,20] Neonates with high seizure burden may have reduced response to ASMs[42]; this suggests that rapid treatment initiation may offer important benefits.

Most ASM treatment guidelines are based on studies of all infants with seizures, regardless of etiology.[43–45] As HIE is the most common cause of neonatal seizures,[1] these guidelines are directly relevant to this patient population. Phenobarbital has a long history of use as a first-line ASM for early-life seizures, supported by observational data and several RCTs.[46–48] Phenobarbital is recommended as a first-line treatment of neonatal seizures because it is easier to use (due to more predictable pharmacokinetics) than phenytoin[48] and has a better response rate and longer duration of seizure-freedom than levetiracetam.[47] Phenobarbital also has stable clearance and does not require dose adjustment with therapeutic hypothermia.[49]

Based on animal and human studies, prolonged use of phenobarbital raises concerns for impaired neurodevelopment.[50] However, as failure to adequately control seizures is associated with poorer survival and worse neurodevelopmental outcomes,[20,21,27] phenobarbital continues to be recommended as the first-line treatment in the acute setting.[43] Importantly, treatment success is likely time-sensitive. Early treatment can result in significantly reduced seizure burden.[51]

Only about 50% of infants with HIE respond to initial phenobarbital doses.[2,4,52] However, due to a paucity of data from RCTs, there is no clear evidence-based recommendation to support a specific second-line ASM. The most recent guidelines, therefore, recommend phenytoin, midazolam, lidocaine, or levetiracetam as second-line medications.[43,48] In the setting of therapeutic hypothermia, additional considerations include drug clearance and comorbid conditions related to other organ injury. Based on limited data, the clearance of midazolam (delivered in a continuous intravenous infusion) and levetiracetam does not appear to be affected by therapeutic hypothermia. Phenytoin clearance may be decreased by therapeutic hypothermia[53] and may be more likely to cause or exacerbate bradycardia in this setting.[54] Both midazolam and phenytoin may contribute to excessive sedation, respiratory depression,[46,55] or hypotension,[46] particularly among infants with severe HIE and end-organ injury.[55] Lidocaine clearance is decreased by therapeutic hypothermia, and dose adjustments are necessary; clinical dosing algorithms are available.[56] Importantly, due to the risk of cardiac arrhythmia, lidocaine is contraindicated for neonates who have received phenytoin.[57]

Based upon concern for side effects and the suggestion that treatment with levetiracetam may be less detrimental to neurodevelopment than prolonged treatment with phenobarbital or phenytoin,[58] levetiracetam has been used more frequently in recent years.[59] However, a high-quality RCT demonstrated clearly that levetiracetam is much less effective than phenobarbital as a first-line ASM (28% seizure cessation with levetiracetam vs 80% with phenobarbital; $P < .001$, relative risk 0.35 [95% confidence interval 0.22–0.56]) and suggested that levetiracetam also has very limited efficacy as a second-line treatment.[47] Therefore, levetiracetam is not recommended as a first-line ASM for neonatal seizures. Additionally, phenytoin/fosphenytoin may be more effective than levetiracetam.[60] When levetiracetam is used, doses of 40 to 60 mg/kg have a better efficacy than lower doses.[61]

Status epilepticus/refractory seizures

When infants with HIE develop seizures that are refractory to first-line and second-line ASMs, continuous infusions are commonly recommended. Options include midazolam, lidocaine, and pentobarbital.

Midazolam. In the United States, a midazolam infusion is the mainstay of treatment of refractory neonatal seizures. Retrospective evidence demonstrates highly variable response rates, with rates of seizure resolution reported to range from essentially 0% up to 100%.[48,54,55] High rates of response to midazolam have been reported specifically in infants with HIE.[62] Notably, studies with better response rates used higher midazolam doses than those with lower reported rates of response.[55]

Lidocaine. A lidocaine infusion may be used as a second-line therapy; however, in practice, it is often initiated after multiple medications have been administered without success. Rates of seizure control using lidocaine range from 20% to 70%.[63] At least one study has reported a higher response rate to lidocaine than to midazolam.[64] However, lidocaine is not recommended for infants with cardiac concerns[43] and is contraindicated if the neonate has previously received phenytoin. While no published data are available, we suggest that neonates who have received lacosamide should also be excluded from exposure to lidocaine due to concerns about induced arrhythmia.

Pentobarbital. Pentobarbital use in neonates has been described in case studies only.[65] This infusion can be considered in an intubated patient whose seizures persist despite other treatment options, including phenobarbital and midazolam.[48]

Based on the studies reviewed earlier, and the International League Against Epilepsy (ILAE) consensus guideline that standard treatment pathways be developed and implemented consistently to facilitate efficient, evidence-based treatment,[43] we provide a suggested treatment algorithm for seizures in the setting of HIE (**Fig. 1**).

Other antiseizure medications with limited evidence

Emerging therapies. There are multiple emerging treatments for neonatal seizures. Of critical importance, none of the ASMs described later in this article currently have sufficient data to support a recommendation for routine clinical practice. Lessons learned from levetiracetam—for which initial noncontrolled and retrospective studies suggested efficacy but an RCT clearly demonstrated the lack of efficacy—should inform a cautious approach to clinical adoption of untested treatments.

Bumetanide An open-label trial (with no control group) of bumetanide as second-line therapy after phenobarbital for infants with HIE was halted prematurely due to

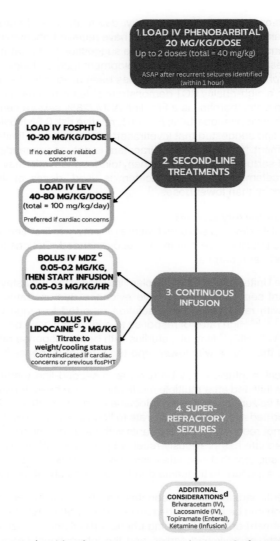

Fig. 1. ASM treatment algorithm for recurrent neonatal seizures[a] after HIE. [a]Recurrent clear clinical seizures later confirmed on EEG *or* electrographic seizures. [b]Follow goal levels 1–2 hours after final loading dose. [c]Secure airway prior to initiating these infusions. [d]Dosing, safety, and efficacy data are not available for these medications. FOSPHT, fosphenytoin; LEV, levetiracetam; MDZ, midazolam.

hearing loss in several treated infants and insufficient evidence for seizure reduction.[66] A subsequent, double-blind, pilot RCT of bumetanide following phenobarbital treatment of infants with seizures (not specific to HIE, although infants with HIE were included) demonstrated no increase in hearing impairment in the bumetanide group compared with controls, despite using a higher dose of bumetanide.[67] Further, this pilot RCT suggested a temporary reduction in seizure burden among neonates with high seizure burden. However, the small sample size and short-term efficacy endpoint do not support current clinical use of bumetanide for neonatal seizure treatment.

Notably, among infants with HIE, bumetanide pharmacokinetics were altered by hypothermia.[67] Overall, bumetanide remains a promising option but requires further investigation before it can be recommended for routine use.

Ketamine Ketamine is used for children and adults with refractory status epilepticus (RSE), with response rates up to 73% in children.[68] A recent study of ketamine for RSE included 19 infants aged less than 30 days, with an overall 46% rate of RSE termination (both in infants and older children) and an additional 28% of patients with seizure reduction. Only 4% of all included patients had adverse effects (ie, hypertension or delirium).[69] Case series have suggested efficacy and safety of ketamine among infants with RSE following HIE.[70] While these preliminary results are promising, further rigorous investigation is advised before administering ketamine for neonates with HIE outside of a research protocol setting.

Brivaracetam Brivaracetam is an analog of levetiracetam and has a Food and Drug Administration (FDA) indication for infants aged older than 1 month. A small (n = 6), single-arm study of newborns suggested that brivaracetam was safe and effective for treatment of refractory seizures, with similar pharmacokinetics to those in older children and adults.[71] Three infants in the study had seizures secondary to HIE. Therefore, brivaracetam is a promising option worthy of additional study but is not currently recommended for routine use.

Lacosamide Lacosamide is a sodium-channel-modulating ASM with an intravenous formulation that can be administered as a loading dose. It is, therefore, being used with increasing frequency among children and infants, although the FDA indication is for children aged 4 years or older. A case series demonstrated safety of lacosamide among newborn infants, with close cardiac monitoring for key side effects.[72] Only a minority (5%) of patients were found to have atrial bigeminy. As animal studies suggest a neuroprotective effect of lacosamide following hypoxic-ischemic injury,[73] further human studies are warranted for this population.

Antiseizure medication cessation
Acute provoked seizures in the setting of neonatal HIE have a predictable timecourse[6] and should resolve within several days. Based on data that demonstrate that stopping ASMs is safe, does not increase the risk for postneonatal epilepsy, and does not harm neurodevelopment,[74] the 2023 ILAE guideline recommends that ASMs be routinely discontinued for neonates with acute provoked seizures prior to hospital discharge. Importantly, this guidance specifies that ASMs may be discontinued after resolution of the acute provoked neonatal seizures regardless of interictal EEG findings or neuroimaging abnormalities. Neonates at high risk for postneonatal epilepsy, including those who had 3 or more days of seizures, a severely abnormal EEG background, and an abnormal tone on discharge neurologic examination, should be closely followed by a child neurologist.[35,75] Families must be counseled about the risk for IESS and linked with appropriate primary care and specialist follow-up.

SUMMARY

Neonatal seizures are common following hypoxic-ischemic brain injury. These acute provoked seizures are often subclinical, which makes cEEG monitoring a vital tool during therapeutic hypothermia. EEG background patterns are important predictors of seizures in the acute period and are associated with later neurodevelopmental outcomes. Timely and effective treatment with ASMs may improve overall outcomes. Phenobarbital remains the recommended first-line therapy, with several options for second-line treatments, and more ASMs currently under investigation. Following acute provoked seizure resolution, early discontinuation of ASMs is safe and does not affect the future risk of epilepsy in infants with HIE.

Best Practices

Best practice/guidelines/care path objectives:

- Duration of EEG monitoring in neonates with HIE
- Using the EEG background to predict long-term outcomes
- Treatment of electrographic and electroclinical seizures
- Neurodevelopmental outcomes following acute provoked seizures in HIE
- Treatment algorithm for neonatal seizures associated with HIE
- Early discontinuation of antiseizure medications following acute provoked seizures in HIE

What changes in current practice are likely to improve outcome?

- Prompt diagnosis of seizures and rapid initiation of effective treatment may improve long-term neurodevelopmental outcomes for neonates with HIE.
- *Clinical algorithm* (see **Fig. 1**)

Pearls/Pitfalls at the point of care

- Accurate diagnosis of seizures with EEG is important to initiate appropriate treatment, evaluate treatment response, and avoid unnecessary exposure to antiseizure medication.
- Delay in seizure treatment may amplify brain injury and worsen neurodevelopmental outcomes.
- Seizures following acute injury in HIE are provoked; continued prophylactic antiseizure medication after hospital discharge does not prevent or delay the onset of epilepsy.

Major recommendations

- CEEG monitoring is recommended for neonates with HIE.
- Early recognition and effective treatment of seizures are key priorities for neonatal neurointensive care.
- Phenobarbital remains the first-line antiseizure medication to treat recurrent seizures, while second-line treatment may include fosphenytoin, levetiracetam, or continuous infusions.
- Early discontinuation of antiseizure medication is safe following cessation of acute provoked seizures in neonates with HIE.

Bibliographic Sources

Shellhaas RA, Chang T, Tsuchida T, et al. The American Clinical Neurophysiology Society's Guideline on Continuous Electroencephalography Monitoring in Neonates. *J Clin Neurophysiol.* 2011;28(6):611 to 617.

Pressler RM, Abend NS, Auvin S, et al. Treatment of seizures in the neonate: Guidelines and consensus-based recommendations—Special report from the ILAE Task Force on Neonatal Seizures. *Epilepsia.* 2023;64(10):2550 to 2570.

DISCLOSURE

Dr R.A. Shellhaas receives royalties from UpToDate for authorship of topics related to neonatal seizures; serves as a consultant for the Epilepsy Study Consortium; and receives a stipend for her role as president-elect of the Pediatric Epilepsy Research Foundation. Drs H.C. Glass, T. Anwar, R.L. Triplett, and A. Ahmed have nothing to disclose.

REFERENCES

1. Glass HC, Shellhaas RA, Wusthoff CJ, et al. Contemporary profile of seizures in neonates: a prospective cohort study. J Pediatr 2016;174:98–103.e1.
2. Shellhaas RA, Chang T, Tsuchida T, et al. The American clinical neurophysiology society's guideline on continuous electroencephalography monitoring in neonates. J Clin Neurophysiol 2011;28(6):611–7.
3. Glass HC, Wusthoff CJ, Shellhaas RA, et al. Risk factors for EEG seizures in neonates treated with hypothermia: a multicenter cohort study. Neurology 2014; 82(14):1239–44.
4. Glass HC, Wusthoff CJ, Comstock BA, et al. Risk of seizures in neonates with hypoxic-ischemic encephalopathy receiving hypothermia plus erythropoietin or placebo. Pediatr Res 2023;94(1):252–9.
5. Benedetti GM, Vartanian RJ, McCaffery H, et al. Early electroencephalogram background could guide tailored duration of monitoring for neonatal encephalopathy treated with therapeutic hypothermia. J Pediatr 2020;221:81–7.e1.
6. Pavel AM, Rennie JM, De Vries LS, et al. Temporal evolution of electrographic seizures in newborn infants with hypoxic-ischaemic encephalopathy requiring therapeutic hypothermia: a secondary analysis of the ANSeR studies. Lancet Child Adolesc Health 2024. https://doi.org/10.1016/S2352-4642(23)00296-1. S2352464223002961.
7. Wusthoff CJ, Dlugos DJ, Gutierrez-Colina A, et al. Electrographic seizures during therapeutic hypothermia for neonatal hypoxic-ischemic encephalopathy. J Child Neurol 2011;26(6):724–8.
8. Low E, Boylan GB, Mathieson SR, et al. Cooling and seizure burden in term neonates: an observational study. Arch Dis Child - Fetal Neonatal Ed 2012;97(4): F267–72.
9. Macdonald-Laurs E, Sharpe C, Nespeca M, et al. Does the first hour of continuous electroencephalography predict neonatal seizures? Arch Dis Child - Fetal Neonatal Ed 2021;106(2):162–7.
10. Orbach SA, Bonifacio SL, Kuzniewicz MW, et al. Lower incidence of seizure among neonates treated with therapeutic hypothermia. J Child Neurol 2014; 29(11):1502–7.
11. Cornet M, Morabito V, Lederer D, et al. Neonatal presentation of genetic epilepsies: early differentiation from acute provoked seizures. Epilepsia 2021;62(8):1907–20.
12. Scher MS, Alvin J, Gaus L, et al. Uncoupling of EEG-clinical neonatal seizures after antiepileptic drug use. Pediatr Neurol 2003;28(4):277–80.
13. Sansevere AJ, Kapur K, Peters JM, et al. Seizure prediction models in the neonatal intensive care unit. J Clin Neurophysiol 2019;36(3):186–94.
14. Worden LT, Chinappen DM, Stoyell SM, et al. The probability of seizures during continuous EEG monitoring in high-risk neonates. Epilepsia 2019;60(12):2508–18.
15. Rothman SM, Glass HC, Chang T, et al. Risk factors for EEG seizures in neonates treated with hypothermia: a multicenter cohort study. Neurology 2014;83(19): 1773–4.
16. Pisani F, Sisti L, Seri S. A scoring system for early prognostic assessment after neonatal seizures. Pediatrics 2009;124(4):e580–7.

17. Nair J, Kumar V. Current and emerging therapies in the management of hypoxic ischemic encephalopathy in neonates. Children 2018;5(7):99.

18. Silverstein FS, Jensen FE. Neonatal seizures. Ann Neurol 2007;62(2):112–20.

19. Miller SP, Weiss J, Barnwell A, et al. Seizure-associated brain injury in term newborns with perinatal asphyxia. Neurology 2002;58(4):542–8.

20. Glass HC, Nash KB, Bonifacio SL, et al. Seizures and magnetic resonance imaging–detected brain injury in newborns cooled for hypoxic-ischemic encephalopathy. J Pediatr 2011;159(5):731–5.e1.

21. Glass HC, Glidden D, Jeremy RJ, et al. Clinical neonatal seizures are independently associated with outcome in infants at risk for hypoxic-ischemic brain injury. J Pediatr 2009;155(3):318–23.

22. Lemmon ME, Boss RD, Bonifacio SL, et al. Characterization of death in neonatal encephalopathy in the hypothermia era. J Child Neurol 2017;32(4):360–5.

23. Uria-Avellanal C, Marlow N, Rennie JM. Outcome following neonatal seizures. Semin Fetal Neonatal Med 2013;18(4):224–32.

24. Chalak LF, Pappas A, Tan S, et al. Association between increased seizures during rewarming after hypothermia for neonatal hypoxic ischemic encephalopathy and abnormal neurodevelopmental outcomes at 2-year follow-up: a nested multisite cohort study. JAMA Neurol 2021;78(12):1484.

25. McBride MC, Laroia N, Guillet R. Electrographic seizures in neonates correlate with poor neurodevelopmental outcome. Neurology 2000;55(4):506–14.

26. Garfinkle J, Shevell MI. Cerebral palsy, developmental delay, and epilepsy after neonatal seizures. Pediatr Neurol 2011;44(2):88–96.

27. Kharoshankaya L, Stevenson NJ, Livingstone V, et al. Seizure burden and neurodevelopmental outcome in neonates with hypoxic–ischemic encephalopathy. Dev Med Child Neurol 2016;58(12):1242–8.

28. Basti C, Maranella E, Cimini N, et al. Seizure burden and neurodevelopmental outcome in newborns with hypoxic-ischemic encephalopathy treated with therapeutic hypothermia: a single center observational study. Seizure 2020;83:154–9.

29. Sewell EK, Shankaran S, McDonald SA, et al. Antiseizure medication at discharge in infants with hypoxic-ischaemic encephalopathy: an observational study. Arch Dis Child Fetal Neonatal Ed 2023;108(4):421–8.

30. Jagadish S, Czech TM, Zimmerman MB, et al. Epilepsy incidence and developmental outcomes after early discontinuation of antiseizure medication in neonatal hypoxic-ischemic encephalopathy. Pediatr Neurol 2024;153:48–55.

31. Trowbridge SK, Condie LO, Landers JR, et al. Effect of neonatal seizure burden and etiology on the long-term outcome: data from a randomized, controlled trial. Ann Child Neurol Soc 2023;1(1):53–65.

32. Van Rooij LGM, De Vries LS, Handryastuti S, et al. Neurodevelopmental outcome in term infants with status epilepticus detected with amplitude-integrated electroencephalography. Pediatrics 2007;120(2):e354–63.

33. Liu X, Jary S, Cowan F, et al. Reduced infancy and childhood epilepsy following hypothermia-treated neonatal encephalopathy. Epilepsia 2017;58(11):1902–11.

34. Abu Dhais F, McNamara B, O'Mahony O, et al. Impact of therapeutic hypothermia on infantile spasms: an observational cohort study. Dev Med Child Neurol 2020;62(1):62–8.

35. Glass HC, Grinspan ZM, Li Y, et al. Risk for infantile spasms after acute symptomatic neonatal seizures. Epilepsia 2020;61(12):2774–84.

36. Tsuchida TN, Wusthoff CJ, Shellhaas RA, et al. American clinical neurophysiology society standardized EEG Terminology and categorization for the description of

continuous EEG monitoring in neonates: report of the American clinical neurophysiology society critical care monitoring committee. J Clin Neurophysiol 2013;30(2): 161–73.

37. Pressler RM, Cilio MR, Mizrahi EM, et al. The ILAE classification of seizures and the epilepsies: modification for seizures in the neonate. Position paper by the ILAE Task Force on Neonatal Seizures. Epilepsia 2021;62(3):615–28.

38. Van Rooij LGM, Toet MC, Van Huffelen AC, et al. Effect of treatment of subclinical neonatal seizures detected with aeeg: randomized, controlled trial. Pediatrics 2010;125(2):e358–66.

39. Srinivasakumar P, Zempel J, Trivedi S, et al. Treating EEG seizures in hypoxic ischemic encephalopathy: a randomized controlled trial. Pediatrics 2015;136(5): e1302–9.

40. Hunt RW, Liley HG, Wagh D, et al. Effect of treatment of clinical seizures vs electrographic seizures in full-term and near-term neonates: a randomized clinical trial. JAMA Netw Open 2021;4(12):e2139604.

41. Srinivasakumar P, Zempel J, Wallendorf M, et al. Therapeutic hypothermia in neonatal hypoxic ischemic encephalopathy: electrographic seizures and magnetic resonance imaging evidence of injury. J Pediatr 2013;163(2):465–70.

42. Numis AL, Glass HC, Comstock BA, et al. Relationship of neonatal seizure burden prior to treatment and response to initial anti-seizure medication. J Pediatr 2024;113957. https://doi.org/10.1016/j.jpeds.2024.113957.

43. Pressler RM, Abend NS, Auvin S, et al. Treatment of seizures in the neonate: guidelines and consensus-based recommendations—special report from the ILAE Task Force on neonatal seizures. Epilepsia 2023;64(10):2550–70.

44. El-Dib M, Soul JS. The use of phenobarbital and other anti-seizure drugs in newborns. Semin Fetal Neonatal Med 2017;22(5):321–7.

45. Zeller B, Giebe J. Pharmacologic management of neonatal seizures. Neonatal Netw 2015;34(4):239–44.

46. Painter MJ, Scher MS, Stein AD, et al. Phenobarbital compared with phenytoin for the treatment of neonatal seizures. N Engl J Med 1999;341(7):485–9.

47. Sharpe C, Reiner GE, Davis SL, et al. Levetiracetam versus phenobarbital for neonatal seizures: a randomized controlled trial. Pediatrics 2020;145(6):e20193182.

48. Slaughter LA, Patel AD, Slaughter JL. Pharmacological treatment of neonatal seizures: a systematic review. J Child Neurol 2013;28(3):351–64.

49. Shellhaas RA, Ng CM, Dillon CH, et al. Population pharmacokinetics of phenobarbital in infants with neonatal encephalopathy treated with therapeutic hypothermia. Pediatr Crit Care Med 2013;14(2):194–202.

50. Farwell JR, Lee YJ, Hirtz DG, et al. Phenobarbital for febrile seizures — effects on intelligence and on seizure recurrence. N Engl J Med 1990;322(6):364–9.

51. Pavel AM, Rennie JM, De Vries LS, et al. Neonatal seizure management: is the timing of treatment critical? J Pediatr 2022;243:61–8.e2.

52. Glass HC, Soul JS, Chu CJ, et al. Response to antiseizure medications in neonates with acute symptomatic seizures. Epilepsia 2019;60(3). https://doi.org/10.1111/epi.14671.

53. Empey PE, Velez De Mendizabal N, Bell MJ, et al. Therapeutic hypothermia decreases phenytoin elimination in children with traumatic brain injury. Crit Care Med 2013;41(10):2379–87.

54. Boylan GB, Rennie JM, Chorley G, et al. Second-line anticonvulsant treatment of neonatal seizures: a video-EEG monitoring study. Neurology 2004;62(3):486–8.

55. Castro Conde JR, Hernández Borges AA, Martínez ED, et al. Midazolam in neonatal seizures with no response to phenobarbital. Neurology 2005;64(5):876–9.

56. Van Den Broek MPH, Rademaker CMA, Van Straaten HLM, et al. Anticonvulsant treatment of asphyxiated newborns under hypothermia with lidocaine: efficacy, safety and dosing. Arch Dis Child - Fetal Neonatal Ed 2013;98(4):F341–5.

57. Weeke LC, Schalkwijk S, Toet MC, et al. Lidocaine-associated cardiac events in newborns with seizures: incidence, symptoms and contributing factors. Neonatology 2015;108(2):130–6.

58. Maitre NL, Smolinsky C, Slaughter JC, et al. Adverse neurodevelopmental outcomes after exposure to phenobarbital and levetiracetam for the treatment of neonatal seizures. J Perinatol 2013;33(11):841–6.

59. Dizon MLV, Rao R, Hamrick SE, et al. Practice variation in anti-epileptic drug use for neonatal hypoxic-ischemic encephalopathy among regional NICUs. BMC Pediatr 2019;19(1):67.

60. Bartha AI, Shen J, Katz KH, et al. Neonatal seizures: multicenter variability in current treatment practices. Pediatr Neurol 2007;37(2):85–90.

61. Khan O, Chang E, Cipriani C, et al. Use of intravenous levetiracetam for management of acute seizures in neonates. Pediatr Neurol 2011;44(4):265–9.

62. Van Leuven K, Groenendaal F, Toet M, et al. Midazolam and amplitude-integrated EEG in asphyxiated full-term neonates. Acta Paediatr 2004;93(9):1221–7.

63. Ziobro JM, Eschbach K, Shellhaas RA. Novel therapeutics for neonatal seizures. Neurotherapeutics 2021;18(3):1564–81.

64. Shany E, Benzaqen O, Watemberg N. Comparison of continuous drip of midazolam or lidocaine in the treatment of intractable neonatal seizures. J Child Neurol 2007;22(3):255–9.

65. Welty TE, Kriel RL. Pentobarbital coma for treating intractable seizures in a neonate. Clin Pharm 1985;4(3):330–2.

66. Pressler RM, Boylan GB, Marlow N, et al. Bumetanide for the treatment of seizures in newborn babies with hypoxic ischaemic encephalopathy (NEMO): an open-label, dose finding, and feasibility phase 1/2 trial. Lancet Neurol 2015;14(5):469–77.

67. Soul JS, Bergin AM, Stopp C, et al. A pilot randomized, controlled, double-blind trial of bumetanide to treat neonatal seizures. Ann Neurol 2021;89(2):327–40.

68. Höfler J, Trinka E. Intravenous ketamine in status epilepticus. Epilepsia 2018; 59(S2):198–206.

69. Jacobwitz M, Mulvihill C, Kaufman MC, et al. Ketamine for management of neonatal and pediatric refractory status epilepticus. Neurology 2022;99(12). https://doi.org/10.1212/WNL.0000000000200889.

70. Pin JN, Leonardi L, Nosadini M, et al. Efficacy and safety of ketamine for neonatal refractory status epilepticus: case report and systematic review. Front Pediatr 2023;11:1189478.

71. Pressler R, Boylan G, Dempsey E, et al. Pharmacokinetics and safety of brivaracetam in neonates with repeated electroencephalographic seizures: a multicenter, open-label, single-arm study. Epilepsia Open 2024;epi4:12875.

72. Bamgbose O, Boyle F, Kean AC, et al. Tolerability and safety of lacosamide in neonatal population. J Child Neurol 2023;38(3–4):137–41.

73. Kim GH, Byeon JH, Eun BL. Neuroprotective effect of lacosamide on hypoxic-ischemic brain injury in neonatal rats. J Clin Neurol 2017;13(2):138.

74. Glass HC, Soul JS, Chang T, et al. Safety of early discontinuation of antiseizure medication after acute symptomatic neonatal seizures. JAMA Neurol 2021;78(7):817.

75. Shellhaas RA, Wusthoff CJ, Numis AL, et al. Early-life epilepsy after acute symptomatic neonatal seizures: a prospective multicenter study. Epilepsia 2021;62(8):1871–82.

Hypothermia for Hypoxic-ischemic Encephalopathy

Second-generation Trials to Address Gaps in Knowledge

Abbot R. Laptook, MD[a],*, Seetha Shankaran, MD[b],
Roger G. Faix, MD[c]

KEYWORDS

- Hypoxic-ischemic encephalopathy • Hypothermia treatment • Premature newborns

KEY POINTS

- Use of deeper (32°C) and/or longer hypothermia (120 hours) for neonates with moderate or severe hypoxic-ischemic encephalopathy (HIE) does not improve outcome and may increase mortality.
- Hypothermia initiated after 6 hours of age in infants with moderate or severe HIE may have a possible treatment benefit, but the results are not conclusive.
- Hypothermia initiated at less than 6 hours of age in infants 33^0 to 35^6 weeks' gestation with moderate or severe HIE does not decrease death or disability at 18 to 22 months' corrected age.

INTRODUCTION

Prior to 2005, the management of hypoxic-ischemic encephalopathy (HIE) among term newborns was limited to intensive supportive care without a specific brain-oriented therapy. Between 2005 and 2011, 6 randomized trials demonstrated that hypothermia for newborns with moderate or severe HIE reduced death or disability or increased survival without neurologic abnormality at 18 to 22 months of age.[1–6] These trials were remarkably homogenous in many key characteristics such as postnatal age, a stepwise process for inclusion, randomization to cooling or usual care, duration of cooling, rate of rewarming, and a similar primary outcome. Almost all enrolled

[a] Department of Pediatrics, Warren Alpert School of Medicine, Women and Infants Hospital of Rhode Island, 101 Dudley Street, Providence, RI 02905, USA; [b] Department of Pediatrics, University of Texas at Austin and Dell Medical School, Wayne State University, 15601 Madriena Way, Austin, TX 78738, USA; [c] Department of Pediatrics, University of Utah School of Medicine, 295 Chipeta Way, Salt Lake City, UT 84108, USA
* Corresponding author.
E-mail address: alaptook@wihri.org

Clin Perinatol 51 (2024) 587–603
https://doi.org/10.1016/j.clp.2024.04.014
0095-5108/24/© 2024 Elsevier Inc. All rights reserved.

infants were $\geq$36 weeks' gestation and either body cooling (target core temperature, Tc, 33.5°C) or head cooling combined with a more modest reduction in Tc (target Tc, 34.5°C) was used. A meta-analysis based on results from these 6 trials and several smaller studies (1344 infants analyzed) indicated a 25% relative risk reduction in death or disability with hypothermia compared to usual care with normothermic temperatures.[7]

Based upon these studies, the *Eunice Kennedy Shriver* National Institute of Child Health and Development (NICHD) convened 2 workshops to identify knowledge gaps for the treatment of HIE with hypothermia.[8,9] Although the initial trials demonstrated a reduction in death or disability at 18 to 22 month follow-up, 40% to 50% of newborns treated with hypothermia still died or survived with serious neurologic disability. The workshops established multiple research priorities, one of which was refinements of hypothermia therapy for newborns with HIE. As a response to these workshops, the NICHD Neonatal Research Network (NRN) performed 3 randomized trials to address selected gaps in our understanding of the use of hypothermia treatment (second-generation trials). These trials include the Optimizing Cooling Trial (NCT 01192776), the Late Hypothermia Trial (00614744), and the Preterm Hypothermia Trial (NCT 01793129) and each will be reviewed in this article.

OPTIMIZING COOLING TRIAL
Rationale

The initial trials of hypothermia for moderate or severe HIE used a Tc of either 33.5°C for whole body cooling or 34.5°C for head cooling over 72 hours.[1–6] These cooling parameters were based on preclinical investigation and pilot human studies and reflected the best estimate of conditions to provide neuroprotection and minimize potential adverse effects. However, multiple observations suggested that neuroprotection could be enhanced by modifying the cooling regimen. Specifically, cooling to a depth greater than 3°C to 6°C below baseline in preclinical studies of timed hypoxia-ischemia demonstrated that cooled animals compared to those maintained normothermic had more histopathological protection,[10] less brain swelling, greater preservation of energy metabolism,[11] differential neuroprotection in white and gray matter,[12] and less reduction in secondary energy failure.[13] In addition, longer cooling was protective against cell necrosis and inflammation initiated during reperfusion and evolving over time.[14,15] Two clinical reports published during the conduct of the Optimizing Cooling (OC) trial are pertinent to the rationale for OC. Noninvasive measurement of brain temperature indicated that neonates with severe HIE had higher brain temperatures than those with moderate HIE during and after hypothermia at 33.5°C for 72 hours.[16] In a second report, despite the expected decrease in brain temperature among neonates with HIE during the first day of cooling, a subsequent increase of brain temperature was noted among those who developed injury on imaging.[17]

Trial design

Based on the above observations, the NICHD NRN undertook the OC randomized controlled trial (RCT) to determine the impact of longer and/or deeper cooling on death or disability of infants with moderate or severe HIE.[18,19] Inclusion and exclusion criteria of the OC RCT were similar to the prior NRN RCT[2] except that infants who were overcooled at screening (Tc <32.5°C for at least 2 hours) were excluded. Neonates at $\geq$36 weeks' gestational age (GA), with severe birth acidosis or need for resuscitation *and* moderate or severe encephalopathy diagnosed by trained and certified physician examiners, were enrolled within 6 hours of age. In a 2 × 2 factorial design, neonates were randomly assigned to 1 of 4 hypothermia groups, 33.5°C for 72 hours, 33.5°C for 120 hours, 32.0°C for 72 hours, and 32.0°C for 120 hours. The cooling and rewarming procedure was similar to the prior NRN trial,[2] except that, to prevent overcooling for the 32.0°C group, the Tc (esophageal) was initially lowered to 33.5°C and once stable for 15 minutes, further lowered to 32.0°C.

The primary outcome was death or moderate or severe disability at 18 to 22 months of age.[11] Death was included as it is a competing outcome for disability. Neurodevelopmental outcomes were assessed by trained examiners, certified to reliability on an annual basis, and were unaware of treatment status. Severe disability included any of the following: Bayley Scales of Infant Development III cognitive score less than 70, a Gross Motor Function Classification System (GMFCS) level of 3 to 5, or blindness or hearing loss despite amplification. Moderate disability was defined as a cognitive score of 70 to 84 and either GMFCS level 2, active seizures, or hearing loss requiring amplification. A sample size of 363 neonates was required for marginal comparison of usual depth (33.5°C) to deeper cooling (32.0°C) and 363 neonates needed for the marginal comparison of usual duration (72 hours) to longer cooling (120 hours, total 726 neonates). The sample size was based on a 2 tailed $\alpha = .05$, a power of 80%, a 5% loss to follow-up to detect a 10% difference in death or disability from 37.5% to 27.5% in the 2 depths and cooling duration groups. The analyses accounted for differential exposure periods (72 hours and 120 hours), controlled for clinical center and level of HIE, and examined interactions between deeper and longer cooling. Prespecified secondary outcomes included mortality, level of disability by stage of encephalopathy, rates of vision, hearing, and multiple disabilities, cognitive and motor scores, cerebral palsy, rehospitalizations, and growth measurements. Interactions between the 2 depths and durations of cooling were assessed for the primary outcome and key secondary outcomes. Predefined severe adverse events included cardiac arrhythmia, persistent acidosis, major vessel thrombosis, and bleeding. The independent data safety and monitoring committee (DSMC) serially evaluated safety after trial initiation in October 2010.

Results

Neonatal intensive care unit mortality and safety

The neonatal intensive care unit (NICU) mortality rate was 7% for the 33.5°C for 72 hours group (n = 95), 14% for the 32.0°C for 72 hours group (n = 90), 16% for the 33.5°C for 120 hours group (n = 96), and 17% for the 32.0°C for 120 hours group (n = 83). The mortality rates were not different between the cooling depths, 33.5°C (12%) and 32.0°C (12%), and the cooling durations, 72 hours (11%) and 120 hours groups (16%), respectively. There was no interaction between depth and duration of cooling and mortality adjusted for center and level of encephalopathy. Safety outcomes were similar between the 2 cooling depths and the 2 cooling durations, except for the following: major bleeding occurred in 1% of the 120 hours group versus 3% in the 72 hours group. The incidence of arrhythmia and anuria was higher and hospital stay was longer for the 120 hours group versus the 72 hours group. During the NICU course, a higher incidence of bradycardia, inhaled nitric oxide and extracorporeal membrane oxygenation use, and more days of oxygen therapy were observed in the 32.0°C group compared with the 33.5°C group. Futility analysis determined that the probability of detecting a statistically significant benefit for longer cooling, deeper cooling, or both for NICU survival was less than 2%. Following the eighth evaluation (in November 2013), the trial was halted because of mortality and safety concerns after

364 neonates had been enrolled, 185 to the 72 hours group, 179 to the 120 hours group, 191 to the 33.5°C group, and 173 to the 32.0°C group.[10]

Outcome at 18 to 22 months

Outcome assessments were completed in January 2016, with data available on 347 of 364 infants (95%).[19] The primary outcome of death or moderate or severe disability was not different between the 2 depth or the 2 cooling duration groups (**Tables 1** and **2**). The primary outcome was also similar between the 2 depth and the 2 cooling duration groups for infants with moderate or severe HIE at randomization. The secondary outcomes were not different between groups except among infants in the 2 cooling duration groups; there were more deaths (19 vs13%, $P = .04$), fewer rehospitalizations after discharge (16 vs 29%, $P = .02$), and fewer infants with motor scores less than 70 (13 vs 19%, $P = .04$) with 120 hours versus 72 hours cooling. The latter reflects lower survival with longer cooling compared to usual duration of cooling. There was an interaction between depth and duration of cooling and the primary outcome ($P = .048$).

The rates of the primary outcome among the 4 hypothermia groups were 29.3% in the 72 hours at 33.5°C group, 34.5% in 72 hours at 32.0°C, 34.5% in 120 hours at 33.5°C, and 28% in the 120 hours at 32.0°C group. Preplanned Bayesian analyses indicated that the probability of increasing death with deeper cooling (32.0°C for 72 hours), longer cooling (33.5°C for 120 hours), or both (32.0°C for 120 hours) compared with usual care cooling (33.5°C for 72 hours) was 66%, 93%, and 89%, respectively (see Late Hypothermia trial: sample size and analytical plan). The OC trial provides important detail regarding early childhood outcomes for infants cooled with usual parameters that are currently used (33.5°C for 72 hours) and maybe helpful for clinicians when counseling families (**Table 3**).

Conclusions

The OC trial confirmed that deeper and longer cooling was not superior to the usual depth of cooling (33.5°C for whole body cooling) and the usual duration of cooling (72 hours). Although the trial may have been underpowered for determination of the primary outcome due to the early closure, the results are consistent with preclinical studies conducted after the initiation of the OC trial that demonstrated longer and deeper cooling were not neuroprotective.[20–22]

An interesting observation was that the rate of death or moderate/severe disability in the OC trial for infants cooled with usual parameters (33.5°C for 72 hours) was 29%.

Table 1			
Outcomes at 18–22 mo of age by the depth of cooling			
	Esophageal Temp 33.5°C	Esophageal Temp 32.0°C	Adjusted Risk Ratio (95% CI)[a]
Death or moderate or severe disability	59/185 (32%)[b]	51/162 (33%)	0.92 (0.68–1.26)
Death	26/185 (14%)	30/162 (19%)	1.17 (0.67–2.04)
Moderate or severe disability	33/159 (21%)	21/132 (16%)	0.71 (0.36–1.39)
Cerebral palsy[c]	26/158 (16%)	21/132 (16%)	0.94 (0.51–1.73)

[a] All models were adjusted for center and severity of encephalopathy. RRs were derived using the 33.5°C group as the reference.
[b] Results are the number of neonates affected divided by the total and expressed as a percent.
[c] Cerebral palsy of any severity.

Table 2
Outcomes at 18–22 mo of age by the duration of cooling

	Duration 72 h	Duration 120 h	Adjusted Risk Ratio (95% CI)[a]
Death or moderate or severe disability	56/176 (32%)[b]	54/171 (32%)	0.92 (0.68–1.25)
Death	23/176 (13%)	33/171 (19%)	1.39 (1.02–1.90)
Moderate or severe disability	33/153 (22%)	21/138 (15%)	0.68 (0.41–1.11)
Cerebral palsy[c]	29/153 (19%)	18/138 (13%)	0.65 (0.36–1.16)

[a] All models were adjusted for center and severity of encephalopathy. RRs were derived using the 72 h group as the reference.
[b] Results are the number of neonates affected divided by the total and expressed as a percent.
[c] Cerebral palsy of any severity.

Table 3
Outcomes at 18–22 mo of neonates cooled to a depth of 33.5°C for 72 h

	No/Total	Percent
Death or moderate or severe disability	27/92	29
Death or moderate/severe disability	—	—
Among neonates with moderate HIE	14/71	20
Among neonates with severe HIE	13/21	62
Death	8/92	9
Among neonates with moderate HIE	4/71	6
Among neonates with severe HIE	4/21	19
Among survivors:	—	—
Severe disability	18/84	21
Moderate disability	1/84	1
Mild disability[a]	16/81	20
No disability[b]	46/81	57
Any cerebral palsy	16/84	19
Disabling cerebral palsy[c]	14/84	17
Bayley III cognitive scores[d]	—	—
Median, interquartile range	90 (80–100)	—
≥85	51	65
70–84	14	18
<70	13	17
Rehospitalization after discharge	16/80	36
Height <10%	19/75	25
Weight <10%	7/78	9
Head circumference <10%	15/76	20

[a] Mild disability: cognitive score of 70 to 80 or a cognitive score of 85 or greater and any of the following: GMFCS level 1 or 2, seizure disorder, or hearing loss not requiring amplification.
[b] No disability: cognitive score of 85 or greater and absence of neurosensory deficits and seizures.
[c] Disabling cerebral palsy: moderate or severe with infants requiring support for sitting, unable to crawl or requiring adult assistance to move.
[d] Bayley III cognitive score normative data, mean ± sd 100 ± 15; data based on 78 infants due to loss to follow-up and inability to test selected infants.

This is considerably lower than death or disability after hypothermia treatment in multiple initial cooling trials (eg, 44% in the NICHD whole body cooling,[2] 45% in the TOBY trial,[3] and 51% for the neo.nEURO.network[4]). An important contributing factor was the lower rate of severe encephalopathy among infants randomized in the OC trial compared to earlier trials. Other variables include earlier recognition of at-risk neonates, improved stabilization, earlier initiation of hypothermia treatment, and more intensive neuromonitoring.[23]

Without the OC trial, enthusiastic clinicians may reason that deeper or longer cooling may provide more neuroprotection than presently achieved with Tc of 33.5°C maintained for 72 hours. The results of the OC trial emphasize the importance of avoiding drifts in practice and adhering to established protocols based on randomized trials.

LATE HYPOTHERMIA TRIAL
Rationale

A key element of hypothermia therapy for neonatal moderate or severe HIE is initiation within 6 hours following birth. The 6 hour interval represents a putative therapeutic window during which hypothermia can be implemented and still favorably alter outcome. The strongest support for a 6 hour therapeutic window is well-done preclinical fetal sheep studies in which 3 groups underwent 72 hours of hypothermia initiated at different times after ischemia (either 1.5, 5.5 or 8.5 hours), and histologic injury was compared to sham controls.[24–26] Neuronal loss was reduced only with the 2 earlier initiation times. Although neuronal loss scores were not lower when hypothermia was initiated at 8.5 hours ($P = .11$), the results were based on a limited sample size (5 hypothermic animals) and cannot exclude the possibility of a longer therapeutic window.[26] Furthermore, direct extrapolation from animals to newborns may be limited given variables of the insult in the clinical setting that cannot be easily replicated in the laboratory (eg, duration, repetitiveness, and severity of hypoxia-ischemia). There is also strong clinical rationale for study of hypothermia beyond 6 hours of age. First, encephalopathy may evolve from absent or mild in extent at less than 6 hours to moderate or severe after 6 hours. Second, preclinical studies employ well-timed hypoxic-ischemic events and the assumption in clinical medicine is that hypoxia-ischemia occurs near or at delivery. However, the frequency of sentinel events at delivery (eg, abruptio placenta, ruptured uterus, prolapsed cord) was approximately 60% in one trial[27] and leaves many neonates with an unclear timing of hypoxia-ischemia. It seems possible that hypoxia-ischemia in some neonates may have its onset hours before birth, and hypothermia treatment initiated within 6 hours after birth may represent a much longer interval from event to treatment. Third, hypothermia treatment may not be initiated within 6 hours of age due to births in remote locations, although controlled cooling on transport may diminish this issue.

Trial Design

The Late Hypothermia trial was designed to estimate the probability that hypothermia initiated at 6 to 24 hours after birth reduced the risk of death or disability at 18 to 22 months among neonates with moderate or severe HIE.[28] This was a randomized trial conducted between April 2008 and June 2016 by 21 centers of the NRN. Inclusion criteria were infants aged 36 weeks' gestation or greater, either severe fetal acidemia or need for resuscitation at birth, and either moderate or severe encephalopathy or a seizure. Encephalopathy or seizure was either recognized between 6 and 24 hours of age or infants arrived at a referral center for cooling after 6 hours. Newborns were randomized to an esophageal temperature of 33.5°C or 37.0°C for 96 hours. A longer duration of hypothermia (96 vs 72 hours) was used based on preclinical data prior to 2008.[29] The primary outcome was death or moderate or severe disability at 18 to 22 months similar to a prior NRN hypothermia trial.[2]

Sample Size and Analytical Plan

A major challenge for this trial was the number of available patients. The sample size was predefined at 168, which was thought to be the largest number of neonates that could be enrolled in a feasible time interval (6 years) using prior experiences.[2,30] A Bayesian analysis was prespecified given the limited sample size and power in conventional frequentist analyses to identify a treatment effect. A Bayesian analysis has been recommended for trials of rare conditions or uncommon features of previously studied disease processes.[31] A Bayesian analysis unlike a conventional frequentist analysis provides a direct assessment of the probability that the hypothesis is true based on the observed data and a prior distribution within a plausible range.

A hypothetical Bayesian analysis is illustrated in **Fig. 1**. Distinct from frequentist analyses, a Bayesian analysis uses pre-existing data from trials to establish a prior distribution that represents the probability of a hypothesized treatment effect. If there is no available information to indicate benefit or harm from the intervention, a neutral prior can be used, centered at a risk ratio (RR) of 1 indicating a 50% probability of

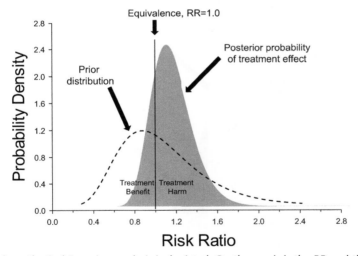

Fig. 1. A hypothetical Bayesian analysis is depicted. On the x-axis is the RR and the y-axis is the probability density, which is the frequency distribution of observed values. For the Late Hypothermia trial, the noncooled group is the reference and an RR of less than 1.0 is the desired outcome indicating a reduction in the outcome of interest in the hypothermic group. In this example, the prior distribution (dashed *line*) is shifted to the left of an RR of 1.0 reflecting encouraging pilot studies in this hypothetical scenario that suggest benefit from the intervention. The prior distribution is asymmetric since a RR less than 1.0 can only go as low as zero but a RR greater than 1.0 can go to infinity. The curve would be symmetric if the x-axis was on a log scale. When combined with the observed trial results, the posterior probability of treatment effect, indicated by the solid gray curve, is shifted to the right of a RR of 1.0. The area under the gray curve less than or greater than a RR of 1.0 provides the posterior probability of benefit and harm, respectively. In this hypothetical case, most of the posterior probability distribution is a RR greater than 1.0 indicating a greater likelihood of harm than benefit.

benefit (RR <1.0 for a reduction in death or disability) and a 50% probability of harm (RR >1.0). Alternatively, the prior can be centered at RR less than 1.0 or greater than 1.0 if existing data suggest benefit or harm, respectively. The prior distribution is described by a 95% credible interval (95% probability that the true RR lies in this interval) reflecting the minimum and maximum likely treatment effects based on effect sizes identified for major outcomes in randomized trials.[32] In the Late Hypothermia trial, a neutral prior was used given the paucity of data for hypothermia initiated beyond 6 hours from birth. The prior distribution is combined with the observed data from the trial to yield a probability of a posterior distribution. The posterior distribution can be characterized by a point estimate, 95% credible intervals, and the area under the curve which is less than RR of 1.0 (treatment benefit) and the area under the curve which is greater than RR of 1.0 (treatment harm). Analyses were adjusted (adjusted RR [aRR]) for age at randomization (≤12 hours, >12 hours) and level of encephalopathy (moderate, severe).

Results

The primary outcome is depicted in **Fig. 2**. Death or disability occurred in 24.4% of the hypothermic group and 27.9% of the noncooled group. Combining the trial results with a neutral prior shifted the distribution to a 76% posterior probability of any reduction in death or disability and a posterior aRR of 0.86 (95% credible intervals, 0.58–1.29). The probability of a treatment benefit for death alone and survival with moderate

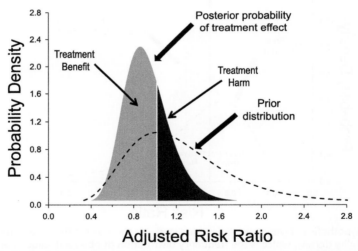

Fig. 2. This figure depicts the results of the primary outcome for the Late Hypothermia trial. A neutral prior (dashed *line*) was used reflecting the absence of other trials examining hypothermia therapy for HIE after 6 hours of age. The neutral prior is asymmetric as described for **Fig. 1**. When the observed results from the trial were combined with a neutral prior distribution, the posterior probability of treatment effect was shifted to the left of an adjusted RR of 1.0 (adjusted for stratifying variables of age at randomization and level of encephalopathy). The area under the curve less than a RR of 1.0, indicated by the gray portion of the posterior distribution, was a 76% probability of any treatment benefit. The area under the curve greater than a RR of 1.0, indicated by the black portion of the posterior distribution, was a 24% probability of any treatment harm. (This figure has been adapted with permission from Figure 2A of Laptook A. et al, JAMA 2017;318(16):1550 to 1560. doi10.1001/jama.2017.14972.)

or severe disability were 73% and 68% with a neutral prior, respectively. When considered as an absolute risk difference (hypothermia minus noncooled), there was a 64% probability of at least a 2% absolute risk difference of less death or disability for hypothermia compared to noncooled treatment. For an absolute risk difference of 2%, hypothermia was associated with a 3.2 fold lower risk of death or disability compared to noncooled neonates assuming a range of risk differences around zero considered equivalent between groups.

Conclusions

The priority for treatment of moderate or severe HIE with hypothermia is to initiate therapy as soon as possible after birth and within 6 hours of age. As discussed, there is strong biologic and clinical rationale to justify study of hypothermia after 6 hours of age. Bayesian analysis provides a probability of benefit or harm even with a limited sample size and results are easily interpretable by clinicians. A 76% probability of any reduction in death or disability, and a 64% probability of at least 2% less death or disability at 18 months with late hypothermia is suggestive but not conclusive evidence. Some clinicians may view the uncertainty as insufficient to justify use of late hypothermia. Alternatively, some clinicians may choose to use late hypothermia in the setting of moderate or severe HIE given the potential for death or a disastrous neurodevelopmental outcome, the absence of harm and lack of any other rigorously tested brain-specific therapy.

PRETERM HYPOTHERMIA
Rationale

All 6 initial trials of hypothermia for HIE were limited to neonates at 36 weeks' GA or greater[1–6] except for one study.[6] The latter trial and one pilot study included an unspecified number of neonates at 35 weeks' GA.[6,33,34] Personal communication with those authors (SE Jacobs, 2014; DJ Eicher, 2014) revealed that there were only 7 neonates enrolled. Based on this group of studies, the Committee on the Fetus and Newborn (COFN) of the American Academy of Pediatrics recommended hypothermia for HIE for infants at 35 GA or greater.[35] Despite the lack of compelling data, many clinicians have adopted the COFN recommendation and provide hypothermia for neonates with HIE at 35 weeks. Furthermore, some centers have elected to provide hypothermia for neonates with HIE below 35 weeks fueled by multiple single-center nonrandomized experiences.[36–40]

Irrespective of the COFN recommendation and ongoing clinical practice, there is a knowledge gap regarding the effectiveness of hypothermia treatment of moderate and severe HIE at 35 weeks' gestation or less. Hypothermia may place preterm neonates at greater risk for initiation and/or exacerbation of prematurity-associated problems (eg, intracranial hemorrhage, necrotizing enterocolitis [NEC], and coagulopathy) compared to more mature neonates.

Trial design

To address this knowledge gap, the *Eunice Kennedy Shriver* NICHD NRN conducted a randomized, controlled trial to determine if hypothermia initiated at less than 6 hours of age among neonates born at 33^0 to 35^6 weeks' gestation with HIE would reduce death or moderate or severe disability at 18 to 22 months' corrected age. This was a randomized trial conducted between July 2015 and December 2022 by 19 centers of the NRN.

Many features of this trial were identical or very similar to previous hypothermia trials conducted by the NRN, including (1) inclusion criteria (severe acidosis and/or perinatal sentinel event with resuscitation at birth, followed by the presence of moderate or severe encephalopathy using modified Sarnat score assessed by certified examiners or clinical seizures at <6 hours), (2) device to achieve whole body hypothermia and monitor esophageal temperature (Tes), (3) randomization to hypothermia (target Tes 33.5°C) or normothermia (target Tes 37.0°C), (4) duration of intervention (72 hours), (5) rewarming rate (0.5°C/h), (6) schedule of Tes surveillance during intervention and rewarming periods, and (7) the primary outcome, death or moderate or severe disability and its definition.[2,18,19,28]

All neonates admitted to the NICUs of participating NRN centers at 33[0] to 35[6] week GA and less than 6 hours postnatal age with a diagnosis of encephalopathy, perinatal asphyxia, neurologic depression, or birth depression were screened for eligibility. Because of concerns about prematurity associated changes in the neurologic examination and Sarnat scoring, an abnormal level of consciousness of moderate or severe degree was required. Similarly, criteria for posture and Moro were adjusted to account for maturational changes between 33 and 35 weeks' GA.[41] Some of the salient exclusion criteria included (1) birthweight less than 1500 g, (2) temperature less than 34°C for greater than 1 hour at screening, (3) paralytic or sedative agents precluding a meaningful examination, and (4) presence of a major anomaly. Passive cooling during transport was discouraged. Because of the association of hyperthermia with adverse outcomes, steps were incorporated to prevent or limit hyperthermia greater than 37.5°C in the normothermia arm.[42-44] Thermal management before and after the intervention and rewarming period as well as other aspects of care such as laboratory and imaging surveillance, respiratory support, sedation, anticonvulsant therapy were per the standards at each center. Infants were not fed during the intervention and rewarming period.

Surveillance was conducted for prespecified safety events as in previous NRN hypothermia trials. In addition, there was surveillance for events pertinent to prematurity (eg, intracranial hemorrhage, NEC, and days of mechanical ventilation). Cranial ultrasounds were to be obtained within 24 hours of randomization and brain MRI at 7 to 21 days of age. The DSMC reviewed accumulating data at 6 intervals during the trial. After its third review of cumulative data on September 17, 2017, the DSMC requested additional measures to prevent or correct Tes less than 32°C. The following steps were implemented: (1) change precooling the blanket prior to the intervention from 5°C to 15°C, (2) immediate notification of research staff if Tes less than 32.0°C, (3) Tes recorded every 10 minutes until target Tes attained, and (4) documentation of corrective actions.

Review of admission records of participating NICUs suggested that a maximum of 168 neonates could be enrolled in a 5 year period. Given the anticipated moderate number of subjects, Bayesian analysis was prespecified. A neutral prior was planned due to absence of randomized studies of hypothermia in this population (see Late Hypothermia trial: sample size and analytical plan). The sample size was preplanned for 168. All analyses were with the intention to treat and were adjusted for level of encephalopathy and study center.

Results

Of the 168 subjects enrolled, 88 were randomized to hypothermia and 80 to normothermia. Demographic and clinical characteristics of mothers and neonates were balanced between groups (**Table 4**). The average GA was 34 weeks and more than 50% of the neonates were outborn. Stabilization interventions at delivery, and the

Table 4
Maternal and neonatal characteristics in the preterm hypothermia trial

	Hypothermia (n = 88) % or Mean ± sd	Normothermia (n = 80) % or Mean ± sd
Maternal		
Age, y	30.9 ± 6.1	28.8 ± 6.4
Black	31	39
Pre-eclampsia/hypertension	37	40
Diabetes	24	29
Abruption	41	46
Intrapartum hemorrhage	20	20
Uterine Rupture	7	1
Intrapartum Temperature >37.5 C	2	4
Fetal deceleration	79	72
Cord mishap	10	9
Emergent C-section	77	84
Infant		
Gestational age, wk	34.0 ± 0.8	34.1 ± 0.8
Birth weight, g	2464 ± 634	2371 ± 608
Male	52	56
Outborn	53	59
Delivery room		
Intubation	64	63
Chest compressions	46	38
Epinephrine	30	33
Apgar Scores ≤5 at 10 min	51	43
pH, cord or postnatal blood gas <1 h	6.90 ± 0.20	6.90 ± 0.20
Randomization		
Age in hours	4.5 ± 1.2	4.5 ± 1.3
Moderate encephalopathy	69	71
Severe encephalopathy	31	29
Seizures alone	0	0

extent of encephalopathy (moderate/severe) at randomization were similar between groups.

The primary outcome was determined beyond 22 months in 52 subjects due to coronavirus disease 2019 center-specific restrictions. Death or moderate/severe disability occurred in 29 of 83 (35%) children in the hypothermia group versus 20 of 69 (29.0%) in the normothermic group. The aRR (hypothermia/normothermia) using a neutral prior probability was 1.11 (95% credibility interval [CrI] 0.74–2.00), resulting in a 74% probability of harm (**Table 5**). When stratified by moderate versus severe encephalopathy at randomization, the primary outcome also revealed no benefit with hypothermia. Stratification by GA revealed a higher incidence of death or disability in hypothermic neonates and of death alone at each GA except for 33 weeks (**Table 6**).

Death alone occurred in 18 (22%) and 9 (13%) neonates randomized to hypothermia and normothermia, respectively. The aRR for death alone was 1.38 (95% CrI 0.79–2.85) with probability of harm of 87% (see **Table 5**). Three deaths occurred after

Table 5
Posterior probabilities of the primary outcome and its components, death alone and survival with disability: neutral prior

	Hypothermic (n = 83)[a]		Normothermic (n = 69)[b]		Bayesian Results	
	n/N	%	n/N	%	aRR (95% credibility interval)	Probability of treatment harm
Death or moderate or severe disability	29/83	35	20/69	29	1.11 (0.74–2.00)	74%
Death	18/83	22	9/69	13	1.38 (0.79–2.85)	87%
Survival with moderate or severe disability	11/83	13	11/69	16	0.86 (0.46–1.63)	32%

[a] The primary outcome was available in 83 of 88 neonates randomized to the hypothermic group. Three neonates were lost to follow-up and 2 had incomplete follow-up.
[b] The primary outcome was available in 69 of 80 neonates randomized to the normothermic group. Seven neonates were lost to follow-up, 2 had incomplete follow-up, and 2 were withdrawn (parental decision) immediately after randomization and prior to initiation of the intervention.

Table 6
Treatment comparison of primary outcome and death alone stratified by gestational age based on best obstetric estimate

	Death or Moderate/Severe Disability n/N (%)		Death n/N (%)	
GA	Hypothermic (N = 83)	Normothermic (N = 69)	Hypothermic (N = 85)	Normothermic (N = 71)
33 wk	13/31 (42)	6/17 (35)	5/31 (16)	4/19 (21)
34 wk	9/24 (38)	10/32 (31)	8/26 (31)	2/32 (6)
35 wk	7/28 (25)	4/20 (20)	5/28 (18)	3/20 (15)

Formal Bayesian analysis to determine aRR and probability of benefit/harm is not reported due to small numbers.

discharge from the initial hospitalization, and all but 2 deaths occurred following decisions to redirect care or withhold resuscitation. Death was attributed to asphyxial brain injury by site investigators in 15 out of 18 (83%) among hypothermic and 5 out of 9 (56%) normothermic neonates and to multiorgan failure in 2 out of 18 (11%) and 2 out of 9 (22%) neonates. Survival with moderate or severe disability occurred in 11 (13%) and 11 (16%) of the hypothermic and normothermic groups, respectively (aRR 0.86, 95% CrI 0.46, 1.63) yielding a 32% probability of harm.

There were no notable differences between groups in prespecified safety events during the intervention (arrhythmia, persistent metabolic acidosis, major bleeding, and skin alterations). Hyperglycemia (serum glucose >180 mg/dL) and thrombocytopenia (platelet count <100,000/mm^3) were noted in greater than 10% of neonates in both groups. Hyperglycemia occurred in 23% and 12% of the hypothermic and normothermic groups, respectively (aRR 1.64, 95% CrI 0.92, 3.27) yielding a 95% probability of harm. The number of neonates with intracranial hemorrhage during the intervention were 6 and 5 for hypothermic and normothermic groups, respectively. The frequency of intracranial hemorrhage was 8% in both groups. MRI results are pending. There were no cases of NEC and rates of pulmonary artery hypertension were 6% and 5% for hypothermic and normothermic groups, respectively.

Conclusions

This study found no evidence of benefit from hypothermia at less than 6 hours among neonates aged at 33^0 to 35^6 weeks' gestation with moderate or severe HIE, unlike previous trials in neonates at 36 weeks' GA or greater. The findings were consistent for both death or moderate/severe disability, and death alone. The 32% probability of harm for survival with moderate or severe disability among the hypothermia group needs cautious interpretation given the higher mortality in the hypothermic group. The sample size was limited but prespecified at 168 reflecting the GA criteria over which a smaller fraction of births occurs compared to trials enrolling neonates at 36 weeks' GA. A traditional frequentist analysis would require a larger sample size despite recruitment at 19 large academic centers that receive transports from a wide community net. Even with the limited sample size, recruitment and follow-up took 7.5 years to complete.

The reasons for lack of benefit from hypothermia for HIE among neonates born at 33^0 to 35^6 GA are unclear. There may be differences in the risk–benefit profile among less mature neonates. However, there were no differences in major bleeding, thrombocytopenia, intracranial hemorrhage, pulmonary hypertension, or NEC compared to normothermic neonates. Interestingly, rates of pulmonary hypertension were lower than the 22% reported in 2 prior NRN hypothermia trials.[45] Maternal complications of pregnancy and the in utero environment may differ compared to hypothermia trials among more mature neonates. Specifically, maternal hypertensive disease and placental abruption were considerably higher compared to the few reports with similar data among more mature neonates.

Many centers provide hypothermia for neonates with HIE at 35 weeks' gestation but the primary outcome and post hoc analysis stratified by GA does not support benefit at any GA. Overall, the results support that targeted normothermia with interventions to prevent or minimize hyperthermia may be the most evidence-based approach for this group of neonates.

SUMMARY

Hypothermia treatment of moderate or severe HIE represents a landmark therapy because it is the first and only treatment to date that has been demonstrated to reduce mortality and improve neurodevelopmental outcome. Randomized trials of hypothermia have laid the groundwork for implementation and dissemination of this treatment. The success of hypothermia has triggered important questions that were not studied in the initial randomized trials. This article has summarized and discussed 3 RCTs for moderate or severe HIE to address the use of longer and/or deeper cooling, initiation of hypothermia after 6 hours of age, and use of hypothermia in preterm neonates. The results of these trials expand the evidence base available to clinicians when using hypothermia to treat moderate or severe HIE.

Best Practices

What is the current practice when using hypothermia treatment of neonatal moderate or severe HIE?

- Hypothermia therapy should be used for the treatment of HIE when there is a reasonable certainty of a hypoxic-ischemic event that occurred at or proximate to birth using inclusion criteria from randomized trials.
- Hypothermia should be initiated within 6 hours after birth but as early as feasible along with stabilization of cardiopulmonary, metabolic, and other critical processes.
- Cooling parameters for whole body hypothermia are a target core temperature (esophageal or rectal) of 33.5°C continued for 72 hours. Rewarming is typically done at 0.5°C/h.

Recommendations:

- Adhere to hypothermia regimens that have been studied in rigorous RCTs.
- For neonates with moderate or severe HIE who meet criteria for hypothermia therapy but are beyond 6 hours of age, late hypothermia can be considered as an option.
- There is no benefit of using hypothermia for moderate or severe HIE among infants at less than 36 weeks' gestation.

DISCLOSURE

The authors have nothing to disclose. Dr A.R. Laptook receives funding support from the National Institutes of Health, United States for project numbers 2UG1 OD 024951, 3 U2 COD 023375-07S2, and 1R61NS126792-01. Dr S. Shankaran receives funding support from the National Institute for Health Research, United Kingdom, United Kingdom for the Cooling in Mild Encephalopathy Randomized Trial (NIHR 152188).

REFERENCES

1. Gluckman PD, Wyatt JS, Azzopardi D, et al. Selective head cooling with mild systemic hypothermia after neonatal encephalopathy: multicentre randomized trial. Lancet 2005;365:663–70.
2. Shankaran S, Laptook AR, Ehrenkranz RA, et al. Whole-body hypothermia for neonates with hypoxic-ischemic encephalopathy. N Engl J Med 2005;353:1574–84.
3. Azzopardi DV, Strohm B, Edwards AD, et al. Moderate hypothermia to treat perinatal asphyxia encephalopathy. N Engl J Med 2009;361:1349–58.
4. Simbruner G, Mittal RA, Rohlmann F, et al, neo.nEURO.network. Systemic hypothermia after neonatal encephalopathy: outcomes of neo.nEURO.network RCT. Pediatrics 2010;126:e771–8.
5. Jacobs SE, Morley CJ, Inder TE, et al. Whole-body hypothermia for term and near term newborns with hypoxic-ischemic encephalopathy: a randomized controlled trial. Arch Pediatr Adolesc Med 2011;165:692–700.
6. Zhou WH, Cheng GQ, Shao XM, et al. Selective head cooling with mild systemic hypothermia after neonatal hypoxic-ischemic encephalopathy: a multicenter randomized controlled trial in China. J Pediatr 2010;157:367–72.e3.
7. Jacobs SE, Berg M, Hunt R, et al. Cooling for newborns with hypoxic ischaemic encephalopathy. Cochrane Database Syst Rev 2013;(1):CD003311.
8. Higgins RD, Raju TNK, Perlman J, et al. Hypothermia and perinatal asphyxia: executive summary of the National Institute of Child Health and Human Development workshop. J Pediatr 2006;148(2):170–5.
9. Higgins RD, Raju T, Edwards AD, et al. Hypothermia and other treatment options for neonatal encephalopathy: an executive summary of the Eunice Kennedy Shriver NICHD workshop. J Pediatr 2011;159(5):851–858 e1.
10. Busto R, DietrichWD Globus MY, Valdés I, et al. GinsbergMD. Small differences in intraischemic brain temperature critically determine the extent of ischemic neuronal injury. J Cerebr Blood Flow Metabol 1987;7(6):729–38.
11. Williams GD, Dardzinski BJ, Buckalew AR, et al. Modest hypothermia preserves cerebral energy metabolism during hypoxia-ischemia and correlates with brain damage: a 31P nuclear magnetic resonance study in unanesthetized neonatal rats. Pediatr Res 1997;42(5):700–8.
12. Iwata O, Thornton JS, Sellwood MW, et al. Depth of delayed cooling alters neuroprotection pattern after hypoxia-ischemia. Ann Neurol 2005;58(1):75–87.
13. Thoresen M, Penrice J, Lorek A, et al. Mild hypothermia after severe transient hypoxia-ischemia ameliorates delayed cerebral energy failure in the newborn piglet. Pediatr Res 1995;37(5):667–70.
14. Lorek A, Takei Y, Cady EB, et al. Delayed (secondary) cerebral energy failure after acute hypoxia-ischemia in the newborn piglet: continuous 48-hour studies by phosphorus magnetic resonance spectroscopy. Pediatr Res 1994;36:699–706.
15. Bennet L, Roelfsema V, Pathipati P, et al. Relationship between evolving epileptiform activity and delayed loss of mitochondrial activity after asphyxia measured by near-infrared spectroscopy in preterm fetal sheep. J Physiol 2006;572:141–54.
16. Wu TW, McLean C, Friedlich P, et al. Brain temperature in neonates with hypoxic-ischemic encephalopathy during therapeutic hypothermia. J Pediatr 2014;165:1129–34.
17. Owji ZP, Gilbert G, Saint. Martin C, et al. Barin temperature is increased during the first days of life in asphyxiated newborns. Developing brain injury despite hypothermia treatment. Am J Neuroradiol 2017;38(11):2180–6.

18. Shankaran S, Laptook AR, Pappas A, et al. Effect of depth and duration of cooling on deaths in the NICU among neonates with hypoxic ischemic encephalopathy: a randomized trial. JAMA 2014;312(24):2629–39.

19. Shankaran S, Laptook AR, Pappas A, et al. Effect of depth and duration of cooling on death or disability at age 18 months among neonates with hypoxic-ischemic encephalopathy: a randomized trial. JAMA 2017;318(1):57–67.

20. Davidson JO, Yuill CA, Zhang FG, et al. Extending the duration of hypothermia does not further improve white matter protection after ischemia in term-equivalent fetal sheep. Sci Rep 2016;6:25178.

21. Alonso-Alconada D, Broad KD, Bainbridge A, et al. Brain cell death is reduced with cooling by 3.5°C to 5°C but increased with cooling by 8.5°C in a piglet asphyxia model. Stroke 2015;46(1):275–8.

22. Wood T, Osredkar D, Puchades M, et al. Treatment temperature and insult severity influence the neuroprotective effects of therapeutic hypothermia. Sci Rep 2016;6(6):23430.

23. Bonifacio S, Van Meurs K, McDonald SA, et al. Differences in patient characteristics and care practices between two trials of therapeutic hypothermia. Pediatr Res 2019 June;85(7):1008–15.

24. Gunn AJ, Gunn TR, de Haan HH, et al. Dramatic neuronal rescue with prolonged selective head cooling after ischemia in fetal lambs. J Clin Invest 1997;99:248–56.

25. Gunn AJ, Gunn TR, Gunning MI, et al. Neuroprotection with prolonged head cooling started before postischemic seizures in fetal sheep. Pediatrics 1998;102:1098–106.

26. Gunn AJ, Bennett I, Gunning MI, et al. Cerebral hypothermia is not neuroprotective when started after postischemic seizures in fetal sheep. Pediatr Res 1999;46:274–80.

27. Shankaran S, Laptook AR, MdDonals SA, et al. Acute perinatal sentinel events, neonatal brain injury pattern, and outcome of infants undergoing a trial of hypothermia for neonatal hypoxic-ischemic encephalopathy. J Pediatr 2017;180:275–8.e2.

28. Laptook AR, Shankaran S, Tyson JE, et al. Effect of therapeutic hypothermia after 6 hours of age on death or disability among newborns with hypoxic-ischemic encephalopathy: a randomized trial. JAMA 2017;318(16):1550–60.

29. Colbourne F, Corbett D. Delayed and prolonged post-ischemic hypothermia is neuroprotective in the gerbil. Brain Res 1994;654(2):265–72.

30. Shalak LF, Laptook AR, Velaphi SC, et al. The amplitude integrated EEG coupled with an early neurological examination enhances prediction of term infants at risk for persistent encephalopathy. Pediatrics 2003;111(2):351–7.

31. Lilford RJ, Thornton JG, Braunholtz D. Clinical trials and rare diseases: a way out of a conundrum. BMJ 1995;311(December):1621–5.

32. Pedroza C, Han W, Truong VTT, et al. Performance of informative priors skeptical of large treatment effects in clinical trials: a simulation study. Stat Methods Med Res 2018;27(1):79–96.

33. Eicher DJ, Wagner CL, Katikaneni LP, et al. Moderate hypothermia in neonatal encephalopathy: efficacy outcomes. Pediatr Neurol 2005;32(1):11–7.

34. Eicher DJ, Wagner CL, Katikaneni LP, et al. Moderate hypothermia in neonatal encephalopathy: safety outcomes. Pediatr Neurol 2005;32(1):18–24.

35. Committee on Fetus, Newborn Papile LA, Baley JE, Benitz W, et al. Hypothermia and neonatal encephalopathy. Pediatrics 2014;133:1146–50.

36. Shipley L, Gale C, Sharkey D. Trends in the incidence and management of hypoxic-ischaemic encephalopathy in the therapeutic hypothermia era: a

national population study. Arch Dis Child Fetal Neonatal Ed 2021 Sep;106(5): 529–34.

37. Rao R, Trivedi S, Vesoulis Z, et al. Safety and short-term outcomes of therapeutic hypothermia in preterm neonates 34-35 weeks gestational age with hypoxic-ischemic encephalopathy. J Pediatr 2017;183:37–42.

38. Herrera TI, Edwards L, Malcolm WF, et al. Outcomes of preterm infants treated with hypothermia for hypoxic-ischemic encephalopathy. Early Hum Dev 2018; 125:1–7, m.

39. Moran P, Sullivan K, Zanelli SA, et al. Single-center experience with therapeutic hypothermia for hypoxic-ischemic encephalopathy in infants with <36 weeks gestation. Am J Perinatol 2024. https://doi.org/10.1055/a-2251-6317.

40. Kim SH, El-Shibiny H, Inder T, et al. Therapeutic hypothermia for preterm infants 34-35 weeks gestational age with neonatal encephalopathy. J Perinatol 2024. https://doi.org/10.1038/s41372-024-01874-x.

41. Volpe JJ. Neurology of the newborn. 5th Edition. Philadelphia PA: Saunders, Elsevier; 2008. Neurological Examination, Chapter 3, p121-153.

42. Wyatt JS, Gluckman PD, Liu PY, et al, Coolcap Study Group. Determinants of outcome after head cooling for neonatal encephalopathy. Pediatrics 2007;119(5): 912–21.

43. Laptook A, Tyson J, Shankaran S, et al. National Institute of Child Health and Human Development Neonatal Research Network. Elevated temperature after hypoxic-ischemic encephalopathy: risk factor for adverse outcomes. Pediatrics 2008;122(3):491–9.

44. Laptook AR, McDonald SA, Shankaran S, et al. Extended hypothermia follow-up SubCommittee of the National Institute of Child Health and Human Development Neonatal Research Network. Elevated temperature and 6- to 7-year outcome of neonatal encephalopathy. Ann Neurol 2013;73(4):520–8.

45. Lakshminrusimha S, Shankaran S, Laptook A, et al. Pulmonary hypertension associated with hypoxic-ischemic encephalopathy0Antecdent characteristics and comorbidities. J Pediatr 2018;196:45–51.

A New Horizon for Understanding the Comparative Effectiveness for Cooling Prospectively Infants with Mild Encephalopathy

Lina F. Chalak, MD, MSCS[a],*, Jonathan L. Slaughter, MD, MPH[b], Wendy C. King, PhD[c], Pollieanna Sepulveda, BS, MSN[a], Stephen R. Wisniewski, PhD[d]

KEYWORDS

- Asphyxia • Mild hypoxic-ischemic encephalopathy (HIE) • Neonate
- Therapeutic hypothermia • Neurodevelopment
- Comparative effectiveness research (CER) • Target trial emulation

KEY POINTS

- The lack of equipoise for the treatment of infants with mild hypoxic-ischemic encephalopathy (HIE) stems from a lack of trial data, the narrow therapeutic window for hypothermia, and fear of disease severity misclassifications due to the dynamic nature of neonatal encephalopathy.
- Despite insufficient data on specific benefits-risks, about half of US institutions offer hypothermia to treat mild neonatal HIE.
- Cooling Prospectively Infants with Mild Encephalopathy,an ongoing (2024–2028) comparative effectiveness research trial, addresses the current conundrum for care of infants with mild HIE by site stratification, leveraging the choice of 2 currently accepted practices: hypothermia and normothermia.

[a] Department of Pediatrics, Neonatal-Perinatal Medicine, University of Texas Southwestern Medical School, 5323 Harry Hines Boulevard, Dallas, TX 75390-9063, USA; [b] Department of Pediatrics and Epidemiology, Center for Perinatal Research, Nationwide Children's Hospital, Colleges of Medicine and Public Health, The Ohio State University, 575 Children's Crossroad, Columbus, OH 43215, USA; [c] Department of Epidemiology, School of Public Health, University of Pittsburgh, Pittsburgh, PA 15260, USA; [d] Department of Epidemiology, School of Public Health, Vice Provost for Budget and Analytics, University of Pittsburgh, Pittsburgh, PA 15260, USA
* Corresponding author.
E-mail address: Lina.chalak@utsouthwestern.edu

Clin Perinatol 51 (2024) 605–616
https://doi.org/10.1016/j.clp.2024.04.003
0095-5108/24/© 2024 Elsevier Inc. All rights are reserved, including those for text and data mining, AI training, and similar technologies.

INTRODUCTION

The World Health Organization reports that birth asphyxia/neonatal hypoxic-ischemic encephalopathy (HIE) accounts for a million deaths annually and represents the most common cause of death and disability in neonates;[1,2] 50% of diagnosed infants in therapeutic hypothermia (TH) are in the understudied mild HIE end of the spectrum, which was excluded from prior large randomized clinical trials (RCTs) demonstrating a reduction in death or disability in moderate to severe HIE following TH.

Over the last decade, there has been compelling evidence that untreated neonates with mild HIE are at significant risk for adverse outcomes. This resulted in a therapeutic drift such that by 2022, half of providers offered TH for mild HIE,[3] with the remainder offering normothermia, reflecting a lack of clear evidence for benefit in this particular population. Another conundrum of the so-called "mild HIE" is rooted in the need to define the severity of HIE within the early therapeutic window of 6 hours postnatal, the time interval at which TH has been demonstrated most effective in clinical trials, despite the evolving nature of HIE in the first week after birth.[3] Physician researchers are divided into 2 camps: the first persisted in the traditional approach of aiming for an ideal RCT,[4] while the second adapted to the necessity of a pragmatic approach to find the best evidence in the real-world setting.[5]

In select neonatal RCTs, lack of equipoise for randomization of fragile newborns due to clinician bias has threatened the external validity (generalizability) of findings and has resulted in nonparticipation, leading to early trial terminations, squandering precious resources.[5] For example, the Prophylactic Phenobarbital After Neonatal Seizures (PROPHENO) RCT met with equipoise challenges that led to termination due to low enrollment. Subsequently, an observational comparative effectiveness research (CER) study in infants with seizures was able to evaluate the risks associated with discontinuation (vs prophylactic use) of antiseizure medication after the resolution of acute symptomatic neonatal seizures and before hospital discharge.[6]

To address the current conundrum of care for infants with mild HIE in a setting of limited equipoise and thus, unwillingness of parents and physicians to randomize treatment in mild HIE, a prospective, observational CER cohort *Cooling Prospectively Infants with Mild Encephalopathy* (COOLPRIME) was designed to determine the safety and effectiveness of hypothermia versus normothermia in infants with mild HIE. Rather than randomizing treatment assignment, participants are treated based on their site's existing local standard of care, either TH or normothermia.

Engagement of Families and Community Affected by Hypoxic-Ischemic Encephalopathy Is Central to Cooling Prospectively Infants with Mild Encephalopathy

As a first step, we engaged the Hope for HIE foundation to advise us on study conceptualization and to create a parent survey to assess the most palatable study design and the most relevant outcomes. Foundations such as "Hope for HIE" and the "Cerebral Palsy Foundation" reach large networks of families who have been affected by asphyxia and are invested in improving outcomes in infants with HIE. These organizations with robust infrastructures (including social media) for parent engagement, knowledge translation, and dissemination are our partners for COOLPRIME. They helped us select an observational CER study design (described in the following sections) and added outcome measures and assessment time points, such as the Infant Behavior Questionnaire-Revised (IBQR) and the Impact on Family Scale-Revised at 9 to 12 months. We continue to partner, leveraging their expertise and their networks beyond design into implementation and dissemination.[7,8]

Study Design Options with Stakeholders Favored Effectiveness over Efficacy Trials

- Efficacy trials: These trials evaluate the effectiveness of an intervention under ideal and controlled conditions. They have limited inclusion criteria to minimize confounding factors resulting in a highly controlled and homogenous study population. The focus of outcomes is on well-defined, objective measures that demonstrate the intervention's safety and efficacy under controlled conditions. The aim is to establish the intervention's optimal performance under ideal circumstances. For example, the first RCT of hypothermia limited inclusion criteria to infants with an acute perinatal event and Apgar scores less than 5 at 10 minutes to minimize confounding factors, resulting in a highly controlled and homogenous study population.
- Effectiveness trials: These trials assess how well an intervention performs under real-world conditions. Broader inclusion criteria (**Fig. 1**) are used to include a broad and diverse population, resembling the real-world scenario. Outcome measures emphasize patient-oriented outcomes and real-world impact, considering factors like quality of life and parent-relevant outcomes (**Fig. 2**). The aim is to determine the intervention's practical utility and generalizability in real life.

Study Design Options with Stakeholders Favored site randomization observational design over standard randomization

- For a standard typical RCT to be deemed successful, there must be equipoise between the implementers of the intervention and its recipients or their representatives.

Observational effectiveness trials

When an RCT is inappropriate (eg, due to ethical reasons) or not feasible (eg, due to lack of equipoise, despite lack of evidence for a superior treatment), an observational study can be used to evaluate competing treatments.

As such, COOLPRIME is CER trial, with an emphasis on practical applicability and understanding how TH performs in everyday clinical settings per clinical centers' standard of care. The aim is to provide evidence-based information on the relative benefits and risks of competing treatments in the care of newborns with mild HIE: a large knowledge gap in the treatment of HIE. The focus is on understanding which intervention, TH or normothermia, works best under real-world conditions to guide health care decisions and improve outcomes for newborns.

Newborns can vary widely in terms of health status, gestational age, Sarnat score, and underlying conditions, such as infection. COOLPRIME will include propensity adjustment for those variables to guide whether an RCT is further needed in a subset of patients.

METHODS

COOLPRIME is a Patient-Centered Outcomes Research Institute–funded multicenter observational CER investigation led by a clinical coordinating center (CCC) at UT Southwestern Medical Center (UTSW), Dallas TX, USA, and a data coordinating center at the University of Pittsburgh, Pittsburgh, PA, USA. A listing of the 15 participating clinical centers, a protocol synopsis, and the trajectory of outcomes are provided in **Box 1** and **Tables 1** and **2**, respectively. Approximately half use normothermia and approximately half use hypothermia as standard of care to treat mild HIE. Data will be reported according to Strengthening the Reporting of Observational Studies in Epidemiology guidelines, as is recommended for observational trials. The ClinicalTrials.gov identifier is NCT04621279.

A

CATEGORY	SIGNS OF HIE		
	NORMAL /MILD HIE	MODERATE HIE	SEVERE HIE
1. LEVEL of CONSCIOUSNESS	1	2 = Lethargic	3 = Stupor/coma
2. SPONTANEOUS ACTIVITY	1	2 = Decreased activity	3 = No activity
3. POSTURE	1	2 = Distal flexion, complete extension	3 = Decerebrate
4. TONE	1	2a = Hypotonia	3a = Flaccid
		2b = Hypertonia	3b = Rigid
5. PRIMITIVE REFLEXES			
Suck	1	2 = Weak or has bite	3 = Absent
Moro	1	2 = Incomplete	3 = Absent
6. AUTONOMIC SYSTEM			
Pupils	1	2 = Constricted	3 = Deviation / dilated /non-reactive to light
Heart rate	1	2 = Bradycardia	3 = Variable HR
Respiration	1	2 = Periodic breathing	3 = Apnea or requires vent 3a=on vent with spont breaths 3b=on vent without spont breaths

B

	Normal = 0	Mild = 1	Moderate = 2	Severe = 3
Level of consciousness	When awake, alert, fixes on visual stimuli	Irritable, hyperalert, poor feeding, excess crying alternating with sleeping	Lethargic	Stupor or coma
Spontaneous activity	Frequent spontaneous movements	Increased and exaggerated movements, jittery	Decreased activity	No activity
Posture	Extremities flexed in toward the trunk	Mild distal or arm flexion with leg abduction or slight extension	Distal flexion, complete extension	Decerebrate
Tone	Normal	Slightly increased	Hypotonia (focal or general)	Flaccid
Primitive reflexes - Suck	Strong coordinated suck	Uncoordinated	Weak/ unsustained/ bite	Absent
- Moro	Complete (full abduction then smooth adduction)	Exaggerated	Incomplete (partial abduction at shoulder and extension of arms)	Absent
Autonomic system - Pupils	Reactive	Dilated, but reactive	Constricted, but reactive	Deviated, dilated, or nonreactive to light
- Respiration	Normal	Irregular and/or tachypneic	Periodic breathing	Apnea or on mechanical ventilation

Fig. 1. (*A*) Modified Sarnat from 2005 to 2015. Notice absent scoring for mild, which was categorized with normal in the screening forms of prior trials. (*B*) COOLPRIME Sarnat. COOLPRIME, cooling prospectively infants with mild encephalopathy; HIE, hypoxic-ischemic encephalopathy; HR, hazard ratio.

Screening Process and Procedures

Subjects will be recruited over 2 years across centers from the delivery room, well-infant nursery, intermediate nursery, or neonatal intensive care unit (NICU) of each participating clinical center. Recruitment can also begin at the time of a request for

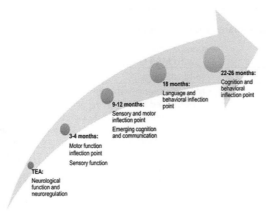

Fig. 2. Cooling Prospectively Infants with Mild Encephalopathy (COOLPRIME) trajectory of outcomes are highlighted to provide a correct classification and facilitate early referrals. School-age outcomes are being planned on follow-up studies.

transport to one of the participating centers. Potential participants will be identified and referred to by the attending neonatologist caring for the infant or in collaboration with the attending neonatologist. Parents or legal guardians of infants meeting eligibility criteria will be approached for consent within 24 hours if the treating neonatologist approves.

Box 1
Cooling prospectively infants with mild encephalopathy sites

Clinical coordinating center
  Principal investigator: Lina F. Chalak
  UT Southwestern Medical Center,
  Dallas, TX

Data coordinating center
  Principal investigator: Stephen Wisniewski
  University of Pittsburgh,
  Pittsburgh, PA

Clinical site
  1. UT Southwestern Medical Center, Dallas, TX
  2. Nationwide Children's Hospital, Columbus, OH
  3. University of California-San Francisco, San Francisco, CA
  4. Children's National Medical Center, Washington, DC
  5. Children's Hospital Los Angeles, Los Angeles, CA
  6. Washington University, St. Louis, MO
  7. Saint Louis University, St. Louis, MO
  8. Seattle Children's, Seattle, WA
  9. Stanford University, Palo Alto, CA
  10. Children's Hospital of Philadelphia, Philadelphia, PA
  11. University of Utah, Salt Lake City, UT
  12. University of Cork, Cork, Ireland
  13. Cincinnati Children's Hospital Medical Center, Cincinnati, OH
  14. Emory University, Atlanta, GA

Table 1 Cooling prospectively infants with mild encephalopathy protocol synopsis	
Title of the Study	Comparative Effectiveness for Cooling Prospectively Infants with Mild Encephalopathy
Indication	Mild HIE
Subject population	Mild HIE identified in the first 6 h of life according to the published PRIME (Prospective Research in Infants With Mild Encephalopathy) study definition: newborn with evidence of encephalopathy (using the validated Sarnat examination) *not* meeting prior cooling trials criteria.
Objectives	1. To compare the effectiveness of TH vs NT in infants with mild HIE at 2 y. 2. To determine the risk of TH vs NT in mild HIE on infant safety composite outcome at discharge. 3. To determine the effect of TH on parental measures of stress and bonding at 3–4 mo of life in infants with mild HIE.
Design	A pragmatic observational CER design based on site predetermined existing practice to assess effectiveness and safety in an unstudied population will bypass the problem of the current loss of equipoise and unwillingness to randomize by physicians.
Comparators	NT, TH
Sample size	326 (163 per group) neonates are needed to have an 80% power of effect sizes (difference of means) of 0.3, accounting for correlation between cognition and language. We have artificially inflated the total sample size to 430 to account for 25% attrition, to ensure that follow-up studies will be adequately powered. Approximately 29 patients will be enrolled at each site across all 15 centers.
Duration	There is 5 y of funding, of which approximately 3 y will be needed to complete enrollment and 2 y will be needed to complete the follow-up for this study. The study will conclude when all enrolled subjects reach 24 - months. Following that, approximately 1 year will likely be required to conduct data management and analysis.
Study centers	15 pediatric hospitals: 7 sites routinely practice TH as standard of care in all mild HIE cases and 8 sites practice NT.
ClinicalTrials.gov Identifier	NCT04621279

Abbreviations: CER, comparative effectiveness research; HIE, hypoxic-ischemic encephalopathy; NT, normothermia; TH, therapeutic hypothermia.

Eligibility Criteria

To be eligible to enroll, an infant must be born ≥35 0/7 weeks of gestation with a weight ≥1800 g, have fetal acidosis and/or an acute perinatal event, and have mild encephalopathy per a COOLPRIME modified Sarnat examination (described in the following sections) within 6 hours of birth, defined as presence of at least 2 signs of mild, moderate, or severe encephalopathy and no more than 2 moderate to severe abnormalities. For COOLPRIME, heart rate was not included in the Sarnat score description of autonomic instability due to concerns of bradycardia, normally listed as a rare sign of HIE, as it is impacted by the hypothermia effect at centers that cool.

Exclusion criteria include infants having a head circumference less than 30 cm, congenital or chromosomal anomalies associated with abnormal neurodevelopment

Table 2
Neurodevelopmental assessments by time point

	Baseline	Hospital Discharge	3–4 mo	9–12 mo	22–26 mo
Study admission vitals and laboratory values	X				
Maternal history	X				
Modified Sarnat examination		X			
Hospital discharge examination		X			
Hammersmith Neonatal Neurologic Examination (HNNE)		X			
Hammersmith Infant Neurologic Examination (HINE)			X		X
Mother-to Infant Bonding Scale (MIBS)		X			
Parenting Stress Index (PSI)		X			
Infant Behavior Questionnaire-Revised (IBQ-R)			X	X	
Impact on Family Scale-Revised (IFS-R)				X	
Bayley Scales of Infant Development IV (Bayley IV)					X
Parent Report of Children's Abilities–Revised (PARCA-R)					X
Child Behavior Checklist (CBCL-Preschool)					X

From time of consent through 22-26 months.

or death, a seizure within the first 6 hours of life, the infant being in foster care, or redirection of the infant's care being considered. Sarnat examinations are performed within 6 hours and scored by trained examiners, and these are video recorded for fidelity evaluation by a neurodevelopmental core.

Treatments

Both treatments must be initiated within 6 hours of birth and carried out for 72 hours, with temperature recorded every 4 hours to ensure the target treatment is achieved.

Normothermia treatment
The normothermia sites will maintain the infant's core temperature at 37.0°C by servo-control of skin temperature and adjustment of the set point based on skin temperature per sites clinical care standard of care practice. A temperature range of 36.5° to 37.5°C is acceptable. If temperature exceeds 37.5°C, steps are taken to prevent hyperthermia and potentially associated adverse effects. For temperatures greater than 37.5°C, active cooling (ie, TH) will be implemented until target temperature range is attained. If the infant progresses to have seizures between 6 and 24 hours, inclusive, cross over to TH treatment is allowed per a published late TH National Institutes of Health trial.[9,10]

Hypothermia treatment
The hypothermia sites will implement whole-body cooling to maintain a core esophageal temperature of 33.5°C by placing infants on a cooling blanket for 72 hours per sites clinical standard of care practice. Temperature will be measured via an esophageal probe placed in the lower third of the esophagus and adjustments are performed based

on published protocols if out of range.[10] At the end of the 72 hours of induced hypothermia, the servo set point is adjusted by an increase of 0.5°C per hour until a temperature of 36.5° is reached.[11]

Neurocognitive Outcomes

Neurodevelopment is a complex continuum and trajectories can change with experience and environmental factors, where infants can develop new functionality.[12,13] A comprehensive and sensitive neurocognitive profile is performed in COOLPRIME to reflect the impact of even mild HIE, which has a subtler outcome than moderate to severe HIE.

Bayley testing at 2 years represents the gold standard and will serve as the primary outcome as it allows comparison with prior hypothermia trials.[9,14] Assessments with a battery of secondary outcomes are also performed just prior to hospital discharge, and at 3 follow-up time points: when the infant is 3 to 4 months, 9 to 12 months, and 22 to 26 months of age. Infants return for an in-clinic follow-up visit at 3 to 4 months and 22 to 26 months, whereas the 9 to 12 month assessment is done remotely via phone or email contact, followed by parent completion of online surveys (ie, the consented parent is emailed or texted a secure survey link that allow them to complete the surveys in their Web browser). See **Table 2** for a listing of all assessments by time point, including the Mother-to-Infant Bonding Scale (MIBS), which was selected by the parents advisory committee to be completed past discharge at 3 to 4 months. Descriptions of each measure follows.

The Hammersmith Neonatal Neurological Examination and the Hammersmith Infant Neurologic Examination: These examinations are standardized reliable and reproducible[15] with measures of tone, motor patterns, observation of movements, reflexes, and visual and auditory attention.[16,17] The examinations have well-studied optimality scores allowing for assessment from birth to 2 years.[18,19]

The *MIBS* is a validated questionnaire with good psychometric properties that assesses the mother's feelings toward the infant (bonding) from birth to 4 months. [20]

The *IBQR* has excellent psychometric properties to measure differences in reactivity and regulation, and the structure of infant temperament and its relation to parental family functioning. [21]

The *Parenting Stress Index, Fourth Edition, Short Form (PSI-4-SF)* is an abbreviated version of the full-length test with 36 items in 3 domains (parental distress, parent-child dysfunctional interaction, and difficult child) that combine to form a Total Stress Scale, which helps identify families that are most in need of support services. Empirical validity has been established and higher scores indicate stress and dyadic dysfunction.[22,23]

The *Child Behavior Checklist*-(parent report) provides a profile of a child's behavior and social functioning in relation to the child's age and gender and in particular internalizing and externalizing tendencies associated with major psychological diagnoses into adolescence.[24]

Secondary Cooling Prospectively Infants with Mild Encephalopathy Studies

At sites where brain monitoring via electroencephalography (EEG) is possible, we recommend EEG monitoring to start as soon as possible after NICU admission for a minimum of 24 hours and up to 96 hours after birth if the infant receives TH. At sites where brain MRI and magnetic resonance spectroscopy (MRS) is standard of care practice, we recommend images be obtained on study days 4 to 5; acceptable range is day 4 to 6 of life to accommodate for holidays. Participating sites send EEG, MRI, and MRS files via a secure electronic data transfer to the CCC (UTSW) for data storage until predetermined secondary studies can be performed. Additionally, after obtaining further funding, we plan to extend follow-up of COOLPRIME to continue our assessment of the neurodevelopmental trajectory. Preschool and school-age follow-up is of interest to all surveyed parents and allows for the assessment of subtle insults which may not be detected until later in life.[25,26]

Sample Size

The study is powered to test the primary aim of comparing the multivariate cognitive and language Bayley-IV scales at 2 years in the 2 treatment groups. We conservatively powered for an effect size of 0.3 (5 points) based on parental surveys feedback that identified 5% improvement as an impactful effect. To achieve 80% power, a sample size of 326 (163 per group) is needed to detect effect sizes (difference of means) of 0.3, accounting for correlation between cognition and language. To ensure adequate power, we inflated the enrollment sample size to 430 to allow for 25% attrition across school-age later follow-up.

Analysis Approach

The analysis will be conducted per intention to treat (per the site's known standard of care for mild HIE treatment). For the primary analysis in aim 1, a 2x1 vector will represent scores across the 2 domains (cognition, language) (Bayley and Parent Report of Children's Abilities-Revised) that are most affected in mild HIE. The rationale for selecting this outcome vector is to avoid averaging of scores and to provide more efficient testing compared to testing each score separately and using Bonferroni correction to adjust for multiplicity. A propensity-adjusted analysis will control for potential confounders.[27] We will include variables measured prior to 6 hours after birth, including risk factors including maternal health and representing total severity of illness, socioeconomic measures, and demographics including sex and race. Site will be included in the model as a fixed effect. A generalized boosted mixed-effects regression model (GBM) will generate a propensity score for each participant. Variables in the GBM will include demographic characteristics, clinical characteristics, and site. From this approach, a propensity score, indicating the probability of having a specific intervention (TH) given the observed characteristics, will be obtained for each subject in COOLPRIME. A multivariate analysis of variance (MANOVA) will then be used to estimate the independent effect of hypothermia on the 2x1 vector of Bayley-IV scores at 2 years. The MANOVA model will include the 2x1 vector of Bayley-IV scores as the dependent variables and an indicator of hypothermia as the independent variable, with the propensity scores used as an inverse probability weight.

SUMMARY

COOLPRIME's observational CER design, rigor, and trajectory of outcomes will allow us to move past the conundrum of care in mild HIE and address the effectiveness of hypothermia for mild HIE, filling an important knowledge gap. The impact will likely be substantial as injury in early life has effects on individual life span and overall quality of life, in addition to large societal impacts. If the results show effectiveness and safety of hypothermia for mild HIE, then dissemination and adoption of TH by non-cooling sites will result in improved outcomes. If no added benefit is detected, then inappropriate cooling will stop and unnecessary separation of parents and infants will be prevented. If propensity shows a possibility of benefit in a subgroup at risk, then the effect size will be determined for future trials. The relevance to public health in mild HIE, a currently understudied population of children, is direct and immediate: comparing widespread clinical practices for mild asphyxia will result in widespread adoption of evidence-based practices, and improve child outcomes in ways that matter to parents.

Best Practices

What is the current practice for mild HIE?

- Normothermia and TH for mild HIE are both currently accepted practices in standardized tertiary care, neonatal intensive care settings.

Best practice/guideline/care path objective(s):

- A prospective comparative effectiveness cohort investigation emulating a clinical pragmatic trial is the solution to compare benefit and risks of these 2 accepted practices.

What changes in current practice are likely to improve outcomes?

- Standardized adoption of TH if superior or normothermia if TH is not shown to be superior.

Is there a clinical algorithm?

- TH is the Standard of care treatment for moderate and severe HIE.
- Avoidance of hyperthermia is recommended following HIE.

Major recommendations:

- A standardized protocol with neuroimaging and neurodevelopmental follow-up is essential when providing care for any infant with HIE, including mild HIE.
- Universal follow-up of infants with mild HIE into school age for early detection of and intervention for neurodevelopmental impairments.

Bibliographic source(s):

- Chalak L. New Horizons in Mild Hypoxic-ischemic Encephalopathy: A Standardized Algorithm to Move past Conundrum of Care. Clin Perinatol. 2022;49(1):279-94.

DISCLOSURE

The authors have no conflicts to disclose.

FUNDING

This work was supported through a Patient-Centered Outcomes Research Institute (PCORI) Program Award (CER-2021C3-24763).

REFERENCES

1. Chalak L. New horizons in mild hypoxic-ischemic encephalopathy: a standardized algorithm to move past conundrum of care. Clin Perinatol 2022;49(1):279–94.
2. Bryce J, Boschi-Pinto C, Shibuya K, et al, WHO Child Health Epidemiology Reference Group. WHO estimates of the causes of death in children. Lancet 2005; 365(9465):1147–52.
3. Mani SLC, Thayyil S, Mehta S, et al, editors. International survey on current practices of therapeutic hypothermia in neonates with mild hypoxic-ischaemic encephalopathy. PAS 2021. Pediatric Academic Societies (PAS); 2021.

4. Chawla S, Bates SV, Shankaran S. Is it time for a randomized controlled trial of hypothermia for mild hypoxic-ischemic encephalopathy? J Pediatr 2020;220: 241–4.

5. Tagin MA, Gunn AJ. Neonatal encephalopathy and potential lost opportunities: when the story fits, please cool. Arch Dis Child Fetal Neonatal Ed 2021;106(5): 458–9.

6. Glass HC, Soul JS, Chang T, et al. Safety of early discontinuation of antiseizure medication after acute symptomatic neonatal seizures. JAMA Neurol 2021;78(7): 817–25.

7. Chalak L, Pilon B, Byrne R, et al. Stakeholder engagement in neonatal clinical trials: an opportunity for mild neonatal encephalopathy research. Pediatr Res 2022; 93(1):4–6.

8. Pappas A, Milano G, Chalak LF. Hypoxic-ischemic encephalopathy: changing outcomes across the spectrum. Clin Perinatol 2023;50(1):31–52.

9. Laptook AR, Shankaran S, Tyson JE, et al, Eunice Kennedy Shriver National Institute of Child Health and Human Development Neonatal Research Network. Effect of therapeutic hypothermia initiated after 6 hours of age on death or disability among newborns with hypoxic-ischemic encephalopathy: a randomized clinical trial. JAMA 2017;318(16):1550–60.

10. Shankaran S, Laptook AR, Pappas A, et al, Eunice Kennedy Shriver National Institute of Child Health and Human Development Neonatal Research Network. Effect of depth and duration of cooling on deaths in the NICU among neonates with hypoxic ischemic encephalopathy: a randomized clinical trial. JAMA 2014; 312(24):2629–39.

11. Chalak LF, Pappas A, Tan S, et al, Eunice Kennedy Shriver National Institute of Child Health and Human Development Neonatal Research Network. Association between increased seizures during rewarming after hypothermia for neonatal hypoxic ischemic encephalopathy and abnormal neurodevelopmental outcomes at 2-year follow-up: a nested multisite cohort study. JAMA Neurol 2021;78(12): 1484–93.

12. Maitre NL. Neurorehabilitation after neonatal intensive care: evidence and challenges. Arch Dis Child Fetal Neonatal Ed 2015;100(6):F534–40.

13. Benninger KL, Inder TE, Goodman AM, et al. Perspectives from the society for pediatric research. neonatal encephalopathy clinical trials: developing the future. Pediatr Res 2020;89(1):74–84.

14. Shankaran S, Laptook AR, Pappas A, et al, Eunice Kennedy Shriver National Institute of Child Health and Human Development Neonatal Research Network. Effect of depth and duration of cooling on death or disability at age 18 months among neonates with hypoxic-ischemic encephalopathy: a randomized clinical trial. JAMA 2017;318(1):57–67.

15. Dubowitz L, Mercuri E, Dubowitz V. An optimality score for the neurologic examination of the term newborn. J Pediatr 1998;133(3):406–16.

16. Novak I, Morgan C, Adde L, et al. Early, accurate diagnosis and early intervention in cerebral palsy: advances in diagnosis and treatment. JAMA Pediatr 2017; 171(9):897–907.

17. Romeo DM, Bompard S, Cocca C, et al. Neonatal neurological examination during the first 6h after birth. Early Hum Dev 2017;108:41–4.

18. Ricci D, Romeo DM, Haataja L, et al. Neurological examination of preterm infants at term equivalent age. Early Hum Dev 2008;84(11):751–61.

19. Ricci D, Romeo DM, Serrao F, et al. Application of a neonatal assessment of visual function in a population of low risk full-term newborn. Early Hum Dev 2008;84(4): 277–80.

20. Taylor A, Atkins R, Kumar R, et al. A new mother-to-infant bonding scale: links with early maternal mood. Arch Womens Ment Health 2005;8(1):45–51.

21. Eeles AL, Anderson PJ, Brown NC, et al. Sensory profiles obtained from parental reports correlate with independent assessments of development in very preterm children at 2 years of age. Early Hum Dev 2013;89(12):1075–80.

22. Spittle AJ, Spencer-Smith MM, Eeles AL, et al. Does the Bayley-III Motor Scale at 2 years predict motor outcome at 4 years in very preterm children? Dev Med Child Neurol 2013;55(5):448–52.

23. Eeles AL, Spittle AJ, Anderson PJ, et al. Assessments of sensory processing in infants: a systematic review. Dev Med Child Neurol 2013;55(4):314–26.

24. Benninger KL, Inder TE, Goodman AM, et al. Perspectives from the Society for Pediatric Research. Neonatal encephalopathy clinical trials: developing the future. Pediatr Res 2021;89(1):74–84.

25. Murray DM, O'Connor CM, Ryan CA, et al. Early EEG grade and outcome at 5 years after mild neonatal hypoxic ischemic encephalopathy. Pediatrics 2016; 138(4). e20160659.

26. Chalak L, Latremouille S, Mir I, et al. A review of the conundrum of mild hypoxic-ischemic encephalopathy: current challenges and moving forward. Early Hum Dev 2018;120:88–94.

27. McCaffrey DF, Ridgeway G, Morral AR. Propensity score estimation with boosted regression for evaluating causal effects in observational studies. Psychol Methods 2004;9(4):403–25.

Key Inflammatory Biomarkers in Perinatal Asphyxia: A Comprehensive Review

Lynn Bitar, MD, MSc[a], Barbara S. Stonestreet, MD[b,c],
Lina F. Chalak, MD, MSCS[a,*]

KEYWORDS

- Hypoxic-ischemic encephalopathy • Therapeutic hypothermia • Perinatal asphyxia
- Biomarkers

KEY POINTS

- Hypoxic-ischemia encephalopathy (HIE) remains a significant cause of neonatal death and disability.
- The role of inflammatory mediators in HIE to prognosticate outcomes is not well-defined.
- Current biomarkers are panels used for research purposes. In the early critical stages of perinatal asphyxia, inflammatory biomarkers may guide clinical decision-making.
- Additional research is required to increase our understanding of the optimal utility of biomarkers to predict the severity, evolution, and developmental outcomes after exposure to HIE.

INTRODUCTION

Perinatal asphyxia resulting in hypoxic–ischemic (HI) brain injury is one of the most common causes of neonatal morbidity and mortality, with nearly 1 million neonatal deaths per year.[1,2] The primary insult is insufficient blood flow, that results in an inadequate supply of oxygen and nutrients necessary to sustain the high-energy metabolic demands of the brain.[3] Reperfusion injury subsequently triggers a cascade of inflammatory mediators, elevating levels of circulating cytokines and chemokines.[4] The following response is associated with epilepsy, cerebral palsy, cognitive impairment, as well as motor and sensory impairment.[5,6]

---

[a] Division of Neonatal-Perinatal Medicine, Department of Pediatrics, University of Texas Southwestern Medical Center, Dallas, TX 75235, USA; [b] Department of Pediatrics, Women & Infants Hospital of Rhode Island; [c] The Alpert Medical School of Brown University, Barrington, RI 02806, USA
* Corresponding author. Buchanan Endowed Chair Professor of Pediatrics and Psychiatry, Division Chief of Neonatal-Perinatal Medicine, Director, Neurological Neonatal Intensive Care Fetal and Neonatal Neurology Fellowship Program, UT Southwestern Medical Center, 5323 Harry Hines Boulevard, Dallas, TX 75390.
E-mail address: lina.chalak@utsouthwestern.edu

Clin Perinatol 51 (2024) 617–628
https://doi.org/10.1016/j.clp.2024.04.004
0095-5108/24/© 2024 Elsevier Inc. All rights reserved.

Therapeutic hypothermia (TH) initiated within the first 6 hours after birth is the current standard of care to treat moderate and severe cases of Hypoxic-Ischemic Encephalopathy (HIE). TH has been shown to attenuate the evolution of cerebral inflammation and improve neurodevelopmental outcomes.[7,8] Although novel anti-inflammatory treatment modalities are currently under investigation, the treatment paradigm for HIE remains the same.[9] In addition to their role in the diagnosis of HIE, inflammatory biomarkers have also been investigated as potential therapeutic targets.[3,9–14]

In this comprehensive article, the authors focus on inflammatory biomarkers: both placental (cord blood) and postnatal blood biomarkers associated with injury to the brain. The authors' aim was to clarify (1) the diagnostic accuracy along the spectrum of HIE, (2) utility in assessing treatment responses, and (3) ability to predict short- and long-term neurodevelopmental outcomes. This work will complement the current efforts in understanding and interpreting inflammatory biomarkers in the early stages of perinatal asphyxia.

PATHOPHYSIOLOGY OF INFLAMMATION IN PERINATAL ASPHYXIA AND ROLE OF BIOMARKERS

In the context of perinatal asphyxia, HIE primarily results from impaired oxygen delivery to the brain parenchyma. This can arise from reduced oxygen-carrying capacity because of the hypoxic component, or from diminished cerebral blood flow because of hemodynamic changes or volume loss.[9] Preclinical experimental models of perinatal injury have demonstrated microglial activation in brain tissue after HI insults.[15] This initiates and contributes to the inflammatory cascade typically seen in HIE.

After the initial injury, cellular energy production is disrupted because of impaired membrane transport, reduced ATP production, and systemic acidosis. Membrane depolarization facilitates calcium entry and activates N-methyl-D-asperate receptors, as well as other excitotoxic neurotransmitters.[9] These processes trigger inflammatory cascades, which generate local and systemic cytokine release that recruit white blood cells to the site of central nervous system injury. The quantity of secondary injury is often influenced by the severity of the immune response,[16] predisposing to cytotoxic edema, excitotoxicity, activation of apoptotic pathways, and ultimately neuronal death.[12,17] Proinflammatory cytokines,[18–20] excitotoxins,[21,22] and reactive oxygen species[23] are considered key contributors to the brain damage resulting from neuroinflammatory processes. Nevertheless, the mechanisms underlying neuroinflammation are not yet completely elucidated.[4,24]

The diagnosis of perinatal asphyxia relies mainly on clinical examination and laboratory findings, within the initial hours after birth, when the critical decision to treat with TH needs to be considered.[25] Imaging plays a crucial role that complements clinical history, physical examination, and neurologic assessment to evaluate the extent of brain damage resulting from asphyxia. Although amplitude electroencephalogram serves as an effective physiologic indicator of neuronal integrity, its predictive value is somewhat reduced during hypothermia.[26,27] Brain MRI has been proposed as the most optimal short-term predictor of early childhood outcomes, despite the challenges with its implementation[28–31] yet MRI has increased sensitivity after the first week of life.[14]

There is a crucial need to identify reliable biomarkers to enable early detection of asphyxia because of the importance of the early diagnosis of brain injury to guide clinical therapy.[13] Biomarkers could contribute information to determine further diagnostic imaging and therapeutic interventions in order to stratify the severity of brain injury. Although neonates with moderate to severe encephalopathy usually require TH to improve outcomes, those with mild encephalopathy may not benefit from TH.[14,32]

INFLAMMATORY BIOMARKERS

Cascades of complex molecular and cellular events are initiated as a result of HI injury to the neonatal brain. Accordingly, it has been suggested that neonatal (cord blood) and postnatal blood biomarkers may identify the presence and severity of HIE. A biomarker driven approach summarized in **Fig. 1** potentially facilitates the timely diagnosis and appropriate interventions.

Placental (Cord Blood) Biomarkers

Cytokines

Cytokine levels in cord blood have been extensively investigated in neonates with HIE to facilitate the timely diagnosis and consequent treatment. Several studies have demonstrated elevated levels of IL-6 and IL-16 in newborns with HIE compared with healthy controls.[33–35] Notably, higher cytokine concentrations were also predictive of the severity of HIE; the most significant elevations were observed in infants with severe HIE.[36] Thus, cord blood measurement of IL-6 and IL-16 may identify neonates at risk of significant morbidity and mortality.[37] Additionally, several other cytokines have been associated with the inflammatory cascade resulting from HI injury to the brain. Bharathi and colleagues reported increased concentrations of TNFα and IL-1β in perinatal asphyxia compared with weight and gender matched healthy neonates.[38]

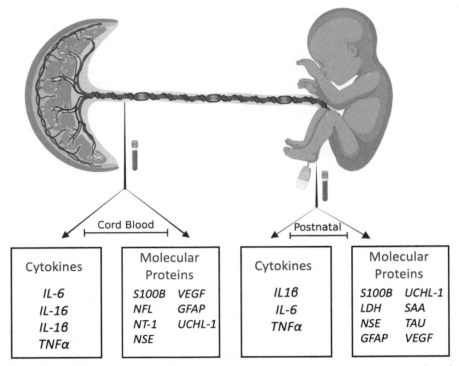

Fig. 1. Placental and postnatal biomarkers in perinatal asphyxia. (Figure created with BioRender.com.)

Molecular proteins

Molecular proteins have also been studied in HIE, in addition to inflammatory cyto-kines. Several studies in neonates exposed to perinatal asphyxia have reported elevated cord blood levels of S100 B, which is a protein with trophic functions in the development of the nervous system.[39–42] Elevations in S100 B drives the activation of nitric oxide (NO) synthase, resulting in excessive production of NO and, consequent death of astrocytes.[43] It is a marker of blood-brain barrier dysfunction and can demonstrate brain damage, but it is not sufficient alone to predict perinatal asphyxia outcomes.[44] This offers a potential rationale for some of the neurotoxicity in cases of HIE.

Neurofilament light chain protein (NFL) serves as an additional biomarker of neuronal injury resulting from perinatal asphyxia.[45] However, NFL levels in contrast to S100 B levels, have not been shown to correlate with the severity of encephalopathy, because the NFL levels were equally high in neonates with and without HIE. Hence, NFL alone may have a role in the diagnosis of asphyxia but cannot quantify the severity of HIE. Consequently, it may not be sufficiently discriminative to determine eligibility for TH in cases of HIE.[36]

In addition, cord blood Netrin-1 (NT-1) and neuron-specific enolase (NSE) were elevated in neonates with HIE compared with healthy controls.[46] Hence, there could be a potential association between NT-1 and NSE levels and neurotoxicity. Consequently, a panel of these biomarkers could potentially more accurately diagnose and stratify the severity of HIE. However, additional research is required to determine the utility of simultaneous measurements of multiple biomarkers to determine the presence and severity of HIE.

Vascular endothelial growth factor (VEGF) and Glial fibrillary acidic protein (GFAP) also exhibit increased levels in neonates with asphyxia, particularly infants who subsequently develop HIE. In addition, higher concentrations of GFAP were detected in infants with severe brain injury (HIE) compared with those with mild injury.[47,48] However, Looney and colleagues and Ennen and colleagues did not identify significant differences in GFAP levels between neonates with HIE and healthy controls.[49,50] Given the variability in the findings regarding GFAP levels in cord blood between different studies, further investigation is warranted.

Similarly, C-terminal hydrolase L1 (UCHL-1) is another molecular protein that is still being investigated. Given its well-established role as a marker for neuronal cells, it has been studied in neonates with HIE to assess brain injury. In a study by Chalak and colleagues, neonates with HIE exhibit higher levels of UCHL-1 levels in cord blood compared with healthy controls. However, there were no distinctions between mild, moderate, and severe HIE groups.[47] Conversely, when evaluating infants with neonatal encephalopathy, Massaro and colleagues found higher cord blood levels of UCHL-1 in those who experienced adverse outcomes, compared with those with more favorable outcomes.[51] Hence, the prognostic role of serum UCHL-1 remains to be determined.[3] All of these placental biomarkers are summarized below in **Table 1**.

Biomarkers Determined in Postnatal Blood Samples

Cytokines

Several potential biomarkers of perinatal asphyxia have been investigated in the blood of neonates during the postnatal period. Studies on serum cytokine levels in newborns with HIE suggested significant increases in IL1β, IL6, and TNFα mRNA levels compared with healthy neonates.[52] Oxygen deprivation triggers the activation of glial cells and the release of inflammatory mediators during an HI insult, ultimately resulting in neuronal death. For instance, adverse neurologic outcomes after HI have been positively correlated with increases in TNF-α levels. TH has been shown to be associated

Table 1
Cord blood biomarkers in perinatal asphyxia

Biomarker	Type	Studies	Origin	Key Findings
IL-6 IL-16	Cytokines	Yoon et al,[37] 1995 Chiesa et al,[33] 2003 Walsh et al,[35] 2013 Bharathi et al,[38] 2015 Walsh et al,[35] 2013 O'Sullivan et al,[34] 2018	Cord blood	IL-6 and IL-16 may be used as diagnostic tools for HIE markers of severity
IL-1β TNFα	Cytokines	Bharathi et al,[38] 2015	Cord blood	IL-1β and TNFα may be useful in the diagnosis of perinatal asphyxia
S100 B	Molecular protein	Lam et al,[43] 2001 Gazzolo et al,[41] 2004 Qian et al,[42] 2009 Mir et al,[39] 2014	Cord blood	S100 B is elevated in perinatal asphyxia and positively correlated with neurotoxicity
NFL	Molecular protein	Toorell et al,[45] 2018 Toorell et al,[36] 2023	Cord blood	NFL could be used in the diagnosis of perinatal asphyxia
NT-1 NSE	Molecular protein	Cakir et al,[46] 2022	Cord blood	Potential association between NT-1, NSE levels, and neurotoxicity
VEGF	Molecular protein	Aly et al,[48] 2009 Chalak et al,[14] 2016	Cord blood	Elevated in perinatal asphyxia
GFAP	Molecular protein	Looney et al,[50] 2015; Chalak et al,[14] 2016 Ennen et al,[49] 2011	Cord blood	Discordant findings for the clinical significance of GFAP
UCHL-1	Molecular protein	Massaro et al,[51] 2013; Chalak et al,[14] 2016	Cord blood	Elevated in perinatal asphyxia but association with the severity of brain injury is still unknown

with reductions in serum TNF-α levels for up to 12 hours after its initiation.[53–55] Similarly, several other in vivo experimental investigations have also demonstrated a decrease in the expression of inflammatory cytokines after the initiation of hypothermia. Consequently, these observations suggest a potential role for TNF-α and related cytokines both in the diagnosis of HI and for the response to treatment.[56,57]

Molecular proteins

Elevated levels of biomarkers have been associated with brain damage in neonates within 12 hours after birth. In addition, it is important to emphasize that these biomarkers were correlated positively with the severity of asphyxia.[58] Concentrations of molecular proteins, including LDH, S100 B, NSE, GFAP, UCH-L1, and serum amyloid A have been quantified in neonates with perinatal asphyxia.[3,48,58] Chalak and colleagues[47] and Toorell and colleagues[36] reported higher levels of GFAP in neonates with moderate or severe HIE compared with those with mild HIE. Traditionally, in children requiring Extracorporeal Membrane Oxygenation, GFAP was also used as a predictor of mortality and poor neurologic outcomes.[59–61]

Table 2
Postnatal biomarkers for perinatal asphyxia

Biomarker	Type	Studies	Origin	Key Findings
IL1β IL-6	Cytokines	Xanthou et al,[52] 2002	Neonatal blood	i. Increased levels in HIE
TNFα	Cytokines	Oygür et al,[53] 1998 Fairchild et al,[56] 2000 Xanthou et al,[52] 2002 Russwurm et al,[57] 2002 Bartha et al,[55] 2004 Aly et al, 2005	Neonatal blood	ii. TNFα correlated with worse adverse outcomes and shows a decrease after TH
S100 B	Molecular protein	Liu et al,[32] 2019 Auriti et al,[4] 2020	Neonatal blood	Potential role in monitoring treatment response
LDH	Molecular protein	Douglas-Escobar et al,[3] 2015 Liu et al,[32] 2019	Neonatal blood	Positively correlated with the degree of asphyxia
NSE	Molecular protein	Celtik et al,[62] 2004 Liu et al,[32] 2019 Caramelo et al,[17] 2023	Neonatal blood	
GFAP	Molecular protein	Pelinka et al,[61] 2004 Vos et al,[59] 2004 Douglas-Escobar et al,[3] 2015 Kaneko et al,[60] 2009 Chalak et al,[47] 2014 Liu et al,[32] 2019	Neonatal blood	Diagnostic marker and predictor of brain severity and mortality
UCHL-1 SAA	Molecular protein Molecular protein	Douglas-Escobar et al,[3] 2015	Neonatal blood Neonatal blood	Positively correlated with the degree of asphyxia
TAU	Molecular protein	Toorell et al,[45] 2018	Neonatal blood	Useful marker for risk stratifying HIE neonates
VEGF	Molecular protein	Sweetman et al,[63] 2017	Neonatal blood	Potential marker for HI events

Given the therapeutic importance of accurate HIE diagnosis, Tau protein has been proposed as a useful biomarker to risk-stratify mild and moderate HIE infants. This informs clinical decision-making and guides management in the first 6 hours of life.[45]

Other potential biomarkers include serum erythropoietin, VEGF, and NSE for HI related events.[17,62,63] Another inflammatory biomarker, the S100 B protein, exhibits significantly reduced concentrations 48 hours after HI insults in neonates. This reduction is more pronounced in those treated with TH,[4] suggesting its potential role in monitoring treatment responses. All of these postnatal biomarkers are summarized below in **Table 2**.

Future promising new inflammatory biomarkers: from bench to bedside

In the last decade, Inter-alpha Inhibitor Proteins (IAIPs) have emerged as promising biomarkers in the diagnosis and management of conditions associated with systemic

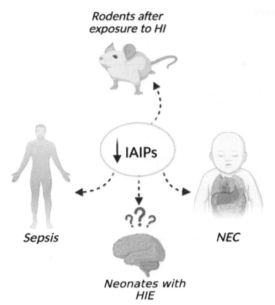

Fig. 2. Key role of IAIPs in inflammatory-related conditions. (Figure created with BioRender. com.)

inflammation. Given the known inflammatory cascade in perinatal asphyxia, IAIPs have also been evaluated in this condition.

Preclinical studies in neonatal rodents exposed to HI insults revealed a lower level of IAIPs compared with healthy controls.[64] In addition to its role as a diagnostic biomarker, Chen and colleagues have investigated its potential therapeutic implications. They evaluated the neuroprotective implications of administering IAIPs to treat neonatal rodents exposed to a HI insult. This therapeutic intervention yielded positive outcomes by reducing neuropathological brain injury and decreasing cell death.[65]

In addition to the preclinical studies, IAIPs were also investigated in neonates with conditions associated with systemic inflammation (**Fig. 2**). Among infants with neonatal sepsis, Baek and colleagues have shown decreased levels of IAIPs suggesting they may be suppressed in inflammatory conditions.[66] Similarly, the predictive value of these proteins were further evaluated in conditions such as Necrotizing Enterocolitis, providing crucial insights that may inform early detection and intervention strategies.[67] Ongoing work at our institution on cord blood levels of IAIPs in HIE has shown a reduction in IAIP levels in moderate or severe cases compared with controls.[68] This provides useful insight into the potential role of IAIPs in risk stratification of neonates with HIE.

SUMMARY

The intricate panel of inflammatory biomarkers in perinatal asphyxia reveals promising avenues for diagnostics and therapeutic strategies. Biomarkers from placental (cord blood) and postnatal blood exhibit potential sensitivity in identifying neonates at risk for perinatal asphyxia. These biomarkers provide valuable insights into neuronal injury and neurotoxicity, emphasizing their role in the inflammatory cascade. Additionally, exploring a panel of biomarkers may offer a more accurate prediction than measuring individual biomarkers alone. Despite significant progress, ongoing research is crucial to fully uncover and validate the diagnostic and prognostic potential of these biomarkers, thereby enhancing outcomes in neonatal care.

Best Practices

What is the current practice?

- Inflammatory Biomarkers are not used at the bedside for clinical decision making in HIE.

What changes in current practice are likely to improve outcomes?

- Additional research is required to increase our understanding of the optimal utility of biomarkers to predict the severity, evolution, and developmental outcomes after exposure to HIE.

Major Recommendations

- None

DISCLOSURE

The authors have nothing to disclose.

REFERENCES

1. Vannucci RC. Hypoxic-ischemic encephalopathy. Am J Perinatol 2000;17(3): 113–20.
2. Ahearne CE, Chang RY, Walsh BH, et al. Cord blood IL-16 is associated with 3-year neurodevelopmental outcomes in perinatal asphyxia and hypoxic-ischaemic encephalopathy. Dev Neurosci 2017;39(1–4):59–65.
3. Douglas-Escobar M, Weiss MD. Hypoxic-ischemic encephalopathy: a review for the clinician. JAMA Pediatr 2015;169(4):397–403.
4. Auriti C, Prencipe G, Inglese R, et al. Mannose binding lectin, S100 B protein, and brain injuries in neonates with perinatal asphyxia. Front Pediatr 2020;8:527.
5. Shankaran S, Pappas A, McDonald SA, et al. Childhood outcomes after hypothermia for neonatal encephalopathy. N Engl J Med 2012;366(22):2085–92.
6. Hill A, Volpe JJ. Perinatal asphyxia: clinical aspects. Clin Perinatol 1989;16(2): 435–57.
7. Azzopardi D, Strohm B, Marlow N, et al. Effects of hypothermia for perinatal asphyxia on childhood outcomes. N Engl J Med 2014;371(2):140–9.
8. Jacobs SE, Berg M, Hunt R, et al. Cooling for newborns with hypoxic ischaemic encephalopathy. Cochrane Database Syst Rev 2013;2013(1):CD003311.
9. Nair J, Kumar VHS. Current and emerging therapies in the management of hypoxic ischemic encephalopathy in neonates. Children (Basel) 2018;5(7):99.
10. Juul SE, Voldal E, Comstock BA, et al. Association of high-dose erythropoietin with circulating biomarkers and neurodevelopmental outcomes among neonates with hypoxic ischemic encephalopathy: a secondary analysis of the heal randomized clinical trial. JAMA Netw Open 2023;6(7):e2322131.
11. Rasineni GK, Panigrahy N, Rath SN, et al. Diagnostic and therapeutic roles of the "omics" in hypoxic-ischemic encephalopathy in neonates. Bioengineering (Basel) 2022;9(10):498.
12. Gunn AJ, Laptook AR, Robertson NJ, et al. Therapeutic hypothermia translates from ancient history in to practice. Pediatr Res 2017;81(1–2):202–9.

13. Cascant-Vilaplana MM, Sánchez-Illana Á, Piñeiro-Ramos JD, et al. Do levels of lipid peroxidation biomarkers reflect the degree of brain injury in newborns? Antioxid Redox Signal 2021;35(17):1467–75.
14. Chalak LF. Inflammatory biomarkers of birth asphyxia. Clin Perinatol 2016;43(3): 501–10.
15. Volpe JJ. Neurology of the newborn. Major Probl Clin Pediatr 1981;22:1–648.
16. Chen Y, Hallenbeck JM, Ruetzler C, et al. Overexpression of monocyte chemoattractant protein 1 in the brain exacerbates ischemic brain injury and is associated with recruitment of inflammatory cells. J Cerebr Blood Flow Metabol 2003;23(6): 748–55.
17. Caramelo I, Coelho M, Rosado M, et al. Biomarkers of hypoxic-ischemic encephalopathy: a systematic review. World J Pediatr 2023;19(6):505–48.
18. Bona E, Andersson AL, Blomgren K, et al. Chemokine and inflammatory cell response to hypoxia-ischemia in immature rats. Pediatr Res 1999;45(4 Pt 1): 500–9.
19. Martin D, Chinookoswong N, Miller G. The interleukin-1 receptor antagonist (rhIL-1ra) protects against cerebral infarction in a rat model of hypoxia-ischemia. Exp Neurol 1994;130(2):362–7.
20. Hedtjärn M, Leverin AL, Eriksson K, et al. Interleukin-18 involvement in hypoxic-ischemic brain injury. J Neurosci 2002;22(14):5910–9.
21. Heyes MP, Saito K, Major EO, et al. A mechanism of quinolinic acid formation by brain in inflammatory neurological disease. Attenuation of synthesis from L-tryptophan by 6-chlorotryptophan and 4-chloro-3-hydroxyanthranilate. Brain 1993; 116(Pt 6):1425–50.
22. Guillemin GJ, Smythe G, Takikawa O, et al. Expression of indoleamine 2,3-dioxygenase and production of quinolinic acid by human microglia, astrocytes, and neurons. Glia 2005;49(1):15–23.
23. Sankarapandi S, Zweier JL, Mukherjee G, et al. Measurement and characterization of superoxide generation in microglial cells: evidence for an NADPH oxidase-dependent pathway. Arch Biochem Biophys 1998;353(2):312–21.
24. Sävman K, Heyes MP, Svedin P, et al. Microglia/macrophage-derived inflammatory mediators galectin-3 and quinolinic acid are elevated in cerebrospinal fluid from newborn infants after birth asphyxia. Transl Stroke Res 2013;4(2):228–35.
25. Davidson JO, Wassink G, van den Heuij LG, et al. Therapeutic hypothermia for neonatal hypoxic–ischemic encephalopathy – where to from here? Front Neurol 2015;6. Available at: https://www.frontiersin.org/articles/10.3389/fneur.2015. 00198. [Accessed 16 January 2024].
26. McAdams RM, Juul SE. The role of cytokines and inflammatory cells in perinatal brain injury. Neurol Res Int 2012;2012:561494.
27. Thoresen M. Hypothermia after perinatal asphyxia: selection for treatment and cooling protocol. J Pediatr 2011;158(2 Suppl):e45–9.
28. Rutherford M, Srinivasan L, Dyet L, et al. Magnetic resonance imaging in perinatal brain injury: clinical presentation, lesions and outcome. Pediatr Radiol 2006;36(7):582–92.
29. Rutherford M, Ramenghi LA, Edwards AD, et al. Assessment of brain tissue injury after moderate hypothermia in neonates with hypoxic-ischaemic encephalopathy: a nested substudy of a randomised controlled trial. Lancet Neurol 2010; 9(1):39–45.
30. Thayyil S, Chandrasekaran M, Taylor A, et al. Cerebral magnetic resonance biomarkers in neonatal encephalopathy: a meta-analysis. Pediatrics 2010;125(2): e382–95.

31. Barkovich AJ, Hajnal BL, Vigneron D, et al. Prediction of neuromotor outcome in perinatal asphyxia: evaluation of MR scoring systems. AJNR Am J Neuroradiol 1998;19(1):143–9.

32. Liu R, Liu Q, He Y, et al. Association between Helicobacter pylori infection and nonalcoholic fatty liver: a meta-analysis. Medicine (Baltimore) 2019;98(44): e17781.

33. Chiesa C, Pellegrini G, Panero A, et al. Umbilical cord interleukin-6 levels are elevated in term neonates with perinatal asphyxia. Eur J Clin Invest 2003;33(4): 352–8.

34. O'Sullivan MP, Sikora KM, Ahearne C, et al. Validation of raised cord blood interleukin-16 in perinatal asphyxia and neonatal hypoxic-ischaemic encephalopathy in the BiHiVE2 cohort. Dev Neurosci 2018;40(3):271–7.

35. Walsh BH, Boylan GB, Livingstone V, et al. Cord blood proteins and multichannel-electroencephalography in hypoxic-ischemic encephalopathy. Pediatr Crit Care Med 2013;14(6):621–30.

36. Toorell H, Carlsson Y, Hallberg B, et al. Neuro-specific and immuno-inflammatory biomarkers in umbilical cord blood in neonatal hypoxic-ischemic encephalopathy. Neonatology 2023;1–9. https://doi.org/10.1159/000533473.

37. Yoon BH, Romero R, Kim CJ, et al. Amniotic fluid interleukin-6: a sensitive test for antenatal diagnosis of acute inflammatory lesions of preterm placenta and prediction of perinatal morbidity. Am J Obstet Gynecol 1995;172(3):960–70.

38. Bharathi B, Bhat BV, Negi VS, et al. Inflammatory mediators as predictors of outcome in perinatal asphyxia. Indian J Pediatr 2015;82(5):433–8.

39. Mir IN, Chalak LF. Serum biomarkers to evaluate the integrity of the neurovascular unit. Early Hum Dev 2014;90(10):707–11.

40. Gazzolo D, Michetti F. Perinatal S100B protein assessment in human unconventional biological fluids: a minireview and new perspectives. Cardiovasc Psychiatry Neurol 2010;2010:703563.

41. Gazzolo D, Marinoni E, Di Iorio R, et al. Urinary S100B protein measurements: a tool for the early identification of hypoxic-ischemic encephalopathy in asphyxiated full-term infants. Crit Care Med 2004;32(1):131–6.

42. Qian J, Zhou D, Wang YW. Umbilical artery blood S100beta protein: a tool for the early identification of neonatal hypoxic-ischemic encephalopathy. Eur J Pediatr 2009;168(1):71–7.

43. Lam AG, Koppal T, Akama KT, et al. Mechanism of glial activation by S100B: involvement of the transcription factor NFkappaB. Neurobiol Aging 2001;22(5): 765–72.

44. Luo Q, Pin T, Dai L, et al. The role of S100B protein at 24 hours of postnatal age as early indicator of brain damage and prognostic parameter of perinatal asphyxia. Glob Pediatr Health 2019;6. https://doi.org/10.1177/2333794X19833729. 2333794X19833729.

45. Toorell H, Zetterberg H, Blennow K, et al. Increase of neuronal injury markers Tau and neurofilament light proteins in umbilical blood after intrapartum asphyxia. J Matern Fetal Neonatal Med 2018;31(18):2468–72.

46. Cakir U, Ceran B, Tayman C. Two useful umbilical biomarkers for therapeutic hypothermia decision in patients with hypoxic ischemic encephalopathy with perinatal asphyxia: netrin-1 and neuron specific enolase. Fetal Pediatr Pathol 2022; 41(6):977–86.

47. Chalak LF, Sánchez PJ, Adams-Huet B, et al. Biomarkers for severity of neonatal hypoxic-ischemic encephalopathy and outcomes in newborns receiving hypothermia therapy. J Pediatr 2014;164(3):468–74.e1.

48. Aly H, Hassanein S, Nada A, et al. Vascular endothelial growth factor in neonates with perinatal asphyxia. Brain Dev 2009;31(8):600–4.

49. Ennen CS, Huisman TAGM, Savage WJ, et al. Glial fibrillary acidic protein as a biomarker for neonatal hypoxic-ischemic encephalopathy treated with whole-body cooling. Am J Obstet Gynecol 2011;205(3):251.e1–7.

50. Looney AM, Ahearne C, Boylan GB, et al. Glial fibrillary acidic protein is not an early marker of injury in perinatal asphyxia and hypoxic-ischemic encephalopathy. Front Neurol 2015;6:264.

51. Massaro AN, Jeromin A, Kadom N, et al. Serum biomarkers of MRI brain injury in neonatal hypoxic ischemic encephalopathy treated with whole-body hypothermia: a pilot study. Pediatr Crit Care Med 2013;14(3):310–7.

52. Xanthou M, Fotopoulos S, Mouchtouri A, et al. Inflammatory mediators in perinatal asphyxia and infection. Acta Paediatr Suppl 2002;91(438):92–7.

53. Oygür N, Sönmez O, Saka O, et al. Predictive value of plasma and cerebrospinal fluid tumour necrosis factor-alpha and interleukin-1 beta concentrations on outcome of full term infants with hypoxic-ischaemic encephalopathy. Arch Dis Child Fetal Neonatal Ed 1998;79(3):F190–3.

54. Aly H, Khashaba MT, El-Ayouty M, et al. IL-1beta, IL-6 and TNF-alpha and outcomes of neonatal hypoxic ischemic encephalopathy. Brain Dev 2006;28(3):178–82.

55. Bartha AI, Foster-Barber A, Miller SP, et al. Neonatal encephalopathy: association of cytokines with MR spectroscopy and outcome. Pediatr Res 2004;56(6):960–6.

56. Fairchild KD, Viscardi RM, Hester L, et al. Effects of hypothermia and hyperthermia on cytokine production by cultured human mononuclear phagocytes from adults and newborns. J Interferon Cytokine Res 2000;20(12):1049–55.

57. Russwurm S, Stonāns I, Schwerter K, et al. Direct influence of mild hypothermia on cytokine expression and release in cultures of human peripheral blood mononuclear cells. J Interferon Cytokine Res 2002;22(2):215–21.

58. Liu B, Lan H, Gao N, et al. The application value of combined detection of serum il-6, ldh, s100, nse, and gfap in the early diagnosis of brain damage caused by neonatal asphyxia. Iran J Public Health 2023;52(11):2363–71.

59. Vos PE, Lamers KJB, Hendriks JCM, et al. Glial and neuronal proteins in serum predict outcome after severe traumatic brain injury. Neurology 2004;62(8):1303–10.

60. Kaneko T, Kasaoka S, Miyauchi T, et al. Serum glial fibrillary acidic protein as a predictive biomarker of neurological outcome after cardiac arrest. Resuscitation 2009;80(7):790–4.

61. Pelinka LE, Kroepfl A, Schmidhammer R, et al. Glial fibrillary acidic protein in serum after traumatic brain injury and multiple trauma. J Trauma 2004;57(5):1006–12.

62. Celtik C, Acunaş B, Oner N, et al. Neuron-specific enolase as a marker of the severity and outcome of hypoxic ischemic encephalopathy. Brain Dev 2004;26(6):398–402.

63. Sweetman DU, Onwuneme C, Watson WR, et al. Perinatal asphyxia and erythropoietin and VEGF: serial serum and cerebrospinal fluid responses. Neonatology 2017;111(3):253–9.

64. Disdier C, Zhang J, Fukunaga Y, et al. Alterations in inter-alpha inhibitor protein expression after hypoxic-ischemic brain injury in neonatal rats. Intl J of Devlp Neuroscience 2018;65(1):54–60.

65. Chen X, Nakada S, Donahue JE, et al. Neuroprotective effects of inter-alpha inhibitor proteins after hypoxic-ischemic brain injury in neonatal rats. Exp Neurol 2019;317:244–59.

66. Baek YW, Brokat S, Padbury JF, et al. Inter-α inhibitor proteins in infants and decreased levels in neonatal sepsis. J Pediatr 2003;143(1):11–5.

67. Chaaban H, Shin M, Sirya E, et al. Inter-alpha inhibitor protein level in neonates predicts necrotizing enterocolitis. J Pediatr 2010;157(5):757–61.

68. Bitar L, Stonestreet BS, Lim YP, et al. Association between decreased cord blood inter-alpha inhibitor levels and neonatal encephalopathy at birth. Early Hum Dev 2024;193:106036.

Advances in Neuroimaging Biomarkers and Scoring

Michelle Machie, MD[a],*, Linda S. de Vries, MD, PhD[b],
Terrie Inder, MBChB, MD[c,d]

KEYWORDS

- Neonatal neuroimaging • MRI score • Biomarker

KEY POINTS

- Neuroimaging, particularly MRI, is widely used as the key modality in the diagnosis of hypoxic-ischemic encephalopathy (HIE) in the setting of neonatal encephalopathy (NE). Although HIE is responsible for the majority of NE, other etiologies, including infectious diseases, metabolic disorders, and congenital disorders, can easily mimic HIE.
- Furthermore, quantification of the degree of brain injury can assist in the prediction of neurodevelopmental outcomes.
- There are a number of additional clinical, laboratory, and electrophysiological biomarkers for adverse neurodevelopmental outcome that have been reported in infants with NE/HIE with an individual's data from each of these assisting in supporting MRI prognostic conclusions in a thorough evaluation of any infant.

INTRODUCTION

Neuroimaging, particularly MRI, is widely used as the key modality in the diagnosis of hypoxic-ischemic encephalopathy (HIE) in the setting of neonatal encephalopathy (NE). Although HIE is responsible for the majority of NE, other etiologies, including infectious diseases, metabolic disorders, and congenital disorders can easily mimic HIE.[1] Furthermore, quantification of the degree of brain injury can assist in the prediction of neurodevelopmental outcomes. There are a number of additional clinical, laboratory, and electrophysiological biomarkers for adverse neurodevelopmental outcome that have been reported in infants with NE/HIE with an individual's data from each of these assisting in supporting MRI prognostic conclusions in a thorough

[a] Division of Pediatric Neurology, Department of Pediatrics, Neurology and Neurotherapeutics, University of Texas Southwestern Medical Center, 5323 Harry Hines Boulevard, Dallas, TX 75390-9063, USA; [b] Department of Neonatology, Leiden University Medical Center, Albinusdreef 2, 2333 ZA Leiden, Netherlands; [c] Department of Pediatric Newborn Medicine, Brigham and Womens Hospital; [d] Children's Hospital of Orange County, University of California Irvine, 1201 W. La Veta, Orange, CA 92868, USA
* Corresponding author. University of Texas Southwestern Medical Center, 5323 Harry Hines Boulevard, Dallas, TX 75390.
E-mail address: michelle.machie@utsouthwestern.edu

evaluation of any infant.[2] With regard to the clinical examination, short-term neurologic improvement, expressed by the Sarnat scale, has been shown to predict neurodevelopmental outcome at 18 to 24 months.[3] Clinical examination using the Thompson scale has also been shown to be helpful in determining adverse prognosis for neurologic development.[4] Of the laboratory investigations, umbilical cord acidemia has been associated with neonatal mortality and HIE.[5] Finally, electrophysiological evaluation has also been associated with outcomes with a persistently abnormal amplitude integrated electroencephalogram (aEEG) at 48 hours or later being associated with an adverse neurodevelopmental outcome.[6] Although these clinical, laboratory, and aEEG biomarkers have proven useful, they have not demonstrated similar singular consistency of high predictive potency similar to that of MRI. However, consideration of all of the clinical, laboratory, and electrophysiological information alongside MRI is helpful.

In considering the value of MRI prognostication, it is important to consider the impact of the information from MRI for the parents of infants with NE/HIE. For these parents, this is a time with an unexpected and life-threatening medical condition for their infant leading to significant levels of anxiety.[7] Being unable to hold their infant, while their infant may be seen uncomfortable in a cold environment adds to parental distress.[8] Communication of prognostic uncertainty is additionally challenging, both for parents and physicians.[9] Targeted communication about the strengths and limitations of MRI in aiding prognostication for an infant is critical in informing parents to assist in reducing anxiety. In a survey with clinical vignettes regarding MRI in guiding prognostication with families of infants with NE/HIE, clinicians reported uncertainty, lack of confidence, and limitations when discussing brain MRI results.[10] Only 27% of the time did clinicians report "always" using MRI results in prognostication discussions.[10] Parents reported struggling with any uncertainty. Parents raised the importance of the setting where the prognostic discussion took place and the importance of informing them as quickly as possible with appreciation of showing the pictures or making representative drawing of the injury, including highlighting the not-injured brains. Clinicians identified strategies to improve these discussions, including interdisciplinary approach, formal training, and standardized approaches to reporting the brain MRI.

EFFICACY OF MRI AS A BIOMARKER IN PERINATAL ASPHYXIA

MRI is widely accepted as the best prognostic biomarker for neurodevelopmental outcomes after NE/HIE. The Food and Drug Administration and National Institutes of Health created working groups to best define and characterize biomarkers.[11,12] In terms of simple definition, a biomarker is "a biological observation that substitutes for and ideally predicts a clinically relevant endpoint or intermediate outcome that is more difficult to observe."[13] Consequently, a biomarker is able to diagnose and monitor biological processes, and/or predict responses to a specific exposure or intervention.[11,14] The use of MRI in NE/HIE meets this definition and informs more than just future risk for neurodevelopmental impairment. Neuroimaging is critical to confirming the nature and severity of the insult, timing, and mechanism of the underlying disease process in perinatal HIE.

As a diagnostic biomarker, MRI is used to confirm the presence of hypoxic-ischemic injury secondary to the asphyxial event. It can also be used in a semiquantitative manner to stratify the severity of brain injury, which may inform early intervention and clinical care.[15–19] A prognostic biomarker is used to identify the likelihood of a clinical event, disease recurrence, or progression in patients with a specific disease.

Commonly MRI is obtained within the first week of life after NE to best provide diagnostic confirmation and prognostication regarding long-term neurodevelopmental outcomes and future risk for neurodevelopmental disability and impairment. In general, a biomarker should be easy to measure, cost-effective, accessible, and noninvasive. To fully optimize the use of MRI as a biomarker in perinatal asphyxia, we must understand the major components that constitute an ideal biomarker (**Fig. 1**).

OPTIMIZING MRI IN THE NEONATAL INTENSIVE CARE UNIT

In terms of cost efficacy, head ultrasound and computed tomographic scans are less expensive but, comparatively, MRI provides the highest degree of sensitivity for hypoxic-ischemic brain injury and is the gold standard for neuroimaging in perinatal HIE.[20] Cranial ultrasound has decreased ability to detect either more subtle MRI changes from mild asphyxia or white matter (WM) predominant injury patterns.[21] MRI acquisition can be complex, and the optimal utility of the study can be subject to both intrasite and intersite variability in acquisition protocols. Within centers, MRI acquisition is often set and run by the MRI technologists undertaking the MRI scans. Optimal acquisition and interpretation require the same MRI sequences being applied to every infant on every imaging session using the same parameters. This requires protocols that are adhered to within the same scanner. A typical neonatal MRI Brain protocol will include T1-weighted (T_1) images, T2-weighted (T_2) images, susceptibility-weighted imaging (SWI), and diffusion-weighted imaging (DWI) on a 1.5 T or 3T scanner. Advanced MRI techniques such as proton MR spectroscopy (^{1}H-MRS) provide in vivo quantitative information regarding energy utilization. These sequences must be optimized to the neonatal brain to account for the incomplete maturation of tissues and small size of cerebral structures that influence soft tissue contrast.[22] Additional mechanisms to optimize signal-to-noise ratio include the use of dedicated coils of appropriate size for the neonatal head.[23] Among centers,

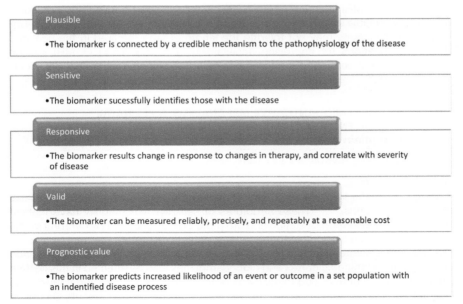

Plausible
- The biomarker is connected by a credible mechanism to the pathophysiology of the disease

Sensitive
- The biomarker sucessfully identifies those with the disease

Responsive
- The biomarker results change in response to changes in therapy, and correlate with severity of disease

Valid
- The biomarker can be measured reliably, precisely, and repeatably at a reasonable cost

Prognostic value
- The biomarker predicts increased likelihood of an event or outcome in a set population with an indentified disease process

Fig. 1. Characteristics of an ideal biomarker.

differences may arise in the brand of MRI machine being used, field strength available, software chosen for data processing, and patient workflow including protocols for immobilization and sedation. In addition, optimal acquisition requires minimal movement of the infant while in the MRI scanner, which is best acquired with experienced neonatal intensive care unit (NICU) trained staff and MRI technicians. Acquisition has been shown to be improved by protocols for immobilization such as "bundle and feed" protocols that avoid sedation, as well as short acquisition and motion tolerant acquisition sequences.[24–26] Finally, experienced neuroradiologists are essential for the accurate interpretation of MRI in newborns with NE/HIE and combined neuroradiological conferences with the clinical teams can further facilitate optimal interpretation and prognostication.

OPTIMIZING MRI IN THERAPEUTIC HYPOTHERMIA PROTOCOLS

The effective use of MRI as a biomarker requires significant harmonization of protocols with standardization of sequence parameters, processing methods and timing of MRI to reduce error and to maximize consistency, as was described recently in the development of the HEAL trial, which assessed the efficacy of high-dose erythropoietin in perinatal asphyxia.[27] The period for therapeutic hypothermia is 72 hours followed by a rewarming period. Thurs, the ideal time for MRI is typically day of life (DOL) 4 to 5, after therapeutic hypothermia is complete, but prior to pseudonormalization of DWI sequences. Pseudonormalization refers to the apparent normalization of mean diffusivity values, even in the presence of brain injury, and commences after DOL6. Pseudonormalization appears to be more prolonged into the second week of life in infants who undergo therapeutic hypothermia[28] and may represent ongoing apoptosis at this late phase.

Barriers to obtaining MRI within the first week of life may include complications such as refractory seizures, respiratory failure, or hemodynamic instability related to the hypoxic-ischemic event and end-organ damage. Most NICUs require transport of infants to a remote MRI scanner, which necessitates transport nursing and additional staff. MRI compatible incubators help to make the transport process more stable. Unstable newborn infants may not tolerate the length of time required in the scanner. Future considerations for improving accessibility and acquisition of MRI include ultra-low magnet strength and portable bedside MRI scanners that are not yet widely implemented.[29,30]

DEVELOPMENT OF SEMIQUANTITATIVE MRI ANALYSIS IN PERINATAL HYPOXIC-ISCHEMIC ENCEPHALOPATHY: FROM THEN TO NOW
Historical Descriptions of Brain Injury Patterns

Historically 2 major patterns of injury were seen in HIE[31] (**Fig. 2**).

Basal ganglia/thalamic pattern
An abrupt decrease in blood flow leads to a central pattern of injury to the basal ganglia and thalamus.[32–34] These structures of selective vulnerability have highest metabolic demand at term gestation and are preferentially supplied by cerebral autoregulation.[35–37] When blood flow to the fetus is acutely disrupted, the normal mechanism of cerebral autoregulation fails, and injury occurs affecting the basal ganglia and thalamus. The perirolandic cortex and hippocampi may also be affected in this pattern of injury. Factors that may lead to such an abrupt decrease in fetal blood flow include placental abruption, uterine rupture, or umbilical cord prolapse. Clinically this brain injury pattern is associated with higher severity of HIE.[38,39]

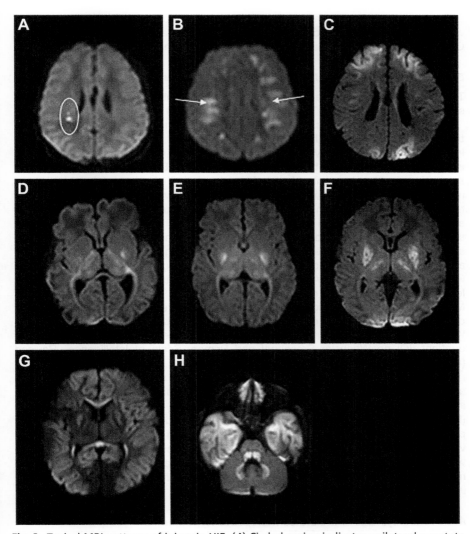

Fig. 2. Typical MRI patterns of injury in HIE. (*A*) Circled region indicates unilateral punctate white matter lesions (PWML) of restricted diffusion (apparent as bright white signal on DWI) in the periventricular WM. (*B*) DWI sequence demonstrates extensive WMI. *White arrows* signify extensive bilateral WMI on DWI sequence. (*C*) Bilateral WS pattern of restricted diffusion. (*D–F*) Restricted diffusion is predominantly shown in the deep gray nuclei (basal ganglia and thalami) with (*D*) focal, (*E*) moderate, and (*F*) extensive deep gray matter involvement. (*G*) Near total or global injury pattern, the diffusion-weighted images demonstrate widespread restricted diffusion throughout both cerebral hemispheres, as well as the bilateral thalami and basal ganglia. (*H*) There is relative sparing of the cerebellum, but there is restricted diffusion present in the dentate nuclei.

White matter/watershed of injury

With a more moderate decrease in cerebral blood flow, the blood flow is shunted preferentially to the posterior circulation to maintain perfusion to high energy structures such as the basal ganglia, cerebellum, and brainstem. In this setting the watershed

(WS) zone between vascular territories is most affected leading to injury in the WS white and gray matter, also described as a parasagittal pattern of brain injury.[33,34,40,41] Clinically, this brain injury pattern is associated with a milder severity of HIE.[38,39,42]

Early Applications of Brain Injury Patterns to MRI Scores

These patterns and observations led to the development of multiple semiquantitative scoring systems over time. These scores are compared in supplemental **Table 1**.

Barkovich and colleagues (1998) developed the first widely used scoring system for the assessment of perinatal asphyxia on MR images.[33] This early score focused on injury affecting the 2 primary patterns of injury: the basal ganglia and WS zones, leading to the development of the basal ganglia/thalamic (BGT) scoring system. Lower scores signified involvement of isolated basal ganglia/thalamic nuclei or cortex, and maximum severity scores were assigned when the MRI demonstrated global or near total injury involving the entire cortex and basal nuclei, with maximum severity score of 4 for the combined BGT score. The BGT score has been validated to predict severely impaired motor and cognitive (Bayley-II) outcome at 30 months of age.[43] This score was recently evaluated in a combined precooling and postcooling era cohort and correlated with the prediction of cerebral palsy diagnoses out to 4 years of age with area under the curve (AUC) (0.895, 0.791–0.998), and with BGT severity scores less than 4 having excellent negative predictive value (94%) for severe disability Gross Motor Function Classification Scale (GMFCS) III or greater.[44] While basal ganglia changes may best predict motor outcomes, it should be noted that increasing WS WM injury severity subscores were associated with decreasing verbal intelligence quotient (IQ) on Wechsler Preschool and Primary Scale of Intelligence- Revised (WPPSI-R).[45]

Rutherford and colleagues (1998) independently at a similar timeframe developed an early nuclear magnetic resonance score that, in addition to the BGT and cortex, included additional specific evaluation of the posterior limb of the internal capsule (PLIC).[39] Abnormal signal intensity (SI) in the PLIC was determined to be an accurate predictor of neurodevelopmental outcomes at 1 year of age with positive predictive value 0.94 (95% confidence interval, 0.88–1.0).[46] This score may be less applicable when MRI is obtained in the first 4 to 5 DOL given that changes in SI in the PLIC may take more than 5 days after the injury to be reliably evident after hypoxia-ischemia.

MRI Scoring Systems in the Era of Therapeutic Hypothermia

The multicenter randomized controlled trials for therapeutic hypothermia required standardized mechanisms to evaluate MRI scans and to increase concordance between centers.

The National Institute of Child Health and Human Development (NICHD) Neonatal Research Network (NRN) developed a score (2005) that was validated in randomized controlled trials of hypothermia and has a 6 step pragmatic escalation ranging from a score of 0 (normal), 1A (focal WM), 1B (extensive WM), 2A (BGT), 2B (BGT and cortex), and up to a maximum severity score of 3 signifying global cerebral devastation.[15,17] This MRI score applied in the first week of life correlated with death or disability at 18 to 22 months of age (odds ratio [OR] 2.4 [1.8–3.3] with MRI as a continuous variable) and also with neurodevelopmental outcomes (death or IQ <70) at 6 to 7 years of age.[15,17]

The Rutherford score (described earlier) was applied to the TOBY and ICE trials of hypothermia and was predictive of death and disability at 18 months of age and 2 years

Table 1
Comparative summary of four scoring systems[17–19,33]

Barkovich Score[1]	NICHD NRN Score[2]	Weeke Score[3] a			Trivedi Score[4] d
0 Normal	0 Normal	Gray matter	6 items	BG, T, PLIC, brainstem, perirolandic cortex, [b]hippocampus / Points possible: 23	Subcortical: • Caudate • Globus pallidus/putamen • Thalamus • PLIC Points possible: 72
1 Abnormal signal in BG or T	1A Minimal ≤3 cerebral lesions without BG, T, ALIC, PLIC, or WS pattern involvement				
2 Abnormal signal in cortex	1 B More extensive cerebral lesions without BGT, PLIC, ALIC, or WS pattern involvement	^{1}H-MRS	2 items	BG NAA, BG Lac / Points possible: 2	WM Points possible: 18
3 Abnormal signal in cortex and BG or T	2A Abnormal BGT, ALIC, PLIC, or WS injury without additional cerebral lesions	WM	6 items	Cortex excluding perirolandic, WM abnormal SI excluding PWML, PMWL, hemorrhage, optic radiation, [c]corpus callosum / Points possible: 21	Cortex Points possible: 18
4 Abnormal signal in entire cortex and BGT	2 B Abnormal BGT, ALIC, PLIC, or WS injury with cerebral lesions	Cerebellum	2 items	Cerebellum abnormal SI or diffusion restriction, cerebellar hemorrhage / Points possible: 8	Cerebellum Points possible: 18
	3 Cerebral hemispheric devastation	Additional subscore	3 items	[d]IVH, [e]SDH, and [c]CVST / Points possible: 3	Brainstem Points possible: 12

The Barkovich and NICHD NRN scores apply a single maximum severity score while the Weeke and Trivedi scores apply a summation of categorical subscores.

There are 138 possible points for this score, and the score can be assigned an MRI injury grade of 0 = no injury, 1–11 = mild injury, 12–32 = moderate injury, and 33–138 = severe injury.

Abbreviations: ALIC, anterior limb of the internal capsule; BG, basal ganglia; BGT, basal ganglia and thalamus; CVST, cerebral sinus venous thrombosis; ^{1}H-MRS, proton MR spectroscopy; IVH, intraventricular hemorrhage; NAA, N acetyl aspartate; PLIC, posterior limb of the internal capsule; PWML, punctate white matter lesions; SDH, subdural hemorrhage; SI, signal intensity; T, thalamus; WM, white matter.

a Weeke Score: Each item receives 1 point if focal injury (<50%) or 2 points if injury is extensive (≥50%), *and* each item also receives 1 point if there is unilateral injury or 2 points if injury is bilateral. There are 4 maximum points per individual item. There are 57 total points possible for this score.

b This item has a maximum point possible of 3.

c This item has a maximum point possible of 1.

d Trivedi score: Each of the subregions is scored based on signal abnormality as either 0 (no injury), 1 (<25% of region), 2 (25%–50% of region), or 3 (>50% of region) in each hemisphere on each of a T1W, T2W, and DWI sequence, culminating in a 6 part score per region. Brainstem is scored 0–2.

of age, respectively, and also determined that therapeutic hypothermia did not diminish the prognostic value of MRI.[16,47]

Recent MRI Scoring Systems

More recently with the recognition of more diverse forms of brain injury than the 2 classic patterns, new MRI scoring systems have been developed that are more comprehensive in the recognition of the presence of any injury, as well as delineating more subtle forms of injury, such as punctate WM injury (WMI). In addition, these scoring systems include newer technologies such as MR spectroscopy.

The Weeke score (2018) was developed in a dual validation and confirmation cohort of infants with moderate-to-severe HIE.[18] The Weeke score is highly detailed ranging from a score of 0 (normal) to a maximum severity score of 57. It is inclusive of the conventional injury scores with DWI evaluation, as well as being the only scoring system to include ^{1}H-MRS. This score has predictive value for outcome at 2 years of age (AUC 0.989, 0.973–1.000) with the inclusion of ^{1}H-MRS and at school age, mean 6 to 7 years of age (AUC 0.935, 0.855–1.000).

The Trivedi score (2018)[19] was adapted from the Bednarek score,[28] and developed in a cohort of infants with NE receiving therapeutic hypothermia. It evaluates SI abnormalities in 5 regions (1) subcortical: caudate nucleus, globus pallidus and putamen, thalamus, and the PLIC; (2) WM; (3) cortex; (4) cerebellum; and (5) brainstem. The subscores are summated with a maximum severity score of 138. This score includes DWI sequences and is weighted specifically for deep nuclear gray matter and PLIC injuries. The Trivedi score has been associated with neurodevelopmental outcomes at 18 to 24 months of age with an AUC of 0.72 (95% confidence interval [CI] 0.57–0.86). This MRI injury scoring system was applied in the evaluation of MRI acquired in the HEAL trial with an association between the score and adverse outcomes at 2 years of life (adjusted odds ratio [aOR] 1.06, 95% CI 1.05, 1.07).[48]

Comparison of MRI Scoring Systems in Perinatal Hypoxic-ischemic Encephalopathy

These scores have since been compared for best efficacy in detecting abnormalities on MRI and prediction of outcomes.

Machie and colleagues compared 44 infants with varying HIE severity levels (mild, moderate, and severe) and found that the Weeke score was most sensitive in detecting brain injury, rating 57% of the MRIs as abnormal, in comparison to the NICHD NRN score (24%) and Barkovich score (7%).[49] This study is one of only a few to apply new MRI scoring systems to infants with mild as well as moderate/severe HIE and additionally found excellent (k 0.90) interrater reliability between expert and trained MRI scorers.

The high sensitivity of the Weeke score for injury detection (Barkovich 40%, NICHD NRN 50%, and Weeke 77%) was confirmed in another study by Ní Bhroin and colleagues, which was inclusive of mild, moderate, and severe HIE, and this study also determined that only the Weeke score was associated with the prediction of Bayley-III language scores, although Bayley-III cognitive and motor scores were significantly associated with all 3 scoring systems.[50] A third study that compared the Barkovich, NICHD, Rutherford, and Weeke scores did not find any difference in MRI score ability to detect injury in a cohort of infants that excluded mild HIE,[51] although they similarly did find that Weeke score best predicted the assigned 2 year neurodevelopmental cognitive outcome, using the Bayley-III scale.

The neuroimaging analysis of PharmaCool evaluated 4 MRI scoring systems for term infants with perinatal asphyxia and found no differences among 4 MRI scoring systems in their ability to predict the composite outcome (death and disability) or adverse outcome at 2 years of age.[52] The 4 scores included were the Rutherford score (including DWI analysis), Trivedi score, Weeke score (without ^{1}H-MRS given the lack of availability), and NICHD NRN score. There was an excellent prediction of death for most scoring systems with AUCs of 0.90 or greater, except for the Rutherford score (AUC 0.84), and all MRI scoring systems had an acceptable prediction of adverse outcome with comparable AUCs between 0.66 and 0.71, and composite outcome with AUCs between 0.79 and 0.86.

In conclusion, the best scoring system selected for a group of patients may need to vary with the degree of brain injury as more detailed and advanced scoring systems may be better at the detection of more subtle brain injury, such as mild WM lesions seen commonly in mild HIE, while all the scoring systems described have proven efficacy in detecting severe brain injury and correlation to long-term outcomes.

CURRENT ADVANCES IN MRI BIOMARKER TECHNOLOGY
Predictive Value of the Signal Intensity of the Posterior Limb of the Internal Capsule

When the landmark article by Rutherford and colleagues was published in 1998, the absence of normal SI of the PLIC could be regarded as an early biomarker for the prediction of an abnormal motor outcome.[46] This was subsequently supported by studies from Martinez-Biarge and colleagues in 2010 and 2011.[32,53] The SI of the PLIC on the T1-weighted sequence could be normal, equivocal, or show an inverted signal. These MRIs were, however, performed well into the second week of life. With the introduction of hypothermia, the MRI was brought forward and is now most often performed on day 4 to 6, soon after rewarming. On this first week MRI, the PLIC still has a normal SI in most infants. The emphasis is now no longer on an abnormal signal of the PLIC, but on the presence of diffusion restriction in the thalami and basal ganglia. In some infants, a repeat MRI will be performed, especially when there is a discrepancy between the early MRI and clinical examination. When a repeat MRI is performed, the PLIC will once again provide important information, in agreement with the data by Rutherford.

The Role of Quantitative ADC

Assessing the extent of brain injury based on the trace map of the DWI may both overestimate and underestimate the abnormalities. There may be a T_2 shine through effect, which can be excluded using the apparent diffusion coefficient (ADC) map. In an infant with a near total pattern of injury, some areas may appear to be unaffected, but when the ADC values are measured, these areas may show reduced ADC values as well (**Fig. 3**). Several studies have shown the use of ADC values as an early biomarker. Bednarek and colleagues have reported that the ADC values are lower in infants undergoing hypothermia and that pseudonormalization of ADC is much slower following therapeutic hypothermia compared with normothermia and may take up to 10 days.[28] Most studies will measure the ADC values using a region of interest (ROI), and this is most often placed in one hemisphere in the region combining the thalamus and the basal ganglia, but making sure that the cerebrospinal fluid from the lateral ventricle is not part of the ROI. It is also possible to perform quantitative ADC measures. In a recent study, volumes with ADC values less than 800×10^{-6} mm^2/s were automatically computed across the whole brain. Volume of acute injury greater than 1 mL (OR, 13.9 [95% CI: 5.93, 32.45]; $P < .001$) and presence of any acute injury in the brain (OR, 4.5 [95% CI: 2.6, 7.8]; $P<.001$) were associated with increased odds of death or any neurodevelopmental impairment (NDI).[54] Quantitative whole-brain acute injury volume was strongly associated with DWI signal abnormalities scored by an expert.

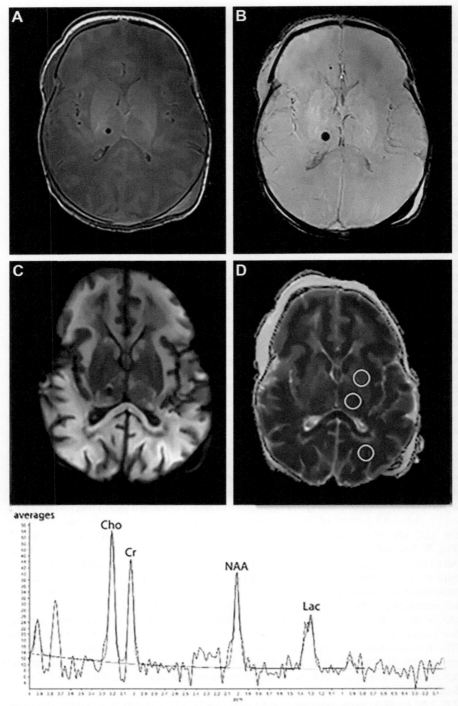

Fig. 3. Severe HIE in a term infant who received hypothermia. MRI performed on day 4. T1-weighted sequence shows a swollen brain with poor gray–white matter differentiation. The PLIC is equivocal. (*A*) The low SI in the right thalamus is a small hemorrhage, confirmed with

MR Spectroscopy

^{1}H-MRS can be used to evaluate brain metabolites in asphyxiated term infants. ^{1}H-MRS can detect impaired cerebral metabolism by measuring the concentration of various chemical compounds such as choline, N-acetyl aspartate (NAA), and lactate (Lac). Elevation of Lac levels and decrease in NAA levels are early indicators of brain injury, seen as early as within hours after birth. Lac/NAA ratio has been shown by several studies to be predictive of an abnormal outcome.[55] In some studies concentrations of NAA were measured, resulting in the highest prediction compared to Lac/NAA ratio.[56] When ^{1}H-MRS data from the first and second week after birth were compared, total NAA concentration had the highest AUC at both time points (AUC 0.97 and 1.00, respectively), with good AUCs of 0.90, 0.95, and 0.97 for ADC values, Lac concentration, and Lac/NAA ratios at 24 to 96 hours of life.[57] Even though ^{1}H-MRS can be obtained on most MR magnets, it is not yet widely used and only part of one of the scoring systems.[18]

Mammillary Bodies to Predict Long-Term Cognitive Outcomes

The mammillary bodies (MBs) are a pair of small round structures located at the under-surface of the diencephalon and are part of the limbic system, and the MBs are known to play an important role in cognitive outcome and memory function. The MBs were only recently recognized to be often affected in infants with HIE. To be able to assess them, thin slices are required, and they are best seen on axial T_2 sequence, using 2 mm slices. In the acute stage, the MBs will have an increased SI and will be swollen on the T_2 sequence and depending on timing of the MRI, there may also be diffusion restriction (**Fig. 4**). On a repeat MRI, there will be atrophy, and this is best seen on a sagittal T_1 or T_2 sequence. They may be the only abnormal finding on an MRI, some-times together with diffusion restriction of the hippocampi, but they can also be affected together with other patterns of brain injury. In a multicenter study of infants receiving hypothermia, abnormal MB SI was seen in approximately 40%.[58] In a retro-spective observational study of neonates with HIE, 76% of the infants with abnormal MBs on the neonatal MRI had MB atrophy at 10 years of age. MB atrophy was seen in 38% of all 10 year old patients.[59] The study also showed that hippocampal volume and MB atrophy were strongly associated with neurocognitive outcome and episodic memory at 10 years of age. These findings at school age were in agreement with another study, where MB atrophy was seen in 34% of the children and an association with cognitive deficits was also noted.[60] In this study, radial diffusivity and fractional anisotropy were measured in the mammillothalamic tract (MTT) and fornix, from diffusion-weighted MRI using deterministic tractography. Increased radial diffusivity was noted in the right MTT ($P = .004$) compared with cases without mammillary body abnormalities.

Volumetric Studies

Since a study with a very small number of infants,[61] there have been a few more volu-metric studies. Subcortical volumes were automatically extracted from T_1-weighted images in 28 newborns.[62] Only 2 infants had basal ganglia injury and none had WS

SWI (*B*). There is widespread diffusion restriction (*C*) but the BGT appear to be relatively spared. (*D*) The *yellow circles* signify 3 areas of measured ADC values, which are very low, including the BG 0.857 × 10³/mm², thalami 0.645 × 10³/mm², and occipital WM 0.55 × 10³/mm². ^{1}H-MRS obtained in the left BGT region shows a clear Lac peak at 1.33 ppm.

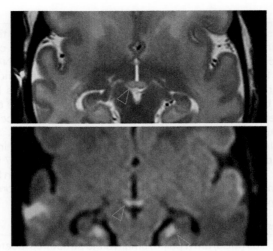

Fig. 4. Term infant with moderate HIE. MRI day 5. T_2 sequence (*top*) shows increased SI and swelling of the MBs (*arrowhead*). DWI shows increased SI in the MBs as well as the hippocampi (*bottom*).

injury. The volumes were compared with those of 28 healthy controls. MRI was performed at a median age of 5 days (4–6). Neonates with HIE had significantly smaller bilateral thalamic, basal ganglia, and right hippocampal and cerebellar volumes compared to controls. This is unexpected as the BGT area tends to be swollen during the first week, but this could be explained as they had only 2 infants with BGT injury.

Another study specifically looked at the volume of acute brain injury as seen on DWI, using quantification of the ADC images. Areas of diffusion restricted were defined as areas where the ADC values were less than $0.8 \times 10^3/mm^2$ and to delineate borders between abnormal low ADC (restricted diffusivity) and noninjured adjacent parenchyma. The areas of acute brain injury were manually traced on serial axial DWI (B1000) images. Higher injury volume was associated with worse 12 month neurodevelopmental outcomes.[63]

FUTURE DIRECTIONS INCLUDE FURTHER OPTIMIZATION OF TIMING OF NEUROIMAGING AFTER PERINATAL ASPHYXIA

Early MR imaging of a newborn with NE in the acute stage, while undergoing therapeutic hypothermia, is an attractive proposition to both the clinician and researcher. Although acquiring MR imaging within 24 hours of birth in NE with ongoing hypothermia has been reported,[64–66] in clinical practice, MRI is not carried out until after hypothermia since most MRI units are located away from the NICU and most commercial cooling blankets are not MRI compatible. One recent report described the use of an in-NICU MRI system with hypothermia blanket during scanning to acquire MRI in the first 24 hours of life.[67] Additional value may exist in MRI at 24 hours to consider "early exit" from hypothermia for milder cases of NE. As hypothermia for NE has been widely adopted and its safety well established, many institutions offering this therapy have broadened their indications to include neonates with milder forms of NE. However, factors such as effects of maternal medications on neonatal arousal state can make the diagnosis of mild encephalopathy in the first 6 hours after birth challenging.

Thus, a pathway for the ongoing evaluation of such mildly affected infants with the possibility of an early exit from hypothermia therapy if HIE is unlikely is desirable. A few studies have addressed this. In one study, 27 out of 208 infants were evaluated with MRI for "early exit" of whom 9 infants (33%) had evidence of injury on MRI that led to the continuation of hypothermia.[68] It is important to realize that an MRI within the first 24 to 48 hours may underestimate the full extent of the injury.[69]

In addition to consideration of a very early (first 24 hours) MRI, there is considerable variation in the timing and number of MRI scans obtained in the setting of NE/HIE. Current guidelines proposed by the American College of Obstetrics and Gynecology suggest performing 2 brain MRIs in the neonatal period following therapeutic hypothermia.[70] These guidelines are based on the notion that early MRI (at 1–4 days) indicates the timing of injury, but later MRI (between 7 and 21 days) more fully defines the extent of the injury. However, disagreement exists regarding whether both are necessary, and which is more valuable in determining injury and prognosis. Although some studies suggest there is no difference between early and late MRI scans,[71] others propose that a late MRI is necessary to appropriately predict prognosis.[72] Conversely, other studies report that the early MRI shows a higher specificity for brain injury than the late MRI and is sufficient to determine prognosis.[73,74] Within this context, the Newborn Brain Society published a review and guideline that recommended that MRI should be performed between 2 and 5 days with repeat MRI being recommended at days 10 to 14 of life when clinical concerns persist, including discrepancies between the early neuroimaging findings and the clinical condition of the infant.[75]

Finally, the value of later infancy and childhood MRI to evaluate prediction of neurodevelopmental disability in NE/HIE remains very understudied. The association of 3 month MRI findings with neurodevelopmental outcome following NE has been demonstrated in several studies, which mainly included noncooled infants. A recent retrospective, single-center study included 63 infants with perinatal asphyxia and NE (n = 28 cooled) with cranial MRI less than 2 weeks and 2 to 4 months after birth applying biometrics, validated injury score for neonatal MRI, and a new score for 3 month MRI, with a WM, deep gray matter (DGM), and cerebellum subscore.[76] The authors concluded that DGM abnormalities on 3 month MRI, preceded by DGM abnormalities on the neonatal MRI, were associated with 18 to 24 month outcome, indicating the utility of 3 month MRI for treatment evaluation in neuroprotective trials. However, the clinical usefulness of 3 month MRI seemed limited compared with neonatal MRI. More data are needed on the value of subsequent neuroimaging after the neonatal intensive care unit period.

SUMMARY

Neuroimaging with MRI is the best prognostic biomarker for NE/HIE and is critical for the diagnosis and confirmation of the timing and extent of brain injury. New more detailed qualitative scoring systems have been introduced to stratify the severity of brain injury, although few are applied systematically in clinical practice. Clinical improvements in the acquisition and interpretation of MRI in the infant with NE/HIE may improve the consistency of communication to parents regarding prognosis. For the future, these imaging evaluative tools can act as short-term biomarkers for outcomes of novel therapeutic agents in NE/HIE and contribute to the design of individualized rehabilitative approaches. Future directions include more widespread implementation of ^{1}H-MRS and more novel advanced imaging methods, such as regional volumes and surface cortical measures. Longitudinal serial imaging, including at a later time point of several months, with such techniques may also more fully inform the extent of the developmental consequences of an early cerebral injury on brain development and outcomes.

Best Practices

What is the current practice for [enter disease/condition(s)]?

- MRI is the current standard of care in neuroimaging for the evaluation of NE/HIE.
- Neonatal MR protocols should include T1-weighted and T2-weighted sequences, DWI with ADC mapping, SWI, in addition to ^{1}H-MRS where available.
- The optimal timing of MRI is at DOL 4 to 6 after therapeutic hypothermia, prior to pseudonormalization of DWI sequences.

What changes in current practice are likely to improve outcomes?

- Application of systematic scoring systems may enhance the definition of the nature and extent of brain injury in NE/HIE.
- ^{1}H-MRS is beneficial as a sensitive biomarker in the evaluation of HIE and is also helpful to identify metabolic mimics of other neonatal encephalopathies. More widespread inclusion of ^{1}H-MRS will be beneficial in identifying those infants at highest risk for poor outcomes.[56]
- If early MRI is obtained during therapeutic hypothermia (DOL 1–3), then an additional MRI after rewarming is indicated as the early MRI may not demonstrate the full extent of the injury.

Bibliographic Source(s): This is important: list current sources/references to support info above

Lally PJ, Montaldo P, Oliveira V, et al. Magnetic resonance spectroscopy assessment of brain injury after moderate hypothermia in neonatal encephalopathy: a prospective multicentre cohort study. *Lancet Neurol.* Jan 2019;18(1):35 to 45. https://doi.org/10.1016/S1474-4422(1830325-9)

Shibasaki J, Niwa T, Piedvache A, et al. Comparison of Predictive Values of Magnetic Resonance Biomarkers Based on Scan Timing in Neonatal Encephalopathy Following Therapeutic Hypothermia. *J Pediatr.* Dec 2021;239:101 to 109.e4. https://doi.org/10.1016/j.jpeds.2021.08.011

Chakkarapani E, Poskitt KJ, Miller SP, et al. Reliability of Early Magnetic Resonance Imaging (MRI) and Necessity of Repeating MRI in Noncooled and Cooled Infants With Neonatal Encephalopathy. *J Child Neurol.* Apr 2016;31(5):553-9. https://doi.org/10.1177/0883073815600865

Wisnowski JL, Wintermark P, Bonifacio SL, et al. Neuroimaging in the term newborn with neonatal encephalopathy. *Semin Fetal Neonatal Med.* Oct 2021;26(5):101304. https://doi.org/10.1016/j.siny.2021.101304

DISCLOSURE

The authors have nothing to disclose.

REFERENCES

1. Sandoval Karamian AG, Mercimek-Andrews S, Mohammad K, et al. Neonatal encephalopathy: etiologies other than hypoxic-ischemic encephalopathy. Semin Fetal Neonatal Med 2021;26(5):101272.
2. Walas W, Wilińska M, Bekiesińska-Figatowska M, et al. Methods for assessing the severity of perinatal asphyxia and early prognostic tools in neonates with

hypoxic-ischemic encephalopathy treated with therapeutic hypothermia. Adv Clin Exp Med 2020;29(8):1011–6.

3. Grass B, Scheidegger S, Latal B, et al. Short-term neurological improvement in neonates with hypoxic-ischemic encephalopathy predicts neurodevelopmental outcome at 18-24 months. J Perinat Med 2020;48(3):296–303.

4. Mendler MR, Mendler I, Hassan MA, et al. Predictive value of thompson-score for long-term neurological and cognitive outcome in term newborns with perinatal asphyxia and hypoxic-ischemic encephalopathy undergoing controlled hypothermia treatment. Neonatology 2018;114(4):341–7.

5. Malin GL, Morris RK, Khan KS. Strength of association between umbilical cord pH and perinatal and long term outcomes: systematic review and meta-analysis. BMJ 2010;340:c1471.

6. Chandrasekaran M, Chaban B, Montaldo P, et al. Predictive value of amplitude-integrated EEG (aEEG) after rescue hypothermic neuroprotection for hypoxic ischemic encephalopathy: a meta-analysis. J Perinatol 2017;37(6):684–9.

7. Pilon B, Craig AK, Lemmon ME, et al. Supporting families in their child's journey with neonatal encephalopathy and therapeutic hypothermia. Semin Fetal Neonatal Med 2021;26(5):101278.

8. Thyagarajan B, Baral V, Gunda R, et al. Parental perceptions of hypothermia treatment for neonatal hypoxic-ischaemic encephalopathy. J Matern Fetal Neonatal Med 2018;31(19):2527–33.

9. Rasmussen LA, Cascio MA, Ferrand A, et al. The complexity of physicians' understanding and management of prognostic uncertainty in neonatal hypoxic-ischemic encephalopathy. J Perinatol 2019;39(2):278–85.

10. Cascio A, Ferrand A, Racine E, et al. Discussing brain magnetic resonance imaging results for neonates with hypoxic-ischemic encephalopathy treated with hypothermia: a challenge for clinicians and parents. eNeurologicalSci 2022;29:100424.

11. Group F-NBW. BEST (Biomarkers, EndpointS, and other Tools) Resource. 2016.

12. Group BDW. Biomarkers and surrogate endpoints: preferred definitions and conceptual framework. Clin Pharmacol Ther 2001;69(3):89–95.

13. Aronson JK, Ferner RE. Biomarkers-a general review. Curr Protoc Pharmacol 2017;76:9231–7.

14. Califf RM. Biomarker definitions and their applications. Exp Biol Med (Maywood) 2018;243(3):213–21.

15. Shankaran S, McDonald SA, Laptook AR, et al. Neonatal magnetic resonance imaging pattern of brain injury as a biomarker of childhood outcomes following a trial of hypothermia for neonatal hypoxic-ischemic encephalopathy. J Pediatr 2015;167(5):987–93.e3.

16. Rutherford M, Ramenghi LA, Edwards AD, et al. Assessment of brain tissue injury after moderate hypothermia in neonates with hypoxic-ischaemic encephalopathy: a nested substudy of a randomised controlled trial. Lancet Neurol 2010;9(1):39–45.

17. Shankaran S, Barnes PD, Hintz SR, et al. Brain injury following trial of hypothermia for neonatal hypoxic-ischaemic encephalopathy. Arch Dis Child Fetal Neonatal Ed 2012;97(6):F398–404.

18. Weeke LC, Groenendaal F, Mudigonda K, et al. A novel magnetic resonance imaging score predicts neurodevelopmental outcome after perinatal asphyxia and therapeutic hypothermia. J Pediatr 2018;192:33–40.e2.

19. Trivedi SB, Vesoulis ZA, Rao R, et al. A validated clinical MRI injury scoring system in neonatal hypoxic-ischemic encephalopathy. Pediatr Radiol 2017;47(11): 1491–9.

20. Groenendaal F, de Vries LS. Fifty years of brain imaging in neonatal encephalopathy following perinatal asphyxia. Pediatr Res 2017;81(1–2):150–5.

21. Cizmeci MN, Wilson D, Singhal M, et al. Neonatal hypoxic-ischemic encephalopathy spectrum: severity-stratified analysis of neuroimaging modalities and association with neurodevelopmental outcomes. J Pediatr 2023;266:113866.

22. Dubois J, Alison M, Counsell SJ, et al. MRI of the neonatal brain: a review of methodological challenges and neuroscientific advances. J Magn Reson Imaging 2021;53(5):1318–43.

23. Hughes EJ, Winchman T, Padormo F, et al. A dedicated neonatal brain imaging system. Magn Reson Med 2017;78(2):794–804.

24. Antonov NK, Ruzal-Shapiro CB, Morel KD, et al. Feed and wrap MRI technique in infants. Clin Pediatr (Phila) 2017;56(12):1095–103.

25. Ibrahim T, Few K, Greenwood R, et al. 'Feed and wrap' or sedate and immobilise for neonatal brain MRI? Arch Dis Child Fetal Neonatal Ed 2015;100(5):F465–6.

26. King R, Low S, Gee N, et al. Practical stepwise approach to performing neonatal brain mr imaging in the research setting. Children (Basel) 2023;10(11). https://doi.org/10.3390/children10111759.

27. Wisnowski JL, Bluml S, Panigrahy A, et al. Integrating neuroimaging biomarkers into the multicentre, high-dose erythropoietin for asphyxia and encephalopathy (HEAL) trial: rationale, protocol and harmonisation. BMJ Open 2021;11(4): e043852.

28. Bednarek N, Mathur A, Inder T, et al. Impact of therapeutic hypothermia on MRI diffusion changes in neonatal encephalopathy. Neurology 2012;78(18):1420–7.

29. Cawley P, Padormo F, Cromb D, et al. Development of neonatal-specific sequences for portable ultralow field magnetic resonance brain imaging: a prospective, single-centre, cohort study. EClinicalMedicine 2023;65:102253.

30. Sien ME, Robinson AL, Hu HH, et al. Feasibility of and experience using a portable MRI scanner in the neonatal intensive care unit. Arch Dis Child Fetal Neonatal Ed 2023;108(1):45–50.

31. Ghei SK, Zan E, Nathan JE, et al. MR imaging of hypoxic-ischemic injury in term neonates: pearls and pitfalls. Radiographics 2014;34(4):1047–61.

32. Martinez-Biarge M, Diez-Sebastian J, Rutherford MA, et al. Outcomes after central grey matter injury in term perinatal hypoxic-ischaemic encephalopathy. Early Hum Dev 2010;86(11):675–82.

33. Barkovich AJ, Hajnal BL, Vigneron D, et al. Prediction of neuromotor outcome in perinatal asphyxia: evaluation of MR scoring systems. AJNR Am J Neuroradiol 1998;19(1):143–9.

34. Parmentier CEJ, de Vries LS, Groenendaal F. Magnetic resonance imaging in (Near-)term infants with hypoxic-ischemic encephalopathy. Diagnostics (Basel) 2022;12(3). https://doi.org/10.3390/diagnostics12030645.

35. Douglas-Escobar M, Weiss MD. Hypoxic-ischemic encephalopathy: a review for the clinician. JAMA Pediatr 2015;169(4):397–403.

36. Barkovich AJ, Truwit CL. Brain damage from perinatal asphyxia: correlation of MR findings with gestational age. AJNR Am J Neuroradiol 1990;11(6):1087–96.

37. Westmark KD, Barkovich AJ, Sola A, et al. Patterns and implications of MR contrast enhancement in perinatal asphyxia: a preliminary report. AJNR Am J Neuroradiol 1995;16(4):685–92.

38. Bobba PS, Malhotra A, Sheth KN, et al. Brain injury patterns in hypoxic ischemic encephalopathy of term neonates. J Neuroimaging 2023;33(1):79–84.
39. Rutherford M, Pennock J, Schwieso J, et al. Hypoxic-ischaemic encephalopathy: early and late magnetic resonance imaging findings in relation to outcome. Arch Dis Child Fetal Neonatal Ed 1996;75(3):F145–51.
40. Rutherford M, Malamateniou C, McGuinness A, et al. Magnetic resonance imaging in hypoxic-ischaemic encephalopathy. Early Hum Dev 2010;86(6):351–60.
41. Volpe JJ, Pasternak JF. Parasagittal cerebral injury in neonatal hypoxic-ischemic encephalopathy: clinical and neuroradiologic features. J Pediatr 1977;91(3): 472–6.
42. Chalak LF, Nguyen KA, Prempunpong C, et al. Prospective research in infants with mild encephalopathy identified in the first six hours of life: neurodevelopmental outcomes at 18-22 months. Pediatr Res 2018;84(6):861–8.
43. Miller SP, Ramaswamy V, Michelson D, et al. Patterns of brain injury in term neonatal encephalopathy. J Pediatr 2005;146(4):453–60.
44. Lambing H, Gano D, Li Y, et al. Using neonatal magnetic resonance imaging to predict gross motor disability at four years in term-born children with neonatal encephalopathy. Pediatr Neurol 2023;144:50–5.
45. Steinman KJ, Gorno-Tempini ML, Glidden DV, et al. Neonatal watershed brain injury on magnetic resonance imaging correlates with verbal IQ at 4 years. Pediatrics 2009;123(3):1025–30.
46. Rutherford MA, Pennock JM, Counsell SJ, et al. Abnormal magnetic resonance signal in the internal capsule predicts poor neurodevelopmental outcome in infants with hypoxic-ischemic encephalopathy. Pediatrics 1998;102(2 Pt 1):323–8.
47. Cheong JL, Coleman L, Hunt RW, et al. Prognostic utility of magnetic resonance imaging in neonatal hypoxic-ischemic encephalopathy: substudy of a randomized trial. Arch Pediatr Adolesc Med 2012;166(7):634–40.
48. Wu YW, Monsell SE, Glass HC, et al. How well does neonatal neuroimaging correlate with neurodevelopmental outcomes in infants with hypoxic-ischemic encephalopathy? Pediatr Res 2023;94(3):1018–25.
49. Machie M, Weeke L, de Vries LS, et al. MRI score ability to detect abnormalities in mild hypoxic-ischemic encephalopathy. Pediatr Neurol 2021;116:32–8.
50. Ní Bhroin M, Kelly L, Sweetman D, et al. Relationship between MRI scoring systems and neurodevelopmental outcome at two years in infants with neonatal encephalopathy. Pediatr Neurol 2022;126:35–42.
51. Kang OH, Jahn P, Eichhorn JG, et al. Correlation of different mri scoring systems with long-term cognitive outcome in cooled asphyxiated newborns. Children (Basel) 2023;10(8). https://doi.org/10.3390/children10081295.
52. Langeslag JF, Groenendaal F, Roosendaal SD, et al. Outcome prediction and inter-rater comparison of four brain magnetic resonance imaging scoring systems of infants with perinatal asphyxia and therapeutic hypothermia. Neonatology 2022;119(3):311–9.
53. Martinez-Biarge M, Diez-Sebastian J, Kapellou O, et al. Predicting motor outcome and death in term hypoxic-ischemic encephalopathy. Neurology 2011; 76(24):2055–61.
54. Calabrese E, Wu Y, Scheffler AW, et al. Correlating quantitative MRI-based apparent diffusion coefficient metrics with 24-month neurodevelopmental outcomes in neonates from the HEAL trial. Radiology 2023;308(3):e223262.
55. Alderliesten T, de Vries LS, Staats L, et al. MRI and spectroscopy in (near) term neonates with perinatal asphyxia and therapeutic hypothermia. Arch Dis Child Fetal Neonatal Ed 2017;102(2):F147–52.

56. Lally PJ, Montaldo P, Oliveira V, et al. Magnetic resonance spectroscopy assessment of brain injury after moderate hypothermia in neonatal encephalopathy: a prospective multicentre cohort study. Lancet Neurol 2019;18(1):35–45.

57. Shibasaki J, Niwa T, Piedvache A, et al. Comparison of predictive values of magnetic resonance biomarkers based on scan timing in neonatal encephalopathy following therapeutic hypothermia. J Pediatr 2021;239:101–9.e4.

58. Lequin MH, Steggerda SJ, Severino M, et al. Mammillary body injury in neonatal encephalopathy: a multicentre, retrospective study. Pediatr Res 2022;92(1): 174–9.

59. Annink KV, de Vries LS, Groenendaal F, et al. Mammillary body atrophy and other MRI correlates of school-age outcome following neonatal hypoxic-ischemic encephalopathy. Sci Rep 2021;11(1):5017.

60. Spencer APC, Lequin MH, de Vries LS, et al. Mammillary body abnormalities and cognitive outcomes in children cooled for neonatal encephalopathy. Dev Med Child Neurol 2023;65(6):792–802.

61. Parikh NA, Lasky RE, Garza CN, et al. Volumetric and anatomical MRI for hypoxic-ischemic encephalopathy: relationship to hypothermia therapy and neurosensory impairments. J Perinatol 2009;29(2):143–9.

62. Kebaya LMN, Kapoor B, Mayorga PC, et al. Subcortical brain volumes in neonatal hypoxic-ischemic encephalopathy. Pediatr Res 2023;94(5):1797–803.

63. Mulkey SB, Ramakrishnaiah RH, McKinstry RC, et al. Erythropoietin and brain magnetic resonance imaging findings in hypoxic-ischemic encephalopathy: volume of acute brain injury and 1-year neurodevelopmental outcome. J Pediatr 2017;186:196–9.

64. Gano D, Chau V, Poskitt KJ, et al. Evolution of pattern of injury and quantitative MRI on days 1 and 3 in term newborns with hypoxic-ischemic encephalopathy. Pediatr Res 2013;74(1):82–7.

65. Shetty AN, Lucke AM, Liu P, et al. Cerebral oxygen metabolism during and after therapeutic hypothermia in neonatal hypoxic-ischemic encephalopathy: a feasibility study using magnetic resonance imaging. Pediatr Radiol 2019;49(2): 224–33.

66. Wintermark P, Labrecque M, Warfield SK, et al. Can induced hypothermia be assured during brain MRI in neonates with hypoxic-ischemic encephalopathy? Pediatr Radiol 2010;40(12):1950–4.

67. Roychaudhuri S, Ersen Y, El-Dib M, et al. The practicality and utility of early and serial MRI in neonatal encephalopathy undergoing therapeutic hypothermia: a brief report. J Perinatol 2024 (In Press).

68. White YN, Grant PE, Soul JS, et al. Early exit from neonatal therapeutic hypothermia: a single institution experience using MRI to guide decision-making. J Neonatal Perinatal Med 2020;13(4):441–7.

69. Barkovich AJ, Westmark KD, Bedi HS, et al. Proton spectroscopy and diffusion imaging on the first day of life after perinatal asphyxia: preliminary report. AJNR Am J Neuroradiol 2001;22(9):1786–94.

70. Executive summary. Neonatal encephalopathy and neurologic outcome, second edition. Report of the American College of Obstetricians and Gynecologists' task force on neonatal encephalopathy. Obstet Gynecol 2014;123(4):896–901. https://doi.org/10.1097/01.AOG.0000445580.65983.d2.

71. Rollins N, Booth T, Morriss MC, et al. Predictive value of neonatal MRI showing no or minor degrees of brain injury after hypothermia. Pediatr Neurol 2014;50(5): 447–51.

72. Chakkarapani E, Poskitt KJ, Miller SP, et al. Reliability of early magnetic resonance imaging (MRI) and necessity of repeating MRI in noncooled and cooled infants with neonatal encephalopathy. J Child Neurol 2016;31(5):553–9.
73. Charon V, Proisy M, Bretaudeau G, et al. Early MRI in neonatal hypoxic-ischaemic encephalopathy treated with hypothermia: prognostic role at 2-year follow-up. Eur J Radiol 2016;85(8):1366–74.
74. O'Kane A, Vezina G, Chang T, et al. Early versus late brain magnetic resonance imaging after neonatal hypoxic ischemic encephalopathy treated with therapeutic hypothermia. J Pediatr 2021;232:73–9.e2.
75. Wisnowski JL, Wintermark P, Bonifacio SL, et al. Neuroimaging in the term newborn with neonatal encephalopathy. Semin Fetal Neonatal Med 2021;26(5): 101304.
76. Parmentier CEJ, Lequin MH, Alderliesten T, et al. Additional value of 3-month cranial magnetic resonance imaging in infants with neonatal encephalopathy following perinatal asphyxia. J Pediatr 2023;258:113402.

Advances in Electroencephalographic Biomarkers of Neonatal Hypoxic Ischemic Encephalopathy

Jacopo Proietti, MD[a,b], John M. O'Toole, PhD[b,c],
Deirdre M. Murray, MD, PhD[b,d], Geraldine B. Boylan, PhD[b,d,*]

KEYWORDS

- EEG • Neonate • Encephalopathy • Biomarker

KEY POINTS

- Electroencephalography (EEG) is an excellent objective biomarker for hypoxic ischemic encephalopathy (HIE), assisting in the assessment of HIE severity, treatment guidance, seizure detection, and outcome prediction.
- An isoelectric EEG pattern or extreme discontinuity is an early objective biomarker of hypoxia ischemia in a neonate with a history of perinatal asphyxia, and can support selection for neuroprotective treatment.
- Electrographic seizures on the EEG in neonates with HIE are a biomarker of moderate–severe injury.
- Delayed re-emergence of continuous normal voltage EEG patterns (>36 hours) is a biomarker of higher risk for poor outcome.
- Real-time conventional EEG interpretation for nonexperts is a challenge in the neonatal intensive care unit and this is being addressed through the development of quantitative EEG biomarkers and advanced machine learning techniques.

INTRODUCTION

Hypoxia ischemia is the most common cause of newborn encephalopathy (NE) in term newborn infants and despite improvements in outcome with therapeutic hypothermia, it remains a major cause of death and disability in childhood worldwide.[1–3] The pathophysiology and resultant encephalopathy of HIE is dynamic and evolves

[a] Department of Engineering for Innovation Medicine, University of Verona, Strada le Grazie, Verona 37134, Italy; [b] INFANT Research Centre, University College Cork, Cork, Ireland; [c] Cergenx Ltd., Dublin, Ireland; [d] Department of Paediatrics & Child Health, University College Cork, Paediatric Academic Unit, Cork University Hospital, Wilton, Cork, T12 DC4A, Ireland
* Corresponding author. Prof Geraldine B Boylan, INFANT Research Centre and Department of Paediatrics and Child Health, University College Cork, Cork T12 DC4A, Ireland
E-mail address: g.boylan@ucc.ie

Clin Perinatol 51 (2024) 649–663
https://doi.org/10.1016/j.clp.2024.04.006   perinatology.theclinics.com
0095-5108/24/© 2024 Elsevier Inc. All rights reserved, including that for text and data mining, AI training, and similar technologies.

over time, presenting significant difficulties for clinicians who must navigate unique challenges in clinical assessment during rapidly changing phases of disease progression.[4]

Neonatal electroencephalography (EEG) is an important diagnostic tool for the evaluation of neurologic function. It is a noninvasive real-time recording of the electrical activity of the brain using electrodes placed on the scalp. It is particularly useful in neonates, as it provides immediate insights into functional neurologic state. By capturing dynamic changes in brain activity, neonatal EEG plays a vital role in guiding therapeutic interventions, assessing the effectiveness of treatments, and predicting neurodevelopmental outcome. However, conventional multichannel EEG monitoring has not been widely adopted in neonatal intensive care units (NICUs), largely due to resourcing challenges and a lack of available out of hours expertise for real-time interpretation. Amplitude integrated EEG (aEEG), which displays a compressed trend of up to 2 channels of EEG, is more widely used due to ease of interpretation by attending neonatologists, lower cost, and higher availability compared to conventional EEG (cEEG), but it does have limitations.[5–7]

Continuous monitoring with cEEG is, without doubt, the best tool available to provide real-time accurate information about neonatal brain health.[8] It involves the placement of 8 or more active EEG electrodes to the scalp covering frontal, central, temporal, and parietal/occipital regions and can be continued for days depending on requirements. For optimal use in the NICU, real-time interpretation is required. Many units are now doing this remotely on a 24 h basis and in-built algorithms for interpretation are coming on stream. In this review, the authors outline the value of neonatal EEG for neonates with suspected HIE and identify advances in specific EEG biomarkers, both qualitative and quantitative.

ELECTROENCEPHALOGRAPHIC BIOMARKERS FOR GRADING THE SEVERITY OF ENCEPHALOPATHY

On admission to the NICU, a neonate with suspected HIE requires confirmation of the diagnosis by carefully considering all clinical information from pregnancy, delivery, and the early postnatal period. This allows the reasonable exclusion of other potential causes of NE so that a diagnosis of probable HIE can be reached.[9] EEG is an invaluable tool to help support the diagnosis of probable HIE and it is important to refer to studies of healthy term neonates when considering HIE. The EEG of the healthy term newborn is continuous, dominated by frequencies in the delta range (up to 4 Hz) with an average amplitude of 50 μV and has clearly identifiable sleep–wake cycling (SWC), even in the first hours after birth[10] (**Fig. 1**).

The severity of the hypoxic ischemic injury is characterized by the temporal evolution of EEG abnormalities.[11] In animal models of neonatal induced hypoxia ischemia, the insult is followed by suppression of the EEG which is proportional to the intensity and duration of the insult[12,13] (**Fig. 2**). After a severe sustained insult, a profound and prolonged suppression of the EEG is seen, called an isoelectric EEG or flat trace. Less severe and shorter insults may produce less pronounced alteration in amplitude, or discontinuity of the background, with a tendency to recover over a variable period.[14] An isoelectric or excessively discontinuous EEG detected in the earliest hours after birth, when consistent with clinical information, is a valuable biomarker of probable HIE.

Once a diagnosis of probable HIE is confirmed, efforts are then focused on the prevention of further injury. Therapeutic hypothermia, effective in reducing death, and improving neurodevelopmental outcomes in survivors, represents the cornerstone of treatment in HIE.[16] The window of opportunity for effective treatment is narrow,

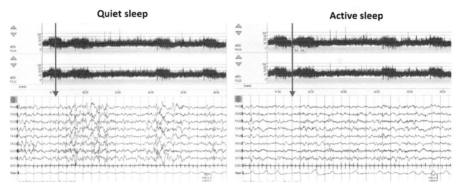

Fig. 1. EEG in a healthy full-term infant within 12 hours of birth.

making it crucial to select which infants are most likely to benefit from treatment quickly.

Clinically, the severity of hypoxic ischemic injury primarily relies on clinical assessment which is better at later timepoints beyond the narrow therapeutic window of 6 hours after birth.[17] The need for complementary methods of assessment in the very early newborn period is well recognized in neonatology. The benefit of EEG for grading the severity of NE early is supported by studies demonstrating a mismatch between clinical grade and EEG grade.[18–20] Clinical grade may underestimate the severity of encephalopathy compared to EEG assessment, and infants with mildly abnormal findings on early neurologic examination but altered EEG patterns can progress to develop acute provoked seizures and abnormalities on MRI.[18,20]

As most EEG assessment in the NICU uses the aEEG trend, simple rules defining what is normal and abnormal have been developed.[21] The altered aEEG patterns considered to indicate moderate or severe encephalopathy are shown in **Fig. 3**. However, the accuracy of aEEG in assessing background activity is lower than conventional EEG, with a higher risk of misinterpretation of findings. Disagreement between individual grades of HIE on the cEEG and aEEG of the same infants has been reported.[5] Muscle activity, interference from the electrocardiogram, high-frequency oscillation, and interelectrode distance can affect the appearance and the interpretation of the aEEG trace. Biological and environmental artifacts in the NICU can produce an elevation of the lower margin of the aEEG lower baseline, and the aEEG can be misinterpreted as being more reassuring than it actually is.[22] Newer digital aEEG machines now display both the impedance and the raw EEG traces, making it possible to inspect the source signal and identify these artifacts.[23]

Conventional EEG monitoring interpreted by a neurophysiologist/board-certified neurologist represents the gold standard for neonatal EEG assessment. Although EEG is better at predicting outcome at later timepoints, it can reliably determine the level of injury within 6 hours and support early management.[14,24] On visual qualitative

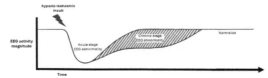

Fig. 2. Changes in EEG activity magnitude seen following an acute hypoxic ischemic insult. (*Adapted from* Kidokoro 2021.[15])

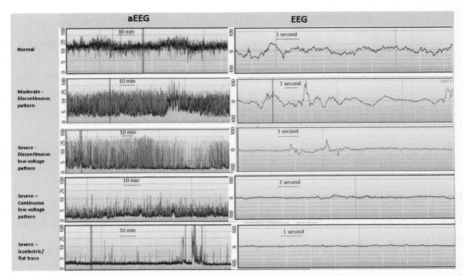

Fig. 3. aEEG patterns from the INNESCO background scale score for grading neonatal encephalopathy.[21] Left shows aEEG examples, right column shows corresponding EEG traces. (*Adapted from* Dilena et al 2021.)

analysis, continuous, symmetric, appropriate amplitude activity with early detectable sleep cycling is recognized as an excellent biomarker of newborn brain health.[10,14] Suppressed or reduced EEG amplitude and discontinuity are biomarkers of encephalopathy secondary to hypoxia ischemia. Nonetheless, how best to accurately grade the EEG in full-term HIE remains unclear.[25] Numerous EEG classification schemes have been published with a varying number of grades, and all incorporate features of amplitude, continuity, symmetry, synchrony, and sleep–wake state but absolute cut-off values for amplitude attenuation and discontinuity differ.[24,26–30] Focal transient waveforms and maturational graphoelements are usually not included in these schemes[28] and descriptions of different grades are subjectively applied. While agreement is high at the extremes of severity, boundaries are blurred for intermediate grades. This ambiguity creates difficulty in interpretation and substantial disagreement even among experienced reviewers.[31] Classifying severity into a restricted number of categories represents a limitation that does not always reflect the continuum of the variability seen in NE (**Fig. 4**).

Furthermore, access to conventional EEG monitoring and the expertise required for interpretation is frequently not available, particularly in the earliest hours immediately after birth. This is the case, for example, at small peripheral units with long transfer times to a tertiary level center. Efforts have been made to develop easy to use EEG sensors, suitable for neonates to enable real-time EEG monitoring with automated or centralized review.[32,33] This will make EEG monitoring more widely available in health care settings.[34]

ELECTROENCEPHALOGRAPHIC BIOMARKERS OF SEIZURES IN HYPOXIC ISCHEMIC ENCEPHALOPATHY

Neonates with HIE are at risk of developing acute provoked seizures and EEG is essential for accurate diagnosis, especially in HIE where many seizures are

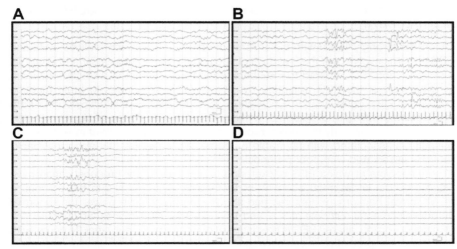

Fig. 4. Background EEG severity.[24] Grade 1—mild abnormalities: the EEG shows some periods of reduced amplitude but continuous activity; sleep cycling is not clearly evident (A). Grade 2—moderate abnormalities: the EEG is discontinuous with interburst periods of flattening less than 10 seconds (B). Grade 3—severe abnormalities: the EEG is highly discontinuous with interburst intervals of 10 to 60 seconds (C). Grade 4—isoelectric: EEG is fully suppressed with no activity above 10 μV or interburst intervals longer than 60 seconds (D).

electrographic only (no clinical expression).[35–37] In the era of hypothermia, the incidence of neonatal seizures has not changed although the overall seizure burden has reduced.[38,39] Seizures represent a symptom of ongoing encephalopathy, and have an independent negative effect on neurodevelopment, with higher seizure burden associated with poorer outcomes.[40–44] Their prompt detection and adequate treatment has the potential to reduce the consequences of encephalopathy.[37,45] EEG plays a role in predicting the risk for seizures and allows for their accurate diagnosis and management.[46–48]

Literature on the temporal characteristic of neonatal seizures has flourished in recent years: the median age at seizure onset in HIE is between 12 and 24 hours of age in most studies, with periods of higher seizure risk in the first 24 to 36 hours and during and after rewarming.[49–53] In addition, the severity of early background abnormalities may predict which neonates will develop seizures,[46] and seizure prediction models combining early EEG background features with readily available clinical data can quantify the risk of seizures hours before they occur and is a useful biomarker.[48,54] This can direct the attention of clinicians and optimize allocation of available resources, allowing targeted EEG monitoring. Automated quantitative EEG (qEEG) background analysis has proved to be as reliable as expert qualitative analysis for predicting seizures, supporting the use of automated assessment tools as biomarkers for early evaluation of HIE, which may have a significant impact for units with less neurophysiology support.[48]

Continuous conventional EEG monitoring represents the gold standard for diagnosing seizures by virtue of the higher spatial and temporal resolution provided compared to the aEEG.[55] It outperforms clinical and aEEG assessment for seizure detection.[56,57] Given the prevalence of seizures during or after rewarming and evidence of their further impact on outcome,[21,52,53] EEG monitoring should continue for up to 24 hours after completion of hypothermia.[21]

ELECTROENCEPHALOGRAPHIC BIOMARKERS OF PROGNOSIS IN HYPOXIC ISCHEMIC ENCEPHALOPATHY

Outcome is strongly linked with the severity of detected EEG abnormalities. EEG and aEEG patterns evolve over the first days of age and the timing of assessment is crucial to interpretation.[25] Compared to EEG background assessment at a single timepoint, the evaluation of the EEG trajectory over time, reflects changes in brain function and helps guide prognostication. EEGs showing normal features within 6 hours of birth are associated with normal outcome. Among neonates with altered background activity on the EEG at an early timepoint, rapid recovery with improvement in voltage and continuity is associated with favorable outcome, while persistently abnormal background is associated with poor prognosis.[43,58]

The timepoints at which EEG background is most useful for prognostication have shifted after the widespread adoption of therapeutic hypothermia. In the precooling era, abnormal background features had shown good predictive power for abnormal neurodevelopmental outcome at 3, 6, and 12 hours after birth, highest at 24 hours.[24,59] In the era of cooling, altered EEG is predictive of poor prognosis only after 24 hours, with highest negative predictive values between 36 and 72 hours.[35,43,58,60] In various studies, the time required to regain continuous background voltage has been highlighted as the best predictor of later neurologic outcome, and neonates who never revert to normal background patterns on EEG have the poorest outcomes.[30,43,61–63] The longer time required by infants that are cooled with good outcome to reach a normal background pattern is partially explained by the effectiveness of hypothermia in reducing the severity of the insult, and possibly due to additional sedative treatment used during hypothermia. A large meta-analysis on the ability of EEG background patterns to anticipate abnormal neurodevelopmental outcome identified discontinuous pattern, low voltage, and flat tracings as the most predictive biomarkers for outcome.[64] However, variability exists between published studies in the definitions used for these background patterns, with different amplitude and duration cut-offs resulting in differing sensitivity and specificity.

Latency to the appearance of SWC also reflects the severity of the encephalopathy and has a predictive value as a biomarker for neurodevelopmental outcome.[24,58] A longer time to onset of SWC has been reported in hypothermia-treated infants compared to nontreated. At the same time, more uncooled neonates than hypothermia-treated never developed SWC, which strongly predicts a poorer outcome, supporting evidence of efficacy of treatment.[60] Even though the time of onset of SWC and time to continuity and voltage recovery tend to correlate, the latter seems to be a better marker for predicting a good outcome. This is suggested by studies reporting normal outcome in infants with early continuity and voltage recovery, despite delayed development of SWC during EEG monitoring.[65]

TRANSLATION OF NEONATAL ELECTROENCEPHALOGRAPHY BIOMARKERS IN THE NEONATAL INTENSIVE CARE UNIT

Despite the usefulness of EEG biomarkers for HIE, their real-time application in neonatal care is hindered by the scarcity of experts, especially out of hours. Efforts are now focused on leveraging qEEG and machine learning (ML) for automated analysis. We now discuss leading qEEG biomarkers for HIE and recent advances in ML.

QUANTITATIVE ELECTROENCEPHALOGRAPHY BIOMARKERS

qEEG uses mathematical measures to summarize EEG characteristics. Advances in signal processing have enabled more sophisticated techniques, that are better suited to neonatal EEG and HIE.[66,67] In contrast to the visual interpretation of the EEG, qEEG features are objective, repeatable, and scalable. EEG is filtered into frequency bands to calculate features like absolute and relative spectral power, capturing EEG power within and between frequency bands (**Fig. 5**). Given the complexity of the EEG, multiple qEEG features, rather than individual features, are required to adequately summarize broad characteristics of the EEG.[66]

qEEG features can be displayed in commercial EEG review software alongside the EEG.[67] The qEEG features are calculated over a short segment of time, (typically tens of seconds), and then compressed and displayed as a trend over hours of EEG recording. A common qEEG feature in review software is the spectrogram, a display of time-varying spectral power. Displaying qEEG features in addition to the raw EEG can assist in the review of the EEG.[68,69] A recent study of qEEG in the pediatric-ICU found that although many centers do use qEEG in review software, many found that the lack of understanding and lack of standardization of qEEG features were a barrier to widespread clinical use.[69]

qEEG has proven useful to advance our understanding of encephalopathy.[14] By summarizing the main attributes of EEG, qEEG can be used to compare different cohorts, for example, to find differences in the EEG for differing grades of HIE. Another active area of research for qEEG, is the study of connectivity in cortical electrophysiology.[70] This is achieved by developing and applying qEEG measures of connectivity between the channels of EEG to provide insight into the activity of cortical networks.

qEEG features are ideally suited as potential biomarkers of HIE (**Fig. 6**). **Table 1** lists more recent qEEG studies in HIE.

MACHINE LEARNING AND DEEP LEARNING BIOMARKERS

A major limitation of qEEG features as biomarkers is the difficulty in selecting the most appropriate features to use. A lack of standard definitions for something as simple as spectral power, for example, can make it difficult to compare research studies or develop trust in clinical applications.[66,69,82,83] The other challenge with multiple features is how to combine them to best represent neonatal EEG, as the goal of qEEG is to summarize the EEG, not to further complicate it.

ML methods combine qEEG features using a data-driven approach. ML models are developed through a training process with classification labels, such as EEG grades of

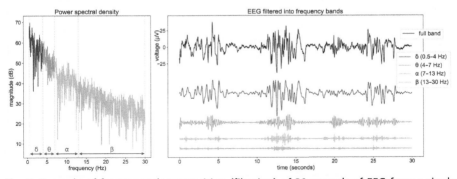

Fig. 5. Example of frequency decomposition (filtering) of 30 seconds of EEG from a single channel (F3–C3). Left: power spectral density of the signal, highlighting the different frequency bands: delta (δ), theta (θ), alpha (α), and beta (β). Right: the signal before and after filtering in the different bands.

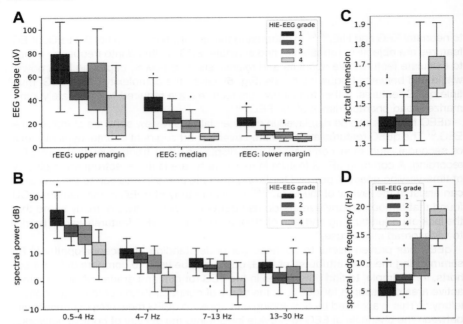

Fig. 6. Difference in qEEG features for different EEG grades of HIE. Features of peak-to-peak amplitude in (*A*) as measured by range EEG, an alternate standardized measure of aEEG; spectral power at different frequency bands in (*B*); and features of fractal dimension in (*C*) and spectral edge frequency in (*D*). " ◆ " Outliers as estimated by the box-plot algorithm. (Adapted with permission from O'Toole et al.[71])

HIE. Feature selection methods, again driven by the data, decide on which features to keep and which to discard. Certain ML methods are robust to features with low predictive value, enabling inclusion of extensive feature sets. This approach allows the ML model to capture the most relevant features for the predictive task.

Table 1
Examples of recent qEEG analysis for neonates with HIE

Author	qEEG Features
Govindan et al,[72] 2017	Spectral power
Kota et al,[73] 2021	Spectral power
Zhang et al,[74] 2021	Spectral power and coherence analysis
Lacan et al,[75] 2021	Spectral power, aEEG, spectral distribution, and burst–suppression ratio
Garvey et al,[14] 2021	NEURAL qEEG feature set—amplitude, spectral distribution, and interhemispheric coherence
Bakheet et al,[76] 2021	Spectral entropy and connectivity (weighted phase–lag index)
Wang et al,[77] 2022; Wang et al,[78] 2022	Phase–amplitude coupling
Keene et al,[67] 2023	Ultra-slow wave (<0.01 Hz) amplitude modulation
O'Toole et al,[71] 2023	NEURAL qEEG feature set—multiple features
Alotaibi et al,[79] 2022	Spectral entropy and connectivity (weighted phase–lag index)
Kim et al,[80] 2022	sLORETA software—low-resolution tomography
Khazaei et al,[70] 2023	Connectivity analysis
Syvälahti et al,[81] 2023	Connectivity analysis

One of the first studies to employ an ML approach to neonatal qEEG was Löfhede and colleagues[84] The authors developed ML models to classify sleep states and burst suppression, comparing a cohort of neonates with birth asphyxia with a healthy control group. Stevenson and colleagues[85] developed an ML classifier to distinguish 4 grades of EEG background activity in a cohort with HIE. Ahmed and colleagues[86] updated this approach by using a different feature set and ML model, with improved results. They also produced a prototype for how the 4-class classifier could be used as a continuous trend over time. Matic and colleagues[87] developed a method with adaptive segmentation, feature extraction, and tensor decomposition to generate a feature set for an ML model. This model was trained as 3-class classifier for background EEG grades in a cohort with HIE. The authors also developed an ML method to extract interburst intervals for grading the EEG.[88] Guo and colleagues[89] and Moghadam and colleagues[90] used qEEG features with an ML model to classify background EEG activity.

More recent background grading studies have applied deep learning (DL) methods.[91–93] DL is a type of ML that eliminates the need for designing and selecting qEEG features. DL methods perform *end-to-end* learning which means the raw EEG and not qEEG features are used to train a classification model. The DL methods then internally generate the features. The main advantage is that this further optimizes the training process which enables more accurate classification models. In almost every other scientific discipline, given sufficient labeled data, DL methods outperform ML methods.

Following the example of Ahmed and colleagues,[86] 2 background grading methods have developed a continuous-valued output score to reflect an estimate of the severity of background abnormalities.[92,93] These continuous-valued scores could be used to assess the temporal evolution of the EEG over time, as other qEEG trends do. O'Sullivan and colleagues[93] updated a previous DL method[91] to output a continuous-value representing the grade of EEG. The approach by Moghadam and colleagues[92] incorporated a sleep-staging algorithm, allowing the trend to oscillate in the presence of sleep–wake cycling. The trend, known as the brain state of the newborn, includes a confidence interval to present more information to enhance clinical decision-making. The trend compared favorably to the aEEG for identifying continuity and SWC. The algorithm is available for research use from a cloud-hosted service called the BabaCloud.[92]

A limitation of all qEEG analysis, including ML and DL methods, is the potential for EEG artifacts to confound analysis. However, methods have been developed that automatically detect multiple types of artifacts associated with neonatal EEG[93,94] and these algorithm can serve as pre- or post-processing for ML/DL methods.93

Despite concerns about their opacity, DL methods surpass current qEEG analysis in capturing essential EEG characteristics effectively. qEEG methods often provide limited insights and can be complex, making DL models a promising alternative for future EEG analysis despite their "black box" nature.

SUMMARY

EEG serves as an excellent objective biomarker of hypoxic ischemic encephalopathy, aiding in assessing severity, guiding treatment, detecting seizures, and predicting outcomes. Neonatal EEG interpretation challenges for nonexperts are mitigated by promising qEEG biomarkers and advanced ML techniques. Some of these innovations are already applied cot-side in NICUs, and further advances in artificial intelligence for automated, continuous EEG interpretation for neonates with HIE are anticipated.

DISCLOSURE

D.M. Murray is the founder of Liltoda Ltd. G.B. Boylan has a consultancy with Nihon Kohden; she is co-founder of Kephala Ltd and CergenX Ltd. J.M. O'Toole is an employee of CergenX Ltd.

Best Practices

- EEG monitoring should be instigated as soon as possible in neonates with clinical encephalopathy. In HIE this should continue for up to 24 hours after completion of hypothermia.
- Conventional EEG is the gold standard for neonatal monitoring in HIE and should be implemented where possible.
- Real-time EEG interpretation must be provided by experienced neonatal neurophysiologists/ neurologists, in-house or remotely through telemedicine strategies.
- Innovative digital EEG and machine learning tools, which allow automated seizure detection and grading of background EEG abnormalities are now available for use at the cot-side and can enhance clinical decision-making.

REFERENCES

1. Azzopardi D, Strohm B, Marlow N, et al. Effects of hypothermia for perinatal asphyxia on childhood outcomes. N Engl J Med 2014;371(2):140–9.
2. Pappas A, Milano G, Chalak LF. Hypoxic-ischemic encephalopathy: changing outcomes across the spectrum. Clin Perinatol 2023;50(1):31–52.
3. Steinmetz JD, Seeher KM, Schiess N, et al. Global, regional, and national burden of disorders affecting the nervous system, 1990–2021: a systematic analysis for the Global Burden of Disease Study 2021. Lancet Neurol 2024;23(4):344–81.
4. Davidson JO, Gonzalez F, Gressens P, et al. Update on mechanisms of the pathophysiology of neonatal encephalopathy. Semin Fetal Neonatal Med 2021;26(5): 101267.
5. Evans E, Koh S, Lerner J, et al. Accuracy of amplitude integrated EEG in a neonatal cohort. Arch Dis Child Fetal Neonatal Ed 2010;95(3):F169–73.
6. Rakshasbhuvankar A, Paul S, Nagarajan L, et al. Amplitude-integrated EEG for detection of neonatal seizures: a systematic review. Seizure 2015;33:90–8.
7. Sakpichaisakul K, El-Dib M, Munster C, et al. Amplitude-integrated electroencephalography evolution and magnetic resonance imaging injury in mild and moderate to severe neonatal encephalopathy. Am J Perinatol 2023. https://doi. org/10.1055/a-2118-2953.
8. El-Dib M, Abend NS, Austin T, et al. Neuromonitoring in neonatal critical care part I: neonatal encephalopathy and neonates with possible seizures. Pediatr Res 2023;94(1):64–73.
9. Gunn AJ, Soul JS, Vesoulis ZA, et al. The importance of not increasing confusion around neonatal encephalopathy and hypoxic-ischemic encephalopathy. Pediatr Res 2024;95(4):871–2.
10. Korotchikova I, Connolly S, Ryan C, et al. EEG in the healthy term newborn within 12 hours of birth. Clin Neurophysiol 2009;120(6):1046–53.
11. Gunn AJ, Thoresen M. Neonatal encephalopathy and hypoxic–ischemic encephalopathy. Handb Clin Neurol 2019;162:217–37.
12. Zayachkivsky A, Lehmkuhle MJ, Ekstrand JJ, et al. Background suppression of electrical activity is a potential biomarker of subsequent brain injury in a rat model of neonatal hypoxia-ischemia. J Neurophysiol 2022;128(1):118–30.

13. Lacan L, Garabedian C, De Jonckheere J, et al. Fetal brain response to worsening acidosis: an experimental study in a fetal sheep model of umbilical cord occlusions. Sci Rep 2023;13(1):23050.

14. Garvey AA, Pavel AM, O'Toole JM, et al. Multichannel EEG abnormalities during the first 6 hours in infants with mild hypoxic–ischaemic encephalopathy. Pediatr Res 2021;90(1):117–24.

15. Kidokoro H. Delta brushes are not just a hallmark of EEG in human preterm infants. Pediatr Int 2021;63(2):130–6.

16. Jacobs S, Hunt R, Tarnow-Mordi W, et al. Cooling for newborns with hypoxic ischaemic encephalopathy. Pediatr Res 2005;58(2):385.

17. Sarnat HB, Sarnat MS. Neonatal encephalopathy following fetal distress: a clinical and electroencephalographic study. Arch Neurol 1976;33(10):696–705.

18. Gagne-Loranger M, Sheppard M, Ali N, et al. Newborns referred for therapeutic hypothermia: association between initial degree of encephalopathy and severity of brain injury (what about the newborns with mild encephalopathy on admission?). Am J Perinatol 2016;33(02):195–202.

19. Weeke LC, Vilan A, Toet MC, et al. A comparison of the Thompson encephalopathy score and amplitude-integrated electroencephalography in infants with perinatal asphyxia and therapeutic hypothermia. Neonatology 2017;112(1):24–9.

20. Natarajan N, Benedetti G, Perez FA, et al. Association between early EEG background and outcomes in infants with mild HIE undergoing therapeutic hypothermia. Pediatr Neurol 2022;134:52–8.

21. Dilena R, Raviglione F, Cantalupo G, et al. Consensus protocol for EEG and amplitude-integrated EEG assessment and monitoring in neonates. Clin Neurophysiol 2021;132(4):886–903.

22. De Vries L, Hellström-Westas L. Role of cerebral function monitoring in the newborn. Arch Dis Child Fetal Neonatal Ed 2005;90(3): F201–FF207.

23. de Vries LS, Toet MC. How to assess the aEEG background. J Pediatr 2009; 154(4):625–6.

24. Murray DM, Boylan GB, Ryan CA, et al. Early EEG findings in hypoxic-ischemic encephalopathy predict outcomes at 2 years. Pediatrics 2009;124(3):e459–67.

25. Walsh B, Murray D, Boylan G. The use of conventional EEG for the assessment of hypoxic ischaemic encephalopathy in the newborn: a review. Clin Neurophysiol 2011;122(7):1284–94.

26. Van Lieshout H, Jacobs J, Rotteveel J, et al. The prognostic value of the EEG in asphyxiated newborns. Acta Neurol Scand 1995;91(3):203–7.

27. Selton D, Andre M. Prognosis of hypoxic-ischaemic encephalopathy in full-term newborns-value of neonatal electroencephalography. Neuropediatrics 1997; 28(05):276–80.

28. Tsuchida TN, Wusthoff CJ, Shellhaas RA, et al. American clinical neurophysiology society standardized EEG terminology and categorization for the description of continuous EEG monitoring in neonates: report of the American Clinical Neurophysiology Society critical care monitoring committee. J Clin Neurophysiol 2013;30(2):161–73.

29. Lamblin M-D, Esquivel EW, Andre M. The electroencephalogram of the full-term newborn: review of normal features and hypoxic-ischemic encephalopathy patterns. Neurophysiologie Clinique/Clinical Neurophysiology 2013;43(5–6):267–87.

30. Glass HC, Numis AL, Comstock BA, et al. Association of EEG background and neurodevelopmental outcome in neonates with hypoxic-ischemic encephalopathy Receiving hypothermia. Neurology 2023;101(22):e2223–33.

31. Wusthoff CJ, Sullivan J, Glass HC, et al. Interrater agreement in the interpretation of neonatal electroencephalography in hypoxic-ischemic encephalopathy. Epilepsia 2017;58(3):429–35.
32. Ibrahim Z, Chari G, Abdel Baki S, et al. Wireless multichannel electroencephalography in the newborn. J Neonatal Perinat Med 2016;9(4):341–8.
33. Poveda J, O'Sullivan M, Popovici E, et al. Portable neonatal EEG monitoring and sonification on an Android device. Int Conf IEEE Eng Med Bio (EMBC) 2017;2018–21.
34. Variane GFT, Dahlen A, Pietrobom RFR, et al. Remote monitoring for seizures during therapeutic hypothermia in neonates with hypoxic-ischemic encephalopathy. JAMA Netw Open 2023;6(11):e2343429.
35. Nash K, Bonifacio S, Glass H, et al. Video-EEG monitoring in newborns with hypoxic-ischemic encephalopathy treated with hypothermia. Neurology 2011; 76(6):556–62.
36. Cornet MC, Morabito V, Lederer D, et al. Neonatal presentation of genetic epilepsies: early differentiation from acute provoked seizures. Epilepsia 2021; 62(8):1907–20.
37. Pavel AM, Rennie JM, de Vries LS, et al. Neonatal seizure management: is the timing of treatment critical? J Pediatr 2022;243:61–8. e2.
38. Low E, Boylan GB, Mathieson SR, et al. Cooling and seizure burden in term neonates: an observational study. Arch Dis Child Fetal Neonatal Ed 2012;97(4): F267–72.
39. Srinivasakumar P, Zempel J, Wallendorf M, et al. Therapeutic hypothermia in neonatal hypoxic ischemic encephalopathy: electrographic seizures and magnetic resonance imaging evidence of injury. J Pediatr 2013;163(2):465–70.
40. Kharoshankaya L, Stevenson NJ, Livingstone V, et al. Seizure burden and neurodevelopmental outcome in neonates with hypoxic–ischemic encephalopathy. Dev Med Child Neurol 2016;58(12):1242–8.
41. Fitzgerald MP, Massey SL, Fung FW, et al. High electroencephalographic seizure exposure is associated with unfavorable outcomes in neonates with hypoxic-ischemic encephalopathy. Seizure 2018;61:221–6.
42. Alharbi HM, Pinchefsky EF, Tran MA, et al. Seizure burden and neurologic outcomes after neonatal encephalopathy. Neurology 2023;100(19):e1976–84.
43. Bourel-Ponchel E, Querne L, Flamein F, et al. The prognostic value of neonatal conventional-EEG monitoring in hypoxic-ischemic encephalopathy during therapeutic hypothermia. Dev Med Child Neurol 2023;65(1):58–66.
44. Trowbridge SK, Condie LO, Landers JR, et al. Effect of neonatal seizure burden and etiology on the long-term outcome: data from a randomized, controlled trial. Annals of the Child Neurology Society 2023;1(1):53–65.
45. Numis AL, Glass HC, Comstock BA, et al. Relationship of neonatal seizure burden before treatment and response to initial Antiseizure Medication. J Pediatr 2024;268:113957.
46. Glass HC, Wusthoff CJ, Shellhaas RA, et al. Risk factors for EEG seizures in neonates treated with hypothermia: a multicenter cohort study. Neurology 2014; 82(14):1239–44.
47. Benedetti GM, Vartanian RJ, McCaffery H, et al. Early electroencephalogram background could guide Tailored duration of monitoring for neonatal encephalopathy treated with therapeutic hypothermia. J Pediatr 2020;221:81–7.e1.
48. Pavel AM, O'Toole JM, Proietti J, et al. Machine learning for the early prediction of infants with electrographic seizures in neonatal hypoxic-ischemic encephalopathy. Epilepsia 2023;64(2):456–68.

49. Shah DK, Wusthoff CJ, Clarke P, et al. Electrographic seizures are associated with brain injury in newborns undergoing therapeutic hypothermia. Arch Dis Child Fetal Neonatal Ed 2014;99(3):F219–24.

50. Mahfooz N, Weinstock A, Afzal B, et al. Optimal duration of continuous video-electroencephalography in term infants with hypoxic-ischemic encephalopathy and therapeutic hypothermia. J Child Neurol 2017;32(6):522–7.

51. Rennie JM, de Vries LS, Blennow M, et al. Characterisation of neonatal seizures and their treatment using continuous EEG monitoring: a multicentre experience. Arch Dis Child Fetal Neonatal Ed 2019;104(5): F493–f501.

52. Chalak LF, Pappas A, Tan S, et al. Association between increased seizures during rewarming after hypothermia for neonatal hypoxic ischemic encephalopathy and abnormal neurodevelopmental outcomes at 2-year follow-up: a nested multisite cohort study. JAMA Neurol 2021;78(12):1484–93.

53. Pavel AM, Rennie JM, de Vries LS, et al. Temporal evolution of electrographic seizures in newborn infants with hypoxic-ischaemic encephalopathy requiring therapeutic hypothermia: a secondary analysis of the ANSeR studies. Lancet Child Adolesc Health 2024;8(3):214–24.

54. Sansevere AJ, Kapur K, Peters JM, et al. Seizure prediction models in the neonatal intensive care Unit. J Clin Neurophysiol 2019;36(3):186–94.

55. Shellhaas RA, Chang T, Tsuchida T, et al. The American clinical neurophysiology Society's Guideline on continuous electroencephalography monitoring in neonates. J Clin Neurophysiol 2011;28(6):611–7.

56. Shellhaas RA, Soaita AI, Clancy RR. Sensitivity of amplitude-integrated electroencephalography for neonatal seizure detection. Pediatrics 2007;120(4):770–7.

57. Murray DM, Boylan GB, Ali I, et al. Defining the gap between electrographic seizure burden, clinical expression and staff recognition of neonatal seizures. Arch Dis Child Fetal Neonatal Ed 2008;93(3):F187–91.

58. Sewell EK, Vezina G, Chang T, et al. Evolution of amplitude-integrated electroencephalogram as a predictor of outcome in term encephalopathic neonates Receiving therapeutic hypothermia. Am J Perinatol 2018;35(3):277–85.

59. Hellström-Westas L, Rosen I, Svenningsen NW. Predictive value of early continuous amplitude integrated EEG recordings on outcome after severe birth asphyxia in full term infants. Arch Dis Child Fetal Neonatal Ed 1995;72(1):F34–8.

60. Thoresen M, Hellström-Westas L, Liu X, et al. Effect of hypothermia on amplitude-integrated electroencephalogram in infants with asphyxia. Pediatrics 2010; 126(1):e131–9.

61. Weeke LC, Boylan GB, Pressler RM, et al. Role of EEG background activity, seizure burden and MRI in predicting neurodevelopmental outcome in full-term infants with hypoxic-ischaemic encephalopathy in the era of therapeutic hypothermia. Eur J Paediatr Neurol 2016;20(6):855–64.

62. Chandrasekaran M, Chaban B, Montaldo P, et al. Predictive value of amplitude-integrated EEG (aEEG) after rescue hypothermic neuroprotection for hypoxic ischemic encephalopathy: a meta-analysis. J Perinatol 2017;37(6):684–9.

63. Ouwehand S, Smidt LC, Dudink J, et al. Predictors of outcomes in hypoxic-ischemic encephalopathy following hypothermia: a meta-analysis. Neonatology 2020;117(4):411–27.

64. Awal MA, Lai MM, Azemi G, et al. EEG background features that predict outcome in term neonates with hypoxic ischaemic encephalopathy: a structured review. Clin Neurophysiol 2016;127(1):285–96.

65. Nyman J, Mikkonen K, Metsäranta M, et al. Poor aEEG background recovery after perinatal hypoxic ischemic encephalopathy predicts postneonatal epilepsy by age 4 years. Clin Neurophysiol 2022;143:116–23.

66. Toole J.M., Boylan G.B., NEURAL: quantitative features for newborn EEG using Matlab. *arXiv preprint arXiv*:1704.05694. 2017.

67. Keene JC, Benedetti GM, Tomko SR, et al. Quantitative EEG in the neonatal intensive care unit: current application and future promise. Annals of the Child Neurology Society 2023;1(4):289–98.

68. Haider HA, Esteller R, Hahn CD, et al. Sensitivity of quantitative EEG for seizure identification in the intensive care unit. Neurology 2016;87(9):935–44.

69. Benedetti GM, Morgan LA, Sansevere AJ, et al. The spectrum of quantitative EEG Utilization across North America: a Cross-Sectional Survey. Pediatr Neurol 2023; 141:1–8.

70. Khazaei M, Raeisi K, Vanhatalo S, et al. Neonatal cortical activity organizes into transient network states that are affected by vigilance states and brain injury. NeuroImage 2023;279:120342.

71. O'Toole JM, Mathieson SR, Raurale SA, et al. Neonatal EEG graded for severity of background abnormalities in hypoxic-ischaemic encephalopathy. Sci Data 2023; 10(1):129.

72. Govindan RB, Massaro A, Vezina G, et al. Does relative or absolute EEG power have prognostic value in HIE setting? Clin Neurophysiol 2017;128(1):14.

73. Kota S, Jasti K, Liu Y, et al. EEG spectral power: a proposed physiological biomarker to classify the hypoxic-ischemic encephalopathy severity in real time. Pediatr Neurol 2021;122:7–14.

74. Zhang Q, Hu Y, Dong X, et al. Clinical significance of electroencephalography power spectrum density and functional connection analysis in neonates with hypoxic-ischemic encephalopathy. Int J Dev Neurosci 2021;81(2):142–50.

75. Lacan L, Betrouni N, Lamblin M-D, et al. Quantitative approach to early neonatal EEG visual analysis in hypoxic-ischemic encephalopathy severity: Bridging the gap between eyes and machine. Neurophysiol Clin 2021;51(2):121–31.

76. Bakheet D, Alotaibi N, Konn D, et al. Prediction of cerebral palsy in newborns with hypoxic-ischemic encephalopathy using multivariate EEG analysis and machine learning. IEEE Access 2021;9:137833–46.

77. Wang X, Liu H, Kota S, et al. EEG phase-amplitude coupling to stratify encephalopathy severity in the developing brain. Comput Methods Programs Biomed 2022;214:106593.

78. Wang X, Liu H, Ortigoza EB, et al. Feasibility of EEG phase-amplitude coupling to stratify encephalopathy severity in neonatal HIE using short time window. Brain Sci 2022;12(7). https://doi.org/10.3390/brainsci12070854.

79. Alotaibi N, Bakheet D, Konn D, et al. Cognitive outcome prediction in infants with neonatal hypoxic-ischemic encephalopathy based on functional connectivity and complexity of the electroencephalography signal. Front Hum Neurosci 2022;15: 795006.

80. Kim KY, Lee J-Y, Moon J-U, et al. Comparative analysis of background EEG activity based on MRI findings in neonatal hypoxic-ischemic encephalopathy: a standardized, low-resolution, brain electromagnetic tomography (sLORETA) study. BMC Neurol 2022;22(1):204.

81. Syvälahti T, Tuiskula A, Nevalainen P, et al. Networks of cortical activity show graded responses to perinatal asphyxia. Pediatr Res 2023;1–9.

82. O'Toole JM, Boylan GB. Quantitative preterm EEG analysis: the need for caution in using modern data science techniques. Front Pediatr 2019;7:174.

83. Roychaudhuri S, Hannon K, Sunwoo J, et al. Quantitative EEG and prediction of outcome in neonatal encephalopathy: a review. Pediatr Res 2024;1–8.
84. Löfhede J, Thordstein M, Löfgren N, et al. Automatic classification of background EEG activity in healthy and sick neonates. J Neural Eng 2010;7(1):016007.
85. Stevenson N, Korotchikova I, Temko A, et al. An automated system for grading EEG abnormality in term neonates with hypoxic-ischaemic encephalopathy. Ann Biomed Eng 2013;41:775–85.
86. Ahmed R, Temko A, Marnane W, et al. Grading hypoxic–ischemic encephalopathy severity in neonatal EEG using GMM supervectors and the support vector machine. Clin Neurophysiol 2016;127(1):297–309.
87. Matic V, Cherian PJ, Koolen N, et al. Holistic approach for automated background EEG assessment in asphyxiated full-term infants. J Neural Eng 2014;11(6): 066007.
88. Matić V, Cherian PJ, Jansen K, et al. Improving reliability of monitoring background EEG dynamics in asphyxiated infants. IEEE Trans Biomed Eng 2015; 63(5):973–83.
89. Guo J, Cheng X, Wu D. Grading method for hypoxic-ischemic encephalopathy based on neonatal EEG. Comput Model Eng Sci 2020;122(2):721–42.
90. Moghadam SM, Pinchefsky E, Tse I, et al. Building an open source classifier for the neonatal EEG background: a systematic feature-based approach from expert scoring to clinical visualization. Front Hum Neurosci 2021;15:675154.
91. Raurale SA, Boylan GB, Mathieson SR, et al. Grading hypoxic-ischemic encephalopathy in neonatal EEG with convolutional neural networks and quadratic time–frequency distributions. J Neural Eng 2021;18(4):046007.
92. Moghadam SM, Airaksinen M, Nevalainen P, et al. An automated bedside measure for monitoring neonatal cortical activity: a supervised deep learning-based electroencephalogram classifier with external cohort validation. The Lancet Digital Health 2022;4(12):e884–92.
93. O'Sullivan ME, Lightbody G, Mathieson SR, et al. Development of an EEG artefact detection algorithm and its application in grading neonatal hypoxic-ischemic encephalopathy. Expert Syst Appl 2023;213:118917.
94. Webb L, Kauppila M, Roberts JA, et al. Automated detection of artefacts in neonatal EEG with residual neural networks. Comput Methods Programs Biomed 2021;208:106194.

Moving the Needle in Low-Resource Settings
Is Hypothermia a Friend or a Foe?

Reema Garegrat, MD, DNB, MRCPCH, Constance Burgod, MRes, PhD,
Pallavi Muraleedharan, MHA, PhD, Sudhin Thayyil, MD, FRCPCH, PhD*

KEYWORDS

- Neonatal encephalopathy • Hypothermia • Magnetic resonance imaging • Mortality

KEY POINTS

- Neonates with hypoxic-ischemic encephalopathy in low resource settings often have short birth depression and different whole genome expression profile from those in high-income countries.
- Although several pilot randomized controlled trials reported benefits, unequivocal evidence from the largest hypothermia trial in the world reports lack of hypothermia neuroprotection and increased mortality in low resource settings.
- Nonacute or distal nature of fetal hypoxia-ischemia may explain lack of hypothermic neuroprotection.
- Careful patient selection and strict adherence to National Neonatology forum guidelines are important prevent harm from induced hypothermia.

INTRODUCTION

Around 2 to 3 million neonates sustain birth-related brain injury or hypoxic ischemic encephalopathy (HIE) every year. At least 30% of these neonates die soon after birth and over 50% of the survivors develop life-changing neurodisabilities including cerebral palsy, deafness, and blindness. Sub-Saharan Africa and South Asia shoulder the highest disease burden of HIE.[1,2] Total disability-adjusted life years, a composite score of years of life lost due to premature mortality and years of healthy life lost due to disability, attributable to HIE in India alone was 7.9 million in 2019, accounting for 60% of the burden among top 10 countries.[3] A recent study estimated the economic value from lost productivity due to HIE at USD63 billion, underscoring the substantial financial and human costs incurred by individuals, health systems, and other

Department of Brain Sciences, Centre for Perinatal Neuroscience, Imperial College London, Du Cane Road, London W12 0NN, UK
* Corresponding author.
E-mail address: s.thayyil@imperial.ac.uk

social support systems given the persistent nature of these disabilities over the lifespan.[4]

Traditionally most of the preclinical and clinical research on HIE is conducted in high-income country (HIC) settings with low disease burden, while the research in low-income and middle-income countries (LMICs) with high disease burden has been rightly focused on the implementation of these research findings and the improvement of health systems. Given the scarcity of resources, such models have several advantages in many situations. However, in this review, we discuss the harms of conducting clinical research in low-burden settings and implementing these in high-burden settings using induced hypothermia as an example. We explain how such approaches might harm the socioeconomically deprived population, thus further worsening health inequalities within LMIC. A paradigm shift in our approach to clinical research and research capacity building in LMIC is required to reduce the burden of HIE.

CLINICAL TRIALS OF INDUCED HYPOTHERMIA FROM HIGH-INCOME COUNTRIES

Preclinical models of HIE are based on a single acute hypoxic-ischemic insult in a healthy animal which is best represented by an acute intra-partum sentinel event in a clinical scenario.[5] Five major multicenter trials of induced hypothermia in neonates with moderate or severe HIE have been reported from HIC to date—1 selective head cooling[6] and 4 whole-body cooling.[7–10] All these trials were well designed and executed with centralized randomization and external data safety monitoring committee. They also had relatively similar inclusion criteria, and 18 month outcome evaluations enabling credible meta-analysis.[6–10] The individual trials varied from 111[10] to 320[8] patients although 2 of these trials accidently recruited neonates with mild encephalopathy[6,9] and 2 were prematurely discontinued.[9,10]

While not all these trials reported a statistically significant benefit in the primary outcome,[6,8] the direction of treatment effect was remarkably similar in terms of reduced mortality and improved neurodevelopmental outcomes at 18 months. Three of these trials reported continued benefits into childhood.[11,12] A less discussed factor is the high occurrence of hyperthermia (>38°C) of 14%[8] to 29%[6] in the control arm of these trials which would have amplified the treatment effect of hypothermia.[13,14]

Nevertheless, therapeutic hypothermia using servo-controlled whole body hypothermia devices for rapid reduction of core body temperature and maintaining this at 33.5 C for 72 hours followed by rewarming at 0.5 C per hour is now the standard of care for moderate or severe HIE in HICs for moderate or severe HIE. Selective head cooling using servo-controlled devices is no longer used in HICs outside the context of research due to the complexity of the intervention and requirement of intensive nursing resources. Initiation of hypothermia after 6 hours of birth was less effective,[15] and deeper hypothermia (32 C) or prolonged hypothermia (120 hours) is likely to cause harm in HICs.[16] A recent pilot randomized controlled trial reported hypothermia did not reduce brain injury in neonates with mild HIE,[17] although a large clinical trial of cooling in mild encephalopathy (COMET NCT05889507) is currently ongoing in the United Kingdom.

CLINICAL TRIALS OF INDUCED HYPOTHERMIA IN LOW-INCOME AND MIDDLE-INCOME COUNTRIES

Meta-analysis of the data from 22 randomized controlled trials (7 selective head cooling and 15 whole-body hypothermia) involving a total of 1979 neonates suggest that induced hypothermia significantly reduces death and neurodisability after HIE in

LMIC.[18,19] However, a careful examination of the individual trials reveals considerable heterogeneity. Most benefit has been reported in selective head cooling trials, particularly using ice. Whole body cooling using ice or phase material reports reduced mortality while servo-controlled devices report increased mortality. A summary of all the induced hypothermia trials is provided later, so that the readers can appreciate that meta-analysis of cooling trials in LMIC is inappropriate and is likely to give inaccurate pooled estimates.[20]

Selective Head Cooling Trials

Single-center trials
Six single-center trials (4 in China, 1 in Turkey, and 1 in India) of selective head cooling trials involving a total of 331 neonates have reported significant reduction in death or disability at 18 months or more after HIE, particularly when ice was used for cooling. One randomized controlled trial from a tertiary neonatal intensive care unit in India involving 60 neonates reported a significant reduction in death or disability at 30 months (risk ratio [RR]: 0.33 [95% CI: 0.15–0.72]; P = .001) using ice over baby's head for 3 days. This trial reported 100% follow-up assessments at 30 months.[21]

Multicenter trials
Only one multicenter trial of selective head cooling has been reported. This trial involved 256 neonates from 12 hospitals in China and reported reduction in death or disability at 18 months (RR 0.47 (95% CI 0.26–0.84); P =.01) using a servo-controlled head cooling device. However, 21 neonates were excluded after randomization, and further 41 were lost to follow up, and hence the primary outcome data were available only from 194 (76%) neonates in this trial.[22]

Selective head cooling requires very complex, expensive servo-controlled cooling caps and intensive nursing monitoring. Hence it is no longer used in HICs. As selective head cooling has no applicability in LMIC, it would not be appropriate to use these data in meta-analysis of induced hypothermia in LMIC.

Whole-Body Hypothermia Trials

Single-center trials
Pooled data from 12 single-center trials (2 China, 1 Egypt, 1 Africa, 10 India) involving 984 neonates suggest whole-body hypothermia using low-cost manual cooling methods like ice, and phase change material significantly reduces mortality at hospital discharge (RR 0.62; 95% CI 0.49–0.8). Of these, 762 (77%) neonates were recruited from the same institution.[23–28] Limited data were available on post-neonatal mortality and neurodevelopmental outcomes. One randomized controlled trial involving 144 neonates from India reported a significant reduction in cerebral palsy and moderate or severe disability at 8 years of age in the hypothermic group, within 1 year of neonatal recruitment.[29] Another trial from China involving 93 neonates reported significant reduction in death and disability at 18 months (18% vs 48%; P = .01) with delayed whole-body hypothermia initiated by 10 hours of age.[30] The data from these two trials are not shown in the forest plot (**Fig. 1**).

Multicenter trials
Only one multicenter trial of whole-body hypothermia (HELIX; Hypothermia for encephalopathy in low and MICs) has been reported from LMIC.[31] This trial randomly allocated 408 neonates with moderate or severe encephalopathy from 7 tertiary neonatal intensive care units (NICUs) in India, Sri Lanka, and Bangladesh to whole-body hypothermia using a servo-controlled cooling device or control (normothermia) using a web-based central randomization system. The primary outcome was death

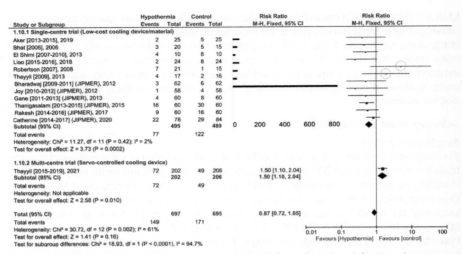

Fig. 1. Mortality at hospital discharge in whole-body hypothermia trials. Recruitment per hospital site is shown in the bar diagram. Of the total 984 neonates recruited to single-center pilot randomized controlled trials, 762 were recruited from one hospital as a part of 6 separate trials. Two pilot trials showed increased mortality (*red circles*).

or disability assessed at 18 months using Bayley III scales of infant development and was available from 399 neonates. Death or moderate or severe disability occurred in 98 (50%) infants in the hypothermia group and 94 (47%) infants in the control group (RR 1·06; 95% CI 0·87–1·30; $P = 0·55$). Eighty infants (42%) in the hypothermia group and 63 (31%; $P = 0·022$) infants in the control group died by 18 months.

It is not uncommon for smaller trials to overestimate treatment effects and for a later definitive trial to show opposite effects.[20] The interim analysis of the data from first 50 neonates recruited to the HELIX trial suggested a benefit from whole-body hypothermia, which gradually disappeared as more neonates were recruited (**Fig. 2**). Nevertheless, the forest plot shown in **Fig. 1** suggests considerable statistical heterogeneity ($I^2 = 95\%$, $P<.0001$) suggesting that data from single pilot trials of low-cost cooling devices cannot be combined with the multicenter HELIX trial data using a servo-controlled device.

In summary, the HELIX trial is the only phase III clinical trial from LMIC and is the largest clinical trial of hypothermia in the world and demonstrated increased mortality with cooling. For 1 in every 10 babies cooled, 1 additional baby died. Hence, the

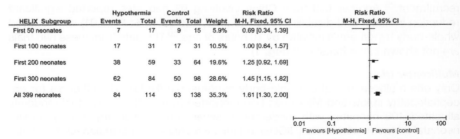

Fig. 2. Multiple interim analysis of the HELIX trial data based on the number of neonates recruited.

continued use of whole-body hypothermia in this population cannot be justified. The subsequent sessions discuss the implication of the HELIX trial results for neuroprotection after HIE in LMIC.

POTENTIAL REASONS FOR LACK OF HYPOTHERMIC NEUROPROTECTION IN THE HELIX TRIAL

When an intervention works in one setting but not in others, it is important to examine whether delivery of the intervention was appropriate and whether these factors could explain the lack of neuroprotection (**Table 1**).

Quality of Supportive Intensive Care

All centers that participated in the HELIX trial were accredited tertiary care intensive care units managed by dedicated neonatologists, 2-tier neonatal trainee doctors and had 1:2 to 4 nursing care (**Fig. 3**). Nevertheless, the overall quality of care and outcome of critically unwell neonates even in the best resourced tertiary intensive care units in LMIC is likely to be lower than tertiary NICU in HICs. In the HELIX trial, hypothermia worsened outcomes of neonates at all participating sites. Any intervention that requires 1:1 nursing care or is unsafe outside a tertiary NICU has no generalizability in LMIC as most HIE occurs in secondary care settings with neonate to nurse ratios of over 1:10.

Place of Birth and Hypothermic Neuroprotection

The hypothermia trials in HIC have included both inborn and outborn neonates, and some of these neonates were born at home. Although the outborn neonates tend to be sicker than inborn neonates in HICs, induced hypothermia improved clinical outcomes irrespective of place of birth in these settings.[32] In contrast, the non-tertiary care centers in LMICs differ from the tertiary care set up in terms of having clinicians with limited neonatal expertise and resources along with a lack of exclusive newborn transport services, adding to suboptimal intra-partum and post-resuscitation care and potential for additional brain injury before arriving at a cooling center.

A sub-group analysis of the HELIX trial suggested whole-body hypothermia did not improve clinical outcomes and brain injury either in inborn neonates or in outborn neonates.[33] Among inborn neonates, the mean (SD) absolute levels of thalamic NAA were 8.04 (1.98) mmol/kg wet weight in the hypothermia group and 8.31 (1.13) mmol/kg wet weight in the control group (odds ratio [OR] -0.28; 95% confidence interval [CI], -1.62–1.07; $P = .68$). Among outborn neonates, the mean (SD) absolute levels of thalamic NAA were 8.03 (1.89) mmol/kg wet weight in the hypothermia group and 7.99 (1.72) in the control group (OR, 0.05; 95% CI, -0.62–0.71; $P = .89$) (**Fig. 4**). There was no difference in brain injury scores or white matter (WM) fractional anisotropy between the hypothermia and control groups among inborn or outborn neonates.[33] Hypothermia also increased mortality by 29% (95% CI, 0.81–2.06; $P = .28$) among inborn and by 38% (95% CI, 1.01–1.89; $P = .01$) among outborn neonates, although the trial was not powered to examine this.[22]

Birth Acidosis and Hypothermic Neuroprotection

As neonatal encephalopathy may occur from a variety of conditions including perinatal hypoxia-ischemia, infection, inborn errors of metabolism, and other genetic conditions, clinical trials of hypothermia used a 2 stage approach to identify neonates with HIE from other causes of encephalopathy. The NICHD NRN trial[7] used an acidosis-based approach and birth acidosis (cord or baby's blood gas pH <7.0)

Table 1
Comparison of the major induced hypothermia trials

Trial Name	HELIX[31]	NICHD NRN[7]	COOLCAP[6]	TOBY[8]
Sample size	408	208	234	325
Extent of birth depression to qualify for recruitment	Apgar score ≤5 or continued resuscitation at 5 min	pH <7.0 AND Apgar score ≤5 or continued resuscitation at 10 min	Either a pH <7.0 OR Apgar score ≤5 or continued resuscitation at 10 min	Either a pH <7.0 OR Apgar score ≤5 or continued resuscitation at 10 min
Severe birth acidosis mandatory	No	Yes[a]	No	No
Blood stream positive sepsis	5%	6%	3%	12%
Funisitis	16%	NA	NA	NA
Proportion of neonates with severe HIE	20%	35%	44%	59%
Birth weight	2.8 kg	3.4 kg	3.4 kg	3.4 kg
Birth weight <2 SD	20%	0	0	0
Hyperthermia	5%	23%	30%	14%
Seizures at randomization	73%	48%	64%	51%
Perinatal sentinel events	10%	62%	NA	74%

[a] If cord pH or blood pH within one of birth was between 7.01 and 7.15, a base deficit was between 10 and 15.9 mmol per liter, or a blood gas was not available, additional criteria of an acute perinatal event and either a 10 min Apgar score of 5 or less or assisted ventilation initiated at birth and continued for at least 10 min was mandatory.

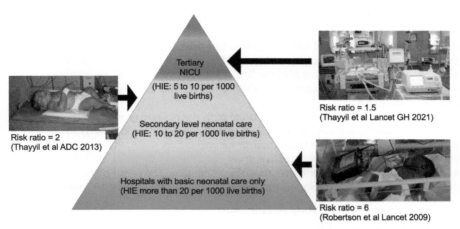

Fig. 3. Diversity of health care in LMICs and potential impact of supportive intensive care on mortality after whole-body hypothermia. The top of the pyramid represents the affluent populations with access to state-of-art health care facilities in selected multispecialty private hospitals.

was an essential criteria alongside clinical evidence of encephalopathy. In contrast, all other HIC cooling trials[6,8–10] used a non-acidosis-based approach where it was not mandatory to have birth acidosis if the neonate had long birth depression defined as Apgar score of less than 7 or need for continued resuscitation at 10 minutes. Both these approaches identified neonates with HIE within 6 hours of birth, and very few had alternative causes of encephalopathy.

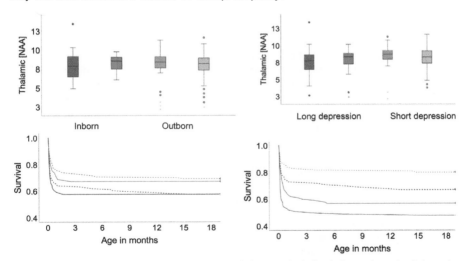

Fig. 4. HELIX trial subgroup analysis. Top panel shows whole-body hypothermia did not increase thalamic [NAA] among inborn or outborn neonates (*left side*) or among those who had long or short depression (*right panel*). Bottom left shows survival among inborn (*straight line*) and outborn (*dotted line*) in the control group (*red*) and hypothermia group (*blue*). Bottom right shows survival among neonates with long depression or acidosis (*straight line*) and short depression (*dotted line*) in the control group (*red*) and hypothermia group (*blue*).

The HELIX trial used Apgar score 5 or less at 5 minutes or continued resuscitation beyond 5 minutes as an inclusion criterion rather than 10 minutes as in HIC hypothermia trials. Thus, of the 408 neonates recruited to the HELIX trial 201 had long birth depression (positive pressure ventilation [PPV] greater than 10 min or Apgar score less than 6 at 10 min or cord pH less than 7.0) similar to the HIC hypothermia trials, and 207 had short birth depression (PPV for 5–10 min or Apgar score<6 at 5 min, but ≥6 at 10 min).[34]

However, no interaction of the duration of birth depression group (long birth depression or short birth depression) on the study group (control or whole-body hypothermia) was seen for any of the MR biomarker or clinical outcomes (death or disability), and hypothermia was not neuroprotective irrespective of the severity of birth depression and acidosis (see **Fig. 4**). Furthermore, 48% of the neonates with long birth depression died and 62% died or developed moderate or severe disability at 18 months.[34]

Cerebral Palsy and Whole-Body Hypothermia

It is important to note that cerebral palsy and survival of neonates with substantial brain injury have an inverse relation. Thus, in the HELIX trial, although one less cerebral palsy occurred for every 10 neonates treated with whole-body hypothermia, this was at the cost of one additional death.[31,33]

Although mortality is an important outcome measure, mortality at hospital discharge is prone to bias in open label interventions due to issues around discharge against medical advice and deaths occurring after hospital discharge. Therefore, it is important that the primary outcome of any neuroprotective intervention for HIE remains the composite of death or disability, and reduction in cerebral palsy should always be considered in the context of shifts in mortality within the same trial and not in isolation.

WHOLE-BODY HYPOTHERMIA IN UPPER MIDDLE-INCOME COUNTRIES AND AFFLUENT POPULATIONS

The HELIX trial was conducted primarily in public sector tertiary care academic centers in South Asia serving low-income populations and did not recruit affluent populations. However, private sector hospitals often tend to have small maternity units with less than 2000 births per year and over 50% elective caesarean section rates. Thus, occurrence of HIE in these settings might be very low. Given the paucity of any published data from neonates born at private sector hospitals,[35] it is difficult to make any recommendations. Adequately powered clinical trials of whole-body hypothermia would be required to establish if induced hypothermia offers any benefits over controlled normothermia in upper middle-income countries.

NATIONAL NEONATOLOGY FORUM (INDIA) GUIDELINES

Following the publication of the HELIX trial, the National Neonatology Forum (NNF) of India published a position statement for curtailing the use of induced hypothermia and recommended it should be offered only to neonates born at 37 weeks or later with a neonatal unit admission temperature 36 to 37.4 C and only if all the following 4 below criteria are met.[36]

1. pH less than 7 or Base Excess greater than -16 on cord or arterial blood gas done within 1 h of birth.
2. Apgar score of 4 or less at 10 minutes or at least 10 minutes of positive pressure ventilation (PPV)

3. Acute perinatal sentinel event such as placental abruption, uterine rupture, cord prolapse.
4. Evidence of moderate or severe encephalopathy

While it is unclear if whole-body hypothermia would be beneficial in this subgroup of neonates, these guidelines are likely to restrict the use of hypothermia and will eventually lead to de-implementation. For example, of the 155 neonates cooled in a public sector hospital in India over a 4 year period, only 8 (5.2%) had an acute sentinel event, and none of the neonates had a 5 min Apgar score less than 5.[37] Another multicenter observational study involving 211 neonates cooled for encephalopathy from 17 Indian hospitals,[35] only 22% had a pH less than 7.0, while Apgar scores and sentinel events were not reported (**Fig. 5**). As only 10% of the neonates with birth acidosis will develop encephalopathy, it is likely that most neonates currently being cooled in LMIC might have no encephalopathy or mild encephalopathy. Of the 392 neonates cooled at single in South Africa 84% had a 5 min Apgar score 4 or greater and 64% had a pH greater than 7.0; Apgar score at 10 minutes were not reported.[38] Adherence to the NNF guidelines might help in minimizing harm and preventing medical litigations, as less than 5% of the neonates with HIE in LMIC will meet these criteria.

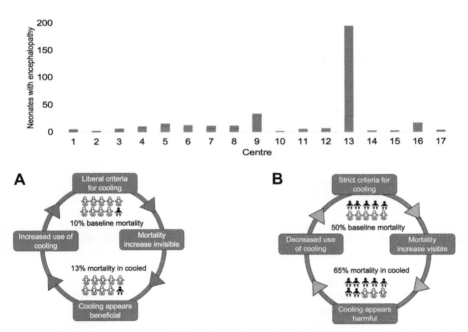

Fig. 5. Variation in occurrence of HIE and use of hypothermia in 17 NICU participating in the Indian neonatal collaborative[37] is shown in the top panel. Neonates who had whole-body hypothermia is shown in blue and those who did not have hypothermia in red. Bottom panel shows a model for de-implementation of whole-body hypothermia. Assuming hypothermia increases death by around 30%, clinicians offering hypothermia to a low-risk population are unlikely to notice an increase in mortality and may feel hypothermia is beneficial leading to wider use (A). On the other hand, if clinicians restrict (B) the use of hypothermia to neonates with moderate or severe encephalopathy meeting the criteria recommended by the National Neonatology Forum of India,[36] the increase in mortality will become more apparent which might lead to de-implementation.

As spontaneous drop in body temperature is proportional to the severity of the initial brain injury,[39] it is unlikely that babies with substantial brain injury have a normal body temperature at admission unless radiant warmers are used during resuscitation and transport. The latter may increase the risk of hyperthermia and increase mortality.

DE-IMPLEMENTATION OF INDUCED HYPOTHERMIA

Although de-implementing inappropriate health interventions is essential to minimizing patient harm, maximizing efficient use of resources, and improving population health it requires a multilevel approach[40] and is often challenging (**Table 2**). Following the original randomized controlled trials reporting benefits,[41] whole-body hypothermia became the standard therapy for neuroprotection in a pediatric and adult cardiac arrest in all HICs. However, the more recent evidence from Targeted Hypothermia versus Targeted Normothermia after Out-of-Hospital Cardiac Arrest trial (TTM2) trial reporting lack of reduction in mortality at 6 (relative risk with hypothermia, 1.04; 95% CI 0.94–1.14; $P = .37$)[42] caused considerable controversy and acrimony.[43] The clinicians and industries who supported induced hypothermia argued TTM2 sites did not have specialist expertise and there were delays in achieving target temperature, nevertheless most centers around the world eventually changed the practice to targeted normothermia, although no harms were reported from induced hypothermia. In LMICs, de-implementation is likely to be more challenging as medical care is much less regulated than HICs, particularly in the private sector.

WHOLE-GENOME EXPRESSION IN HYPOXIC ISCHEMIC ENCEPHALOPATHY

Whole-blood transcriptomics has been used for disease stratification in several conditions including tuberculosis,[44] Kawasaki disease,[45] and viral infections. Transcriptomics holds the potential to provide valuable information before the initiation of hypothermia and to detect molecular subgroups of HIE for targeted neuroprotection. Neonates with HIE have a different whole-genome expression profile birth than healthy neonates or those with infection,[46] and can help in prediction of later outcomes.[47] The HELIX trial investigators compared the transcriptomic profiles of neonates with HIE from a HIC with neonates recruited to the HELIX trial. A total of 1793 and 99 significant genes were identified when comparing neonates with adverse and good outcomes after HIE in HICs and LMICs, respectively. Furthermore, 11 genes were in common between the HICs and LMICs analyses and all had opposite directions in fold change. Biological mechanisms identified within 6 hours after birth also differed between neonates with HIE born in Italy and South Asia. In the Italian dataset, the eIF2-signaling pathway was downregulated soon after birth in infants with adverse outcomes, which is consistent with previous research indicating that eIF2 phosphorylation occurs rapidly following neonatal hypoxia ischemia.[48] This phosphorylation leads to the inhibition of transcription and translation, causing the repression of protein synthesis shortly after the hypoxic-ischemic insult.[49] Upon reoxygenation, phosphorylation is reversed, resulting in the resumption of protein synthesis.[49] Conversely, aldosterone signaling was identified as the most significant pathway in the South Asian dataset within 6 hours after birth. It has been associated with obstructive sleep apnea, a chronic condition resulting in intermittent hypoxia, leading to activation of the renin–angiotensin–aldosterone system.[50] The trends in gene expression were also identified over the first 72 hours after birth, and expression profiles were found to remain significantly different between 35 neonates with HIE and 14 healthy controls from HICs.[51]

Disease mechanisms identified within 6 hours after birth associated with adverse outcomes after HIE were linked to acute hypoxia in HICs, and non-acute hypoxia in

Table 2
Approach to de-implementation of induced hypothermia in low-income and middle-income countries

Multilevel Factors	Characteristics	Questions
Intervention	Strength of evidence	When is the trial evidence from high-income country not generalizable to LMIC? What happens if the strength of the evidence for an intervention change?
Patient	Information	Are parents aware of the potential harms (increased death) of the intervention? Was consent sought for administering cooling outside the local (eg, NNF) guidelines?
Health professionals	Negative past events	Does negative past events affect de-implementation?
	Cognitive dissonance	Is there any evidence of cognitive dissonance?
	Malpractice	Does offering cooling outside of national (eg, NNF) guidelines increase litigation risk?
Organization	Revenue	Is de-implementation of revenue-generating interventions more difficult?
	Competitive advantage	What happens to competitors in the market if de-implementation is partial?
	Liability	Would de-implementation increase risk of liability from past recipient of the intervention?
Policy level	Generalizability	How does interventions that might cause harm outside tertiary NICU inform policy decision in LMIC? Will induced hypothermia increase or decrease inequalities within LMIC?

Actions for De-implementation of Induced Hypothermia	
1. Restrict	Offer cooling only as recommended by local academic bodies (National Neonatology Forum)
2. Reduce	Audit the data on cooled neonates to examine if the intervention was provided according to guideline. Ensure clinicians are trained and certified on modified Sarnat staging for encephalopathy
3. Replace	Change target temperature of the cooling device to 37 C from 33.5 C (targeted normothermia)
4. Remove	Remove cooling devices from neonatal units

Unintended Consequences of De-implementation of Induced Hypothermia	
Hyperthermia	Will de-implementation of hypothermia increase the risk of iatrogenic hyperthermia?
Reduced monitoring	Would de-implementation lead to reduced monitoring and less intensive treatment of neonates?
Reduced resources	Would de-implementation reduce the funding allocations?

Hypothermia Audit as per the National Neonatology Forum (India) Position Statement on Restricting Use of Cooling (All of the Below Should Be Yes)	
1. Was the neonate born at or after 36 wk	Yes/no
2. Was the admission temperature 36–37.4 C	Yes/no
Was the neonate <6 h of age at the start of cooling	Yes/no
3. Was there any acute intra-partum sentinel event	Yes/no
4. Was the umbilical cord pH or an arterial blood gas pH within 1 h or birth <7.0	Yes/no
5. Did the neonate required continued positive pressures ventilation beyond 10 min or have an Apgar score of <4 at 10 min?	Yes/no
6. Did the neonate have moderate or severe encephalopathy on clinical assessment?	Yes/no
7. Was informed parental consent obtained before induced hypothermia?	Yes/no
8. If "no" to any of the above, explain why induced hypothermia was used.	

South Asia. Although these observations are based on a small number of neonates, if proven in subsequent studies, it could open a new avenue for rapid disease stratification using a point of care test and personalized neuroprotection in HIE.

HELIX HYPOTHESIS: THE COMPROMISED BABY IN THE WOMB

The unexpected results of the HELIX trial have challenged many of our current assumptions about HIE. The HELIX trial investigators reported several subtle differences in clinical and neuroimaging data from South Asia and HICs. First, acute intra-partum events were reported in less than 13% of the cases. This observation is supported by the emerging data from the Prevention of Epilepsy from Neonatal Encephalopathy involving 80,000 women from South India where such events occurred in less than 10% of the neonates with encephalopathy. Second, the average birth weight of the neonates in the HELIX trial was much lesser than HIC trials and 18% were growth restricted. None of the major HIC trials had growth restricted neonates. Third, clinical seizures were reported soon after birth in the HELIX trial suggesting the hypoxia-ischemic injury occurred during the labor process and not too distant to birth. Forth, even a short birth depression was associated with encephalopathy and major adverse outcomes suggesting either lower fetal reserve or occurrence of hypoxia-ischemia remote to birth. Recent data from 170 children in the Canadian cerebral registry reported that only 15% of the children with MRI evidence of hypoxia-ischemia had neonatal encephalopathy, suggesting that the fetus might have recovered from intra-uterine hypoxia before birth.[52]

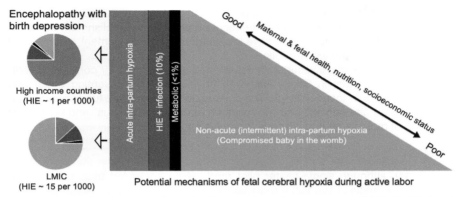

Fig. 6. A schematic of the HELIX hypothesis explaining why occurrence of HIE is high in South Asia and response to whole-body hypothermia is poor. The neonates who had a nonacute or intermittent intrapartum hypoxia are likely to be less depressed at birth but may have substantial brain injury, encephalopathy, and adverse outcomes. Nonacute intrapartum hypoxia may be predictable and preventable by better quality ante-natal and intra-partum care, while the acute intra-partum hypoxia may be more difficult to predict or prevent.

Fifth, most neonates had WM injury on MRI than injury to basal ganglia/thalami (BGT) suggesting sub-acute or chronic hypoxia-ischemia.[53] However, it is possible that the neonates with BGT injury died before MRI. Finally, whole genome expression data suggest non-acute hypoxia providing a biological basis for these clinical observations.

Based on this constellation of findings, the HELIX trial investigators proposed a new hypothesis of "compromised baby in the womb." Thus, the unborn baby is already compromised in the womb from undernutrition and sub-optimal intrauterine milieu. Hence hypoxia from the normal labor process, especially if it is augmented with uterotonics leads to intermittent cerebral hypoxia and HIE[54] occurs without a single well-defined hypoxic event (**Fig. 6**). Such neonates may not have the typical progression of primary and secondary energy failure following intrauterine hypoxia-ischemic and hence hypothermic neuroprotection is likely to be ineffective. A careful examination of the previously published data from all cooling studies from LMIC suggest a similar clinical phenotype confirming the HELIX hypothesis—most neonates with moderate or severe HIE are less depressed at birth than in HICs but tend to have substantial brain injury and adverse outcomes.

There are no preclinical models of such a mechanism, although fetal lamb models of intermittent umbilical cord occlusion may be the closest to this scenario.[55] Unfortunately, such pre-clinical models would require large sample sizes due to the variably of brain injury. If this hypothesis is proven in future mechanistic and clinical studies, it might explain the high occurrence of HIE in LMIC and may lead to novel avenues for prevention and treatment that does not involve induced hypothermia.

COLLABORATIVE NEONATAL NEUROPROTECTION TRIAL PLATFORM IN SOUTH ASIA (CONNECTIONS)

Evaluation of one drug at a time is a highly inefficient way to develop neuroprotective therapies in South Asia given the huge disease burden. Platform trials can be defined as a type of clinical trial aimed at simultaneously evaluating multiple interventions, with the flexibility of addition or removal of treatment arms, against a common control arm and a single master protocol.[16,17] Platform trials like RECOVERY, PANORAMIC, and

PRINCIPLE were instrumental in developing new treatments for COVID-19. However, such trials are complex to design and execute and require establishment of robust research infrastructure alongside active involvement, and engagement of families of affected babies and the wider public.

Hence, the HELIX trial investigators established a consortium for conducting well-designed platform trial in South Asia with an intention of preventing death and disability after HIE in these settings. The consortium is based on 2 fundamental principles "leave no one behind" and "no research about us without us" and will enable evaluation of multiple neuroprotective therapies after HIE.

SUMMARY

In summary, although single-center pilot randomized controlled trials using ice or phase change material suggest a reduction in mortality at hospital discharge in neonates with hypoxic HIE, the increased mortality reported in the largest hypothermia trial conduced in South Asia is unambiguous. Subgroup analysis of the HELIX trial reported hypothermia was not neuroprotective irrespective of the location of birth (inborn or outborn) or duration of birth depression and acidosis. For every 10 cooled neonates, one cerebral palsy was prevented, but one additional death occurred. Low occurrence of perinatal sentinel events, early seizure onset, frequent growth restriction and WM injury, and involvement of aldosterone pathways on whole-genome expression profile suggest that HIE among socioeconomically deprived population in LMIC may be related to intermittent intra-partum hypoxia. Hence continued and indiscriminate use of whole-body hypothermia in LMIC cannot be justified, particularly outside the recommendation of the NNF in India.

Best Practices

- Updated National Neonatology Forum (NNF) position statement recommends induced hypothermia should be offered to term/near term neonates with hypoxic-ischemic encephalopathy ONLY if they have a neonatal unit admission temperature 36–37.4 C, and if they fulfill ALL of the 4 following criteria: (1) pH less than 7 or BE greater than -16 on cord or arterial blood gas done within 1 h of life AND (2) Apgar score less than 5 at 10 minutes or at least 10 min of PPV AND (3) history of acute perinatal event AND (4) evidence of moderate or severe encephalopathy.

- Clinicians should be aware that less than 5% of the neonates with hypoxic-ischemic encephalopathy in low resource settings will meet the NNF criteria.

- Indiscriminate use of induced hypothermia outside these guidelines may cause patient harm and increase medicolegal litigations.

- Ensuring targeted normothermia (36.5–37.5 C) and avoidance of hyperthermia is likely to improve outcomes of neonates with hypoxic-ischemic encephalopathy in low-resourced settings.

ACKNOWLEDGMENTS

The authors thank Dr Paolo Montaldo for preparing the forest plots of the hypothermia trials.

DISCLOSURE

The authors acknowledge funding from the National Insititute of Health and Care Reseaerch (NIHR), UK.

REFERENCES

1. World Health Organization, Newborns: improving survival and well-being. 2020, Available at: https://www.who.int/news-room/fact-sheets/detail/newborns-reducing-mortality2024. Accessed March 1, 2024.

2. Institute for Health Metrics and Evaluation (IHME), GBD Compare. 2023, Available at: http://vizhub.healthdata.org/gbd-compare.2024. Accessed March 1, 2024.

3. K M, R V. Valuing disease burden due to neonatal encephalopathy and birth Trauma: a health economic evaluation. Washington: Pediatric Academic Soceity; 2023.

4. Eunson P. The long-term health, social, and financial burden of hypoxic-ischaemic encephalopathy. Dev Med Child Neurol 2015;57(Suppl 3):48–50.

5. Thoresen M, Penrice J, Lorek A, et al. Mild hypothermia after severe transient hypoxia-ischemia ameliorates delayed cerebral energy failure in the newborn piglet. Pediatr Res 1995;37:667–70.

6. Gluckman PD, Wyatt JS, Azzopardi D, et al. Selective head cooling with mild systemic hypothermia after neonatal encephalopathy: multicentre randomised trial. Lancet 2005;365:663–70.

7. Shankaran S, Laptook AR, Ehrenkranz RA, et al. Whole-body hypothermia for neonates with hypoxic-ischemic encephalopathy. N Engl J Med 2005;353:1574–84.

8. Azzopardi D, Strohm B, Edwards A, et al. Moderate hypothermia to treat perinatal asphyxial encephalopathy. N Engl J Med 2009;361:1349–58.

9. Jacobs SE, Morley CJ, Inder TE, et al. Whole-body hypothermia for term and near-term newborns with hypoxic-ischemic encephalopathy: a randomized controlled trial. Arch Pediatr Adolesc Med 2011;165:692–700.

10. Simbruner G, Mittal RA, Rohlmann F, et al. Systemic hypothermia after neonatal encephalopathy: outcomes of neo.nEURO.network RCT. Pediatrics 2010;126:e771–8.

11. Shankaran S, Pappas A, McDonald SA, et al. Childhood outcomes after hypothermia for neonatal encephalopathy. N Engl J Med 2012;366:2085–92.

12. Azzopardi D, Strohm B, Marlow N, et al. Effects of hypothermia for perinatal asphyxia on childhood outcomes. N Engl J Med 2014;371:140–9.

13. Laptook A, Tyson J, Shankaran S, et al. Elevated temperature after hypoxic-ischemic encephalopathy: risk factor for adverse outcomes. Pediatrics 2008;122:491–9.

14. Laptook AR, McDonald SA, Shankaran S, et al. Elevated temperature and 6- to 7-year outcome of neonatal encephalopathy. Ann Neurol 2013;73:520–8.

15. Laptook AR, Shankaran S, Tyson JE, et al. Effect of therapeutic hypothermia initiated after 6 hours of age on death or disability among newborns with hypoxic-ischemic encephalopathy: a randomized clinical trial. JAMA 2017;318:1550–60.

16. Shankaran S, Laptook AR, Pappas A, et al. Effect of Depth and duration of cooling on death or disability at age 18 Months among neonates with hypoxic-ischemic encephalopathy: a randomized clinical trial. JAMA 2017;318:57–67.

17. Montaldo P, Cirillo M, Burgod C, et al. Whole-body hypothermia for 48 or 72 hours versus targeted normothermia in mild encephalopathy: a multicenter pilot randomised controlled trial. JAMA Netw Open 2024;7(5):e249119.

18. Abate BB, Bimerew M, Gebremichael B, et al. Effects of therapeutic hypothermia on death among asphyxiated neonates with hypoxic-ischemic encephalopathy: a systematic review and meta-analysis of randomized control trials. PLoS One 2021;16:e0247229.

19. Mathew JL, Kaur N, Dsouza JM. Therapeutic hypothermia in neonatal hypoxic encephalopathy: a systematic review and meta-analysis. J Glob Health 2022;12: 04030.

20. Roberts I, Ker K. How systematic reviews cause research waste. Lancet 2015; 386:1536.

21. Das SK, Sarkar N, Bhattacharya M, et al. Neurological outcome at 30 Months of age after mild hypothermia via selective head cooling in term neonates with perinatal asphyxia using low-cost CoolCap: a single-center randomized control pilot trial in India. J Pediatr Neurol 2017;15(04):157–65.

22. Zhou WH, Cheng GQ, Shao XM, et al. Selective head cooling with mild systemic hypothermia after neonatal hypoxic-ischemic encephalopathy: a multicenter randomized controlled trial in China. J Pediatr 2010;157:367–72.

23. Catherine RC, Bhat BV, Adhisivam B, et al. Neuronal biomarkers in predicting neurodevelopmental outcome in term babies with perinatal asphyxia. Indian J Pediatr 2020;87:787–92.

24. Gane BD, Nandhakumar S, Bhat V, et al. Effect of therapeutic hypothermia on chromosomal aberration in perinatal asphyxia. J Pediatr Neurosci 2016;11:25–8.

25. Joy R, Pournami F, Bethou A, et al. Effect of therapeutic hypothermia on oxidative stress and outcome in term neonates with perinatal asphyxia: a randomized controlled trial. J Trop Pediatr 2013;59:17–22.

26. Bharadwaj SK, Vishnu Bhat B. Therapeutic hypothermia using Gel Packs for term neonates with hypoxic ischaemic encephalopathy in resource-limited settings: a randomized controlled trial. J Trop Pediatr 2012;58:382–8.

27. Rakesh K, Vishnu Bhat B, Adhisivam B, et al. Effect of therapeutic hypothermia on myocardial dysfunction in term neonates with perinatal asphyxia - a randomized controlled trial. J Matern Fetal Neonatal Med 2018;31:2418–23.

28. Tanigasalam V, Bhat V, Adhisivam B, et al. Does therapeutic hypothermia reduce acute kidney injury among term neonates with perinatal asphyxia?–a randomized controlled trial. J Matern Fetal Neonatal Med 2016;29:2545–8.

29. Jose S, Ismael M. Effect of hypothermia for perinatal asphyxia on childhood outcomes. International Journal of Contemporary Pediatrics 2018;5:86–91.

30. Li T, Xu F, X C, et al. Systemic hypothermia induced within 10 hours after birth improved Neurological outcome in newborns with hypoxic-ischemic encephalopathy. Hosp Pract 2009;37:147–52.

31. Thayyil S, Pant S, Montaldo P, et al. Hypothermia for moderate or severe neonatal encephalopathy in low-income and middle-income countries (HELIX): a randomised controlled trial in India, Sri Lanka, and Bangladesh. Lancet Glob Health 2021;9(9):e1273-e1285.

32. Natarajan G, Pappas A, Shankaran S, et al. Effect of inborn vs. outborn delivery on neurodevelopmental outcomes in infants with hypoxic-ischemic encephalopathy: secondary analyses of the NICHD whole-body cooling trial. Pediatr Res 2012;72:414–9.

33. Thayyil S, Montaldo P, Krishnan V, et al. Whole-body hypothermia, cerebral Magnetic Resonance biomarkers, and outcomes in neonates with moderate or severe hypoxic-ischemic encephalopathy born at tertiary care centers vs other facilities: a Nested study within a randomized clinical trial. JAMA Netw Open 2023;6: e2312152.

34. Burgod C, Mazlan M, Pant S, et al. Duration of birth depression and neurodevelopmental outcomes after whole-body hypothermia for hypoxic ischemic encephalopathy in India, Sri Lanka and Bangladesh - an exploratory analysis of the HELIX trial. Lancet Reg Health Southeast Asia 2024;20:100284.

35. Kumar C, Peruri G, Plakkal N, et al. Short-term outcome and Predictors of survival among neonates with moderate or severe hypoxic ischemic encephalopathy: data from the Indian neonatal collaborative. Indian Pediatr 2022;59:21–4.

36. National Neonatology Forum (NNF), Position statement and guidelines for the use of therapeutic hypothermia(TH) to treat neonatal hypoxic ischemic encephalopathy(HIE) in India, Available at: http://www.nnfi.org/assests/pdf/NNF_Position_statement_and_Guidelines_for_TH%20_Final_(10112021)-converted. pdf, (Accessed March 1, 2024). 2021.

37. Mascarenhas D, Goyal M, Nanavati R, et al. Short-term outcome and complications of therapeutic hypothermia in neonates with moderate-to-severe hypoxic ischaemic encephalopathy: a single-centre retrospective observational study in a hospital in Mumbai, India. Paediatr Int Child Health 2022;42:117–26.

38. Nakwa FL, Sepeng L, van Kwawegen A, et al. Characteristics and outcomes of neonates with intrapartum asphyxia managed with therapeutic hypothermia in a public tertiary hospital in South Africa. BMC Pediatr 2023;23:51.

39. Enweronu-Laryea C, Martinello KA, Rose M, et al. Core temperature after birth in babies with neonatal encephalopathy in a sub-Saharan African hospital setting. J Physiol 2019;597:4013–24.

40. Norton WE, Chambers DA. Unpacking the complexities of de-implementing inappropriate health interventions. Implement Sci 2020;15:2.

41. Bernard SA, Gray TW, Buist MD, et al. Treatment of comatose survivors of out-of-hospital cardiac arrest with induced hypothermia. N Engl J Med 2002;346: 557–63.

42. Dankiewicz J, Cronberg T, Lilja G, et al. Targeted hypothermia versus targeted Normothermia after out-of-hospital cardiac arrest (TTM2): a randomized clinical trial-Rationale and design. Am Heart J 2019;217:23–31.

43. Fernando SM, Lascarrou JB, Sandroni C, et al. Sweeping TTM conclusion may deprive many post-arrest patients of effective therapy. Author's reply. Intensive Care Med 2021;47:1511–2.

44. Berry MP, Graham CM, McNab FW, et al. An interferon-inducible neutrophil-driven blood transcriptional signature in human tuberculosis. Nature 2010;466: 973–7.

45. Jackson H, Menikou S, Hamilton S, et al. Kawasaki disease patient stratification and pathway analysis based on Host transcriptomic and Proteomic profiles. Int J Mol Sci 2021;22.

46. Montaldo P, Kaforou M, Pollara G, et al. Whole blood gene expression reveals Specific transcriptome changes in neonatal encephalopathy. Neonatology 2019;115:68–76.

47. Montaldo P, Cunnington A, Oliveira V, et al. Transcriptomic profile of adverse neurodevelopmental outcomes after neonatal encephalopathy. Sci Rep 2020;10: 13100.

48. Carloni S, Albertini MC, Galluzzi L, et al. Increased autophagy reduces endoplasmic reticulum stress after neonatal hypoxia-ischemia: role of protein synthesis and autophagic pathways. Exp Neurol 2014;255:103–12.

49. Koumenis C, Naczki C, Koritzinsky M, et al. Regulation of protein synthesis by hypoxia via activation of the endoplasmic reticulum kinase PERK and phosphorylation of the translation initiation factor eIF2alpha. Mol Cell Biol 2002;22:7405–16.

50. Fletcher EC, Orolinova N, Bader M. Blood pressure response to chronic episodic hypoxia: the renin-angiotensin system. J Appl Physiol 2002;92:627–33.

51. Montaldo P, Burgod C, Herberg J, et al. Whole-blood gene expression profile after hypoxic-ischemic Encepahlopathy. JAMA Netw Open 2024;7(2):e2354433.

52. Fortin O, Husein N, Oskoui M, et al. Risk factors and outcomes for cerebral palsy with hypoxic-ischemic brain injury Patterns without Documented neonatal encephalopathy. Neurology 2024;102:e208111.
53. Miller SP, Ramaswamy V, Michelson D, et al. Patterns of brain injury in term neonatal encephalopathy. J Pediatr 2005;146:453–60.
54. Burgod C, Pant S, Morales MM, et al. Effect of intra-partum Oxytocin on neonatal encephalopathy: a systematic review and meta-analysis. BMC Pregnancy Childbirth 2021;21:736.
55. Wassink G, Bennet L, Davidson JO, et al. Pre-existing hypoxia is associated with greater EEG suppression and early onset of evolving seizure activity during brief repeated asphyxia in near-term fetal sheep. PLoS One 2013;8:e73895.

Long-Term Outcomes Following Hypoxic Ischemic Encephalopathy

Simone L. Huntingford, BComm/BSc, MBBS, FRACP[a,b,c],*,
Stephanie M. Boyd, BSc (Med), MPHTM, FRACP[d,e],
Sarah J. McIntyre, PhD, MPS[f,1], Shona C. Goldsmith, PhD[f,1],
Rod W. Hunt, PhD, FRACP, FRCP(UK)[a,b,f], Nadia Badawi, AM[d,f]

KEYWORDS

- Hypoxic ischemic encephalopathy (HIE) • Neonatal
- Neurodevelopmental (ND) outcome • Long-term • Cerebral palsy (CP) • Cognition
- Therapeutic hypothermia (TH)

KEY POINTS

- Hypoxic ischemic encephalopathy (HIE) remains a significant cause of neonatal death and disability.
- Therapeutic hypothermia (TH) has reduced rates of death and disability for term infants with moderate to severe HIE.

Continued

BACKGROUND

In term infants, perinatal hypoxia–ischemia (HI) is a well-established cause of brain injury with an associated syndrome known as hypoxic ischemic encephalopathy (HIE). HIE is the most common cause of neonatal encephalopathy and results in significant morbidity and mortality in the term population.[1] Moderate to severe HIE affects around 0.5 to 3 per 1000 live births in high-income countries.[2] The burden of

[a] Department of Paediatrics, Monash University, 246 Clayton Road, Clayton, Victoria 3168, Australia; [b] Monash Newborn, Monash Health, 246 Clayton Road, Clayton, Victoria 3168, Australia; [c] Paediatric Infant Perinatal Emergency Retrieval, Royal Children's Hospital, 50 Flemington Road, Parkville, Victoria 3052, Australia; [d] Grace Centre for Newborn Intensive Care, The Children's Hospital at Westmead, Hawkesbury Road, Westmead, New South Wales 2145, Australia; [e] Faculty of Medicine and Health, University of Sydney, Campderdown, New South Wales 2006, Australia; [f] CP Alliance Research Institute, Specialty of Child and Adolescent Health, Sydney Medical School, Faculty of Medicine and Health, The University of Sydney, Sydney, New South Wales, Australia
[1] Present address: PO Box 171, Forestville, New South Wales 2087, Australia.
* Corresponding author. Department of Paediatrics, Monash University, 246 Clayton Road, Clayton, Victoria 3168, Australia.
E-mail address: Simone.huntingford@monashhealth.org

Clin Perinatol 51 (2024) 683–709
https://doi.org/10.1016/j.clp.2024.04.008
0095-5108/24/Crown Copyright © 2024 Published by Elsevier Inc. All rights reserved.
perinatology.theclinics.com

Continued

- There are established and evolving concerns about adverse neurodevelopmental (ND) outcomes for infants with mild HIE. Randomized controlled trials (RCTs) of TH for this group are ongoing.
- The role of HIE in modulating ND outcome in the preterm infant is less well understood.
- There is no evidence that adjuvant therapies in combination with TH improve long-term outcomes; RCTs are continuing.

disease in preterm infants is less well studied. Incidence varies across studies from 1.3 to 9/1000 preterm births[3–5] with differing HIE definitions, severities, and gestational ages contributing to these statistics. Of note, there are no studies reporting the incidence of HIE in infants born less than 31 weeks.

The long-term neurodevelopmental (ND) outcomes in HIE are of great interest to both clinicians and families. Established HIE grading criteria have long existed.[6] For term infants with moderate to severe HIE, therapeutic hypothermia (TH) has been shown to reduce death and ND disability[7–10] with the number needed to treat for additional beneficial outcome being 7 infants.[7] Outcomes have shifted in the era of TH, with new studies investigating the effects of adjunctive neuroprotective and neuroregenerative therapies.[11] While many studies report ND outcomes at around 2 years of age, evidence is emerging on later outcomes.[12,13] Additionally, there is growing interest regarding the outcomes of mild HIE and preterm infants with HIE. This article summarizes the currently available evidence on outcomes in the precooling and postcooling eras and identifies areas where further research is needed.

OUTCOMES
Moderate-to-Severe Hypoxic Ischemic Encephalopathy

Prior to the advent of TH, ND sequelae were observed in 6% to 21% of surviving children following moderate HIE.[14,15] Additionally, learning difficulties were identified at school age in a significant proportion of children who were not otherwise considered to have disability.[15–17] Mortality rates following severe encephalopathy were high,[14] and 42% to 100% of survivors of severe HIE experienced ND impairment (NDI).[14–18] There are, however, significant limitations to the literature in the pre-TH era, with ND outcomes research dominated by cohort studies with variability in their enrollment criteria, assessment tools, outcome variables, and duration of follow-up. It is also worth noting that several studies, particularly from the prehypothermia era, reported on neonatal encephalopathy, which incorporates a broad differential diagnosis. The spectrum of ND outcomes differs for this more general population compared with infants with HIE defined according to stringent diagnostic criteria.

The earliest studies on outcomes following HIE focused largely on mortality and developmental assessment in infancy and at preschool age.[19] The mortality rate for severe HIE in a prospective cohort study of 167 infants born between 1974 and 1979 with varying degrees of encephalopathy was 50% in-hospital or 75% including deaths postdischarge,[14] and 100% of survivors had disability. Of survivors with moderate HIE, 20.7% developed NDI.[14] The most frequent sequelae observed among HIE survivors included cognitive delay, cerebral palsy (CP) (with spastic quadriplegia being the most common subtype), seizure disorder, visual impairment, and deafness.[14] CP was also a predominant cause of major disability in other contemporaneous cohorts.[15,16,18]

Studies from the pre-TH era also identified the risk of later onset and less severe cognitive impairments in HIE survivors without an early childhood diagnosis of disability. Robertson and colleagues published results of school performance at 8 years of age in 145 children with neonatal HIE from the original 1974 to 1979 cohort, compared with 155 unaffected peers.[17] Survivors of moderate HIE who were free from disability (CP, severe cognitive impairment, and/or major hearing or visual deficit) performed more poorly on psychoeducational testing and fine motor skill assessment compared with their peers with no or mild HIE.[17] A second cohort study of 71 children with a history of moderate HIE without disability revealed school-readiness delay in 44%.[20] At 8 to 11 years, deficits in language comprehension, reading accuracy, and working memory were observed in infants with encephalopathy compared with infants without encephalopathy.[21] In a systematic review of 352 infants with HIE spanning the pre-TH and post-TH eras (53 treated with TH), cognitive impairment was identified in 25% to 63% of children.[22] Even among cooled infants without CP, a significant proportion go on to have motor and cognitive impairment at school age,[23,24] emphasizing the need for assessment beyond early childhood.

Fueled by the preclinical evidence for TH providing neuroprotection after HI,[25–27] randomized controlled trials (RCTs) of TH commenced for term infants with moderate to severe HIE. The National Institute of Child Health and Human Development (NICHD) Neonatal Research Network trial conducted an RCT comparing whole-body TH with standard care. The primary outcome of death or severe disability at 18 to 22 months was available for 205 infants and occurred in 44% of the hypothermia group compared with 62% in the control group (risk ratio, 0.72; $P = .01$). Mortality rates were 24% and 37%, respectively.[8] Concerns about the risk of increasing disability in survivors were not borne out in this study, with CP reported in 19% in the hypothermia group and 30% of the control group. This cohort subsequently underwent assessment of neurologic outcomes, as well as cognition, attention, and visuospatial and executive function at 6 to 7 years of age. There was no significant difference in moderate or severe disability between the 2 groups; however, the combined outcome of death or severe disability occurred in 41% of the hypothermia group compared with 60% of the control group ($P = .03$).[13]

The Cool Cap trial was the first large RCT comparing selective head cooling with conventional care.[9] The study recruited term infants with moderate to severe encephalopathy and abnormal amplitude-integrated electroencephalography (EEG). Outcome data were available for 218 infants. At 18 months, death or severe disability occurred in 66% versus 55% of the conventional care group (odds ratio, 0.61; $P = .1$).[9] The TOBY trial[10] included 325 infants who were randomized to TH (as per NICHD) or standard care. Mortality rates were similar between the 2 groups, at 26% and 27%, respectively. There was no difference between groups in the combined outcome of death or severe disability; however, increased survival without neurologic abnormality was observed in the TH (relative risk [RR], 1.57; $P = .003$).[10] The TH group had reduced rates of CP (RR, 0.67; $P = .03$) and improved scores on the Mental Developmental Index and Psychomotor Developmental Index of the Bayley Scales of Infant Development II and the Gross Motor Function Classification System (GMFCS). At 6 to 7 year follow-up, the TH group also demonstrated greater rates of survival with an intelligence quotient (IQ) score of 85 or greater (52% vs 39%; relative risk [RR], 1.31; $P = .04$).[12]

Further TH trials have demonstrated consistent findings of a reduction in the risk of death or severe disability.[28–30] A 2013 Cochrane systematic review of 11 RCTs, including 1505 term and late preterm infants with moderate/severe encephalopathy and evidence of intrapartum asphyxia found that TH resulted in a significant reduction in the combined outcome of mortality or major ND disability (typical risk ratio, 0.75).[7]

The number need to treat for an additional beneficial outcome was 7 infants, and statistically significant reductions in both mortality and ND disability in survivors were also observed.

Mild Hypoxic Ischemic Encephalopathy

Comparisons of contemporary cohorts with mild HIE with infants from the pre-hypothermia era are challenging. The original Sarnat classification[6] incorporated serial neurologic assessment over the first postnatal week, in addition to EEG findings. Infants enrolled in the large trials of TH were included based on evidence of moderate to severe encephalopathy in the first 6 hours after birth, with exclusion of infants with features of only mild HIE within this time period. Clinical features of encephalopathy are known to evolve over the first few days after hypoxic ischemic insult.[6,31] It is possible that infants regarded as having mild HIE in the TH trials may have been classified as having moderate encephalopathy historically, when assessment was longitudinal and not limited by the therapeutic window for initiation of hypothermia. In addition to the lack of universally accepted diagnostic criteria for mild HIE,[32] the evolution of developmental assessment tools over time has been identified as an additional potential confounder.[33] Thus, although infants with mild HIE were regarded as being at low risk for NDI in the precooling era, supported by the seminal Robertson study,[14] the evidence is less reassuring in the contemporary context.

In mild HIE, there has been a practice creep toward TH with marked regional and institutional variation. In a cohort from England and Wales, 24.9% of infants with mild HIE received TH between 2011 and 2013, compared to 2014 to 2016, when this figure was 35.8% ($P<.001$).[1] In California, the proportion of 1364 infants with mild HIE receiving TH increased from 46% in 2010 to 79% in 2018.[34] A Canadian study of 215 infants referred for TH between 2008 and 2012 reported use of TH in 16% of infants with mild HIE,[35] whereas a UK national survey of cooling practices for infants with mild HIE published in 2017 found that 75% of centers included in the analysis offered TH for this population.[36]

Contributing to this practice creep is the accumulating evidence that infants with mild HIE are at an increased risk of adverse outcomes. A report by Walsh and colleagues from a single center, where TH was offered based on biochemical evidence of perinatal asphyxia irrespective of HIE grade, described 33 of 64 cooled infants (51.5%) as having mild HIE.[37] MRI evidence of brain injury occurred in 54% infants with mild HIE.[37] Overall rates of MRI abnormality were the same in the moderate and mild HIE groups. Further, infants who are screened for but not treated with TH due to minimal or absent features of encephalopathy may still display MRI evidence of brain injury,[38] the consequences of which are yet to be fully elucidated. The prospective, multicenter PRIME (Prospective Research in Infants with Mild Encephalopathy) study assessed a small cohort of infants with mild HIE and identified disability in 16% at 18 to 22 months of age, with affected children more likely to have abnormalities on discharge examination and cerebral MRI.[39] Based on the Bayley Scales of Infant and Toddler Development, Third Edition (BSID-III) and GMFCS, 7% had disabilities classified as severe.[39]

Consistent with findings from the PRIME study, an analysis of pooled data from 4 prospective cohort studies between 2007 and 2015 identified no significant difference in the mean cognitive composite scores on the BSID-III at age 2 years between untreated children with mild HIE ($n = 47$), whose scores were lower than those of the control group, and surviving children with moderate HIE ($n = 53$) who received TH.[40] A recently published population-based cohort study with a median follow-up time of 3.3 years after birth found that infants with mild HIE were 4 times more likely to be diagnosed with the composite outcome of CP, epilepsy, cognitive impairment, and death up to 6 years of age compared with infants without HIE.[41] Survivors of mild HIE also have a higher rate of cognitive impairment than their peers at school age, with a lower full-scale IQ, verbal IQ, and performance IQ at 5 years reported in a prospective cohort study.[42] Van Handel and colleagues additionally identified higher rates of problem behaviors at 9 to 10 years in children with a history of mild HIE, with higher scores for social and attention problems,[43] noting that the behavioral implications of HIE at all stages remain underinvestigated.

Following inclusion of a small proportion of infants with mild HIE in several of the cooling trials and additional observational data, a systematic review by Conway and colleagues combining RCT and non-RCT studies reported on a total of 341 infants with mild HIE, of whom 25% had an abnormal outcome.[44] A meta-analysis was conducted for the 4 included RCTs, with data available for 91 infants with mild HIE: 45 who received TH and 46 who did not. In the cooled group, 29% had an abnormal outcome versus 37% in the non-cooled group (odds ratio, 0.67, $P = .59$).[44] A further systematic review and meta-analysis by Kariholu and colleagues examined whether TH reduced the composite outcome of death or moderate or severe disability at or beyond 18 months of age.[45] Data on 117 infants recruited to 5 hypothermia trials of moderate and severe encephalopathy were included, of whom 56 received TH. Adverse outcomes in the 2 groups were similar, affecting 11 of 56 (19%) of cooled infants and 12 of 61 (19.7%) of the non-cooled infants.[45] A number of randomized trials of TH in mild HIE are ongoing,[46–48] the outcomes of which are awaited.

Preterm Hypoxic Ischemic Encephalopathy

HIE in the *preterm* infant is less well understood. "Encephalopathy of prematurity" (EOP) is a term used to capture brain dysfunction in preterm infants due to a variety of destructive and dysmaturational processes.[49] It is hypothesized that HI and systemic inflammation may be key drivers of the injury.[49,50] Acute HI may pose a particular threat to the preterm brain due to its population of preoligodendrocytes susceptible to oxidative stress and subsequent white matter injury.[51] However, delineating the effect of acute peripartum hypoxic ischemic events from the multifactorial contributors to EOP is challenging. Furthermore, establishing clinical encephalopathy in preterm infants presents additional complexity. For term infants, established criteria to grade HIE have long existed[6]; however, challenges exist in applying these tools to preterm infants.[52] Even seizures, an important manifestation of brain dysfunction, may be more subtle or subclinical than those in term infants. Seizure onset and evolution in preterm infants differs from those born at term.[53,54] Given these challenges, it is not surprising that there is no universally accepted definition of preterm HIE, and outcome data must be interpreted in the context of populations unique to each study.

A single-center retrospective cohort study investigated the outcomes of 30 infants born 33 to 35 weeks GA after receiving TH for HIE. Criteria for TH followed local practice based on the NICHD cooling trial criteria. Clinical encephalopathy was graded as severe ($n = 6$), moderate ($n = 14$), mild ($n = 3$), or abnormal prior to transfer with subsequently normal/mild examination at the study center ($n = 7$). Twenty-six infants survived to discharge and 18 had outcome data at 18 to 24 months. Infants lost to follow-up had lower rates of complications during TH and morbidities at discharge. Death or moderate–severe disability occurred in 11 of 22 (50%) infants. Secondary outcomes included the proportion of infants with Bayley scores less than 85 (33.3%), CP (29.5%), hearing impairment (23.5%), and visual impairment ($\leq$16.7%).

In another single-center retrospective study, MRI reports of infants $\leq$36 weeks GA were reviewed to identify patterns of brain injury in cases of suspected HIE.[55] Essential inclusion criteria included major resuscitation at birth and depressed Apgar scores (<5 at 1 minute, <7 at 5 minutes). Outcome was classified as normal, mild, moderate, severe, or death based on Griffiths scales and neurologic examination. Fifty-five infants were included with outcome data available for 52. Death or moderate to severe disability occurred in 30 of 52 (58%) infants (death in 15, severe in 13, and moderate in 2 infants). Disability outcomes included quadriplegic CP (13), diplegic CP (2), minor motor delay (3), and isolated cognitive impairment (1).

In a single-center retrospective cohort study of infants born 33 to 35 weeks gestational age, 9 infants were identified as having perinatal acidosis (NICHD study criteria) and HIE.[3] Modified Sarnat staging was mild ($n = 2$), moderate ($n = 4$), and severe ($n = 3$). ND assessment was performed at 12 months with the BSID-III. Outcome was considered normal for all infants with mild and moderate HIE and abnormal for all infants with severe HIE (2 deaths and one infant with severe disability).

Finally, a single-center retrospective study of infants 32 to 36 weeks GA identified 12 infants with suspected HIE as defined by depressed Apgar score, biochemical criteria, encephalopathy (seizures or hypotonia), and presence of a sentinel event. Poor outcome was considered to be death, CP, NDI, bilateral deafness, or bilateral blindness. If no outcome data were available, outcome was considered to be normal. A poor outcome was reported in 7 of 12 (58%) infants.

Evidence on Adjuvant Therapies

Since TH has become the standard of care for infants with moderate to severe HIE, interest has turned to investigating adjuvant therapies which may provide additional benefit beyond TH alone. Twenty-four clinical trials have been published testing adjuvant therapies ($n = 12$) (**Tables 1** and **2**). Only one trial is a phase 3 study[56] with the remaining trials being small phase 1 and larger phase 2 studies. A further 14 trials are registered and either currently recruiting or have completed recruitment. Four of these new trials are investigating novel adjuvants yet to be studied in humans (see **Table 1**). There is only one other phase 3 trial currently recruiting and that is for allopurinol + TH versus TH alone.[57]

The only phase 3 trial published compares erythropoietin (Epo) and TH versus TH alone. There was no significant difference between groups on any of the short- or long-term outcomes measured.[56] There are another 3 phase 3 trials of Epo + TH versus TH alone registered[58–60]; two have completed recruitment and all aim to report on long-term outcomes.

A number of other adjuvant therapies have shown promise in phase 1 and 2 trials, including darbepoetin, magnesium sulfate, melatonin, topiramate, human cord tissue mesenchymal stromal cells (hCT-MSC), and autologous umbilical cord blood (UCB). These are yet to be examined in phase 3 trials with long-term outcomes. Xenon trials seem to have ceased, with no new trials registered. A further 5 adjuvant therapies are registered for the first time in humans: CL2020 cells, dexmedetomidine, RLS-0071, caffeine, and metformin.

Despite early interest and promising results in preclinical, phase 1 and phase 2 trials, there is currently no evidence to suggest that TH plus an adjuvant therapy provides improved long-term ND outcomes compared with TH alone. No studies at any phase have reported significantly less CP. Part of the challenge may relate to the efficacy of TH making incremental benefits difficult to demonstrate with statistical significance. The field awaits the outcomes of the remaining phase 3 Epo and Allopurinol trials, while new adjuvant treatments undergo early investigation. Furthermore, it may be possible to investigate the effect of many of these agents as alternatives rather than adjuvants. This may be useful in contexts where TH has been less successful (eg,

Table 1
Adjuvant therapies to therapeutic hypothermia[8,56,61–82]

Reference Lead Author and Year of Publication	Publication Title	Phase (Number of Participants)	Length of Follow-up	Selected Outcomes Comparisons Are for Trial Versus Placebo/Standard Care
TH + Darbepoetin				
Baserga et al,[61] 2015 and Roberts et al,[62] 2015	Darbepoetin administration to neonates undergoing cooling for encephalopathy: a safety and pharmacokinetic trial / Population pharmacokinetics of darbepoetin alfa in conjunction with hypothermia for the treatment of neonatal hypoxic-ischemic encephalopathy	Phase 1/2 (30)	1 mo	Mortality: 1/10 placebo vs 1/10 lose-dose darbepoetin vs 0/10 high-dose darbepoetin. Deaths were attributed to multiorgan failure rather than study participation.
TH + Erythropoietin				
Wu et al,[56] 2022	Trial of erythropoietin for hypoxic-ischemic encephalopathy in newborns	Phase 3 (500)	22–36 mo	Mortality: 14.4% vs 11.5%, RR 1.24, CI 0.78–1.99; death or NDI: 52.5% vs 49.5%, RR 1.03, CI 0.86–1.24, P = .74; survival free of disability: 47.5% vs 50.5%; NDI combined: 43.8% vs 42.3%, RR 0.97, CI 0.77–1.23; CP: 15.4% vs 12.4%, RR 1.1, CI 0.7–1.73.

(continued on next page)

Table 1
(continued)

Reference Lead Author and Year of Publication	Publication Title	Phase (Number of Participants)	Length of Follow-up	Selected Outcomes Comparisons Are for Trial Versus Placebo/Standard Care
Wu et al,[63] 2016 and Mulkey et al,[64] 2017	High-dose erythropoietin and hypothermia for hypoxic-ischemic encephalopathy: A Phase II trial High-dose erythropoietin population pharmacokinetics in neonates with hypoxic-ischemic encephalopathy receiving hypothermia	Phase 2	12 mo	Death during neonatal admission: 8% vs 19%, P = .42; death or moderate to severe NDI: 16.7% vs 38.5%, P = .12; moderate to severe NDI: 8% vs 19%; P = .42; motor performance on Alberta Infant Motor Scale (AIMS) 53.2 vs 42.8, P = .03.
Wu et al,[65] 2012	Erythropoietin for neuroprotection in neonatal encephalopathy: safety and pharmacokinetics	Phase 1	Neonatal outcomes only	Mortality: no deaths reported.
Lv et al,[66] 2017	Effect of erythropoietin combined with hypothermia on serum tau protein levels and neurodevelopmental outcome in neonates with hypoxic-ischemic encephalopathy	Phase 2 equivalent (41)	9 mo	Mortality: no deaths reported; neurodevelopment assessed on Gesell scale: not significantly different between groups, P > .05.
TH + Magnesium sulfate				
Kumar et al,[67] 2023	Magnesium sulfate as an adjunct to therapeutic hypothermia in the management of term infants with hypoxic-ischemic encephalopathy: A randomized, parallel-group, controlled trial	Phase 2 equivalent (134)	1 y	Mortality: 11.9% vs 19.4%, RR 0.61, CI 0.27–1.39, P = .23; mortality or NDI: 24% vs 33%, RR 0.72, CI 0.40–1.30, P = .30; NDI combined: 11.5% vs 13.6%, RR 0.84, CI 0.29–2.43, P = .76.

Study	Title	Phase (N)	Follow-up	Outcomes
Abdel-Aziz et al,[68] 2021	Outcome of infants with hypoxic-ischemic encephalopathy treated by whole body cooling and magnesium sulfate	Phase 1 equivalent (30)	Neonatal outcomes only	Mortality: no deaths reported.
Rahman et al,[69] 2015	Multicenter randomized controlled trial of therapeutic hypothermia plus magnesium sulfate vs therapeutic hypothermia plus placebo in the management of term and near-term infants with hypoxic ischemic encephalopathy (The Mag Cool Study): A pilot study	Phase 1 equivalent (60)	Neonatal outcomes only	Mortality: 6.9% vs 16.1%, P = .426, RR 0.43, CI 0.10–1.75.
TH + Erythropoietin + Magnesium sulfate				
Nonomura et al,[70] 2019	Combination therapy with erythropoietin, magnesium sulfate and hypothermia for hypoxic-ischemic encephalopathy: an open-label pilot study to assess the safety and feasibility	Phase 1 equivalent (9)	18 mo	Mortality: no deaths reported; survival free of disability: 5/8 (62%); NDI combined: 3/8 (38%); CP: 2/8 (25%): GMFCS V.
TH + Melatonin				
Aly et al,[71] 2015	Melatonin use for neuroprotection in perinatal asphyxia: a randomized controlled pilot study	Phase 1/2 (45)	6 mo	Mortality: 1/15 (6.7%) vs 4/15 (26.7%), P = .33; survival free of disability: 10/14 (71.4%) vs 3/11 (27.3%), P<.001.
Balduini Weiss et al,[72] 2019	Melatonin pharmacokinetics and dose extrapolation after enteral infusion in neonates subjected to hypothermia	Early phase 1 (5)	Pharmacokinetics only	Pharmacokinetic data only.

(continued on next page)

Table 1
(continued)

Reference Lead Author and Year of Publication	Publication Title	Phase (Number of Participants)	Length of Follow-up	Selected Outcomes Comparisons Are for Trial Versus Placebo/Standard Care
Jerez-Calero et al,[73] 2020	Hypothermia plus melatonin in asphyctic newborns: A randomized-controlled pilot study	*Phase 2 (25)*	18 mo	Mortality: no deaths reported; NDI combined: Bayley cognitive score 101.25 $\pm$ 21.51 vs 85.56 $\pm$ 17.40, $P =$ .05. No significant difference Bayley motor score.
TH + Xenon				
Dingley et al,[74] 2014	Xenon ventilation during therapeutic hypothermia in neonatal encephalopathy: a feasibility study	*Phase 2 equivalent (14)*	18–20 mo	Mortality: $n = 3/14$; survival free of disability: 6/14; mortality or NDI: 8/14, NDI combined: 5/14 if BDI < 70 MDI and/or PDI or sensory impairment.
Azzopardi et al,[75] 2019; Azzopardi et al,[76] 2016	Moderate hypothermia within 6 h of birth plus inhaled xenon vs moderate hypothermia alone after birth asphyxia (TOBY-Xe): a proof-of-concept, open-label, randomized controlled trial Prospective qualification of early cerebral biomarkers in a randomized trial of treatment with xenon combined with moderate hypothermia after birth asphyxia	*Phase 1 and 2 equivalent (92)*	2019 paper: 2–3 y	From 2019 data, mortality: 26.08% vs 21.74%, RR 1.2, CI 0.577–2.498; CP GMFCS (Any Level): 25% vs 26.7%; CP GMFCS Level 3–5 18.8% vs. 10% (RR 1.875, CI 0.514–6.834).

TH + Topiramate				
Filippi et al,[77] 2018	Safety and efficacy of topiramate in neonates with hypoxic ischemic encephalopathy treated with hypothermia (NeoNATI): a feasibility study	Phase 2 Equivalent (44)	18–24 mo	Mortality: 3/21 vs 2/23; mortality or NDI: 33.3% vs 30.4%, RR 1.095, CI 0.46–2.60, $P = .841$; CP: 35.0% vs 27.3%, RR 1.167, CI 0.476–2.861, $P = .599$.
Nunez-Ramiro et al,[78] 2019	Topiramate plus Cooling for Hypoxic-Ischemic Encephalopathy: A Randomized, Controlled, Multicenter, Double-Blinded Trial	Phase 2 equivalent (110)	Neonatal outcomes only	Mortality: 9.2% vs 19.2%, $P<.123$.
TH+hCT-MSC				
Cotten et al,[79] 2023	A Pilot Phase I Trial of Allogeneic Umbilical Cord Tissue-Derived Mesenchymal Stromal Cells in Neonates With Hypoxic-Ischemic Encephalopathy	Phase 1 (6)	1 y (12–17 mo)	Mortality: No deaths reported; mortality or NDI: All participants survived and developmental assessment scores were within average to low average range for age.
TH + Autologous Umbilical Cord Blood				
Cotten et al,[80] 2014	Feasibility of autologous cord blood cells for infants with hypoxic-ischemic encephalopathy	Phase 1 equivalent (23)	1 y	Mortality (neonatal): 0/23 vs 11/83, no significant. Mortality (15 mo) 2/18 vs 11/36, $P = .25$; mortality or NDI: OR 0.27, CI 0.08–0.92; survival with all 3 Bayley scores <85: 28% vs 59%, $P = .05$.

(continued on next page)

Table 1
(continued)

Reference Lead Author and Year of Publication	Publication Title	Phase (Number of Participants)	Length of Follow-up	Selected Outcomes Comparisons Are for Trial Versus Placebo/Standard Care
TH+2-Iminobiotin				
Favie et al,[81] 2020	Pharmacokinetics and short-term safety of the selective NOS inhibitor 2-iminobiotin in asphyxiated neonates treated with therapeutic hypothermia	*Phase 1 equivalent (12)*	Neonatal outcomes only	Mortality: 2/12. Deaths considered related to severe perinatal asphyxia and not to study medication.
TH + Phenobarbital				
Meyn et al,[82] 2010	Prophylactic phenobarbital and whole-body cooling for neonatal hypoxic-ischemic encephalopathy	*Retrospective*	18 mo (range 18–49 mo)	Mortality: 0% vs 14%, $P = .3$; NDI: 23% vs 45%, $P = .3$.
Sarkar et al,[83] 2012	Does phenobarbital improve the effectiveness of therapeutic hypothermia in infants with hypoxic-ischemic encephalopathy?	*Retrospective: PB-loading dose prior to TH*	Neonatal outcomes only	Mortality: 17% vs 12%, OR 1.4, CI 0.35–5.49, $P = .739$.

Abbreviations: CI, confidence interval; CP, cerebral palsy; NDI, neurodevelopmental impairment; OR, odds ratio; PB, phenobarbital; RR, relative risk; TH, therapeutic hypothermia.

Table 2
Adjuvant therapy trials[5,6]

Reference/Trial Registration	Trial Name	Trial Number	Phase (n)	Research Update	Length of Follow-up	Outcomes: Survival Free of Disability	Outcomes: Mortality	Outcomes: Mortality + NDI	Outcomes: NDI Combined	Outcomes: Cerebral Palsy	NDI Measures Used
TH + Darbepoetin											
Thayyil[a,84]	Darbepoetin in Neonatal Encephalopathy Trial	NCT04432662	Phase 2	Clinicaltrials.gov: recruiting	Trial registration only						
Baserga 2015[61] (also Roberts 2015)[62]	Darbe Administration in Newborns Undergoing Cooling for Encephalopathy	NCT01471015	Phase 1/2 (30)	Completed/ published	1 mo only		1/10 placebo vs 1/10 lose-dose Darbe vs 0/10 high-dose Darbe (attributed to multiorgan failure, not to study participation)				
TH + EPO											
Mohamed[a,60]	Effect of Erythropoietin and Hypothermia on Management of Neonatal Hypoxic Ischemic Encephalopathy	NCT03163589	Phase 3	Clinicaltrials.gov: unknown status	Trial registration only						
Patkai[a,59]	Efficacy of Erythropoietin to Improve Survival and Neurologic Outcome in Hypoxic Ischemic Encephalopathy	NCT01732146	Phase 3	Clinicaltrials.gov: completed	Trial registration only						
Liley[a,58]	Erythropoietin for Hypoxic Ischaemic Encephalopathy in Newborns	NCT03079167	Phase 3	Clinicaltrials.gov: active (completed recruiting)	Trial registration only						
Wu et al,[56] 2022	High-dose Erythropoietin for Asphyxia and Encephalopathy	NCT02811263	Phase 3 (501)	Completed/ published	22–36 mo	47.5 vs 50.5%	14.4 vs 11.5%; 1.24 (0.78–1.99)	52.5% vs 49.5%; 1.03 (0.86–1.24) $P =.74$[a]	43.8% vs 42.3%; 0.97 (0.77–1.23)	15.4% vs 12.4%; 1.1 (0.7–1.73)	

(continued on next page)

Table 2
(continued)

Reference/Trial Registration	Trial Name	Trial Number	Phase (n)	Research Update	Length of Follow-up	Outcomes: Survival Free of Disability	Outcomes: Mortality	Outcomes: Mortality + NDI	Outcomes: NDI Combined	Outcomes: Cerebral Palsy	NDI Measures Used
Wu et al,[63] 2016 (also Mulkey et al,[64] 2017)	Neonatal Erythropoietin and Therapeutic Hypothermia Outcomes in Newborn Brain Injury	NCT01913340	Phase 2	Completed/published	12 mo		Neonatal hospitalization death at 12 mo: no additional deaths): 8% vs 19%; P = .42	Death or moderate/severe NDI at 12 mo; 16.7 vs 38.5%; P = .12	Moderate-to-severe NDI 8% vs 19%; P = .42	Not reported; motor performance Alberta Infant Motor Scale (53.2 vs 42.8, P = .03)	ªModerate to severe neurodevelopmental impairment at 12 mo was defined as an AIMS score less than the fifth percentile for age, or a Warner Initial Developmental Evaluation (WIDEA) score >2 SDs below the mean based on normative data from typically developing infants at 12.9 mo of age (ie, WIDEA <76.4)
Wu et al,[65] 2012	Neonatal Erythropoietin in Asphyxiated Term Newborns	NCT00719407	Phase 1	Completed/published	Neonatal outcomes only		No neonatal deaths				
Lv et al,[66] 2017			*Phase 2 equivalent (41)*	Published	9 mo (and neonatal neurologic measures)	52.3 vs 50.0% "Good neurodevelopment" on gross motor assessment of Gesell's (P > .05).	No deaths reported?	Not reported	19.1% vs 30.0% "neurodevelopmental retardation" on gross motor scale of Gesell's assessment (P > .05)	Not reported	
TH + MgSO₄											
Kumar et al,[67] 2023		CTRI/2018/06/014594	*Phase 2 equivalent (134)*	Completed/published	1 y		11.9% vs 19.4%; RR 0.61 (0.27–1.39); P = .23	24% vs 33%; RR 0.72 (0.40–1.30); P = .30	11.5% vs 13.6%; RR 0.84 (0.29–2.43); P = .76	Not reported	Developmental Assessment Scale for Indian Infants (DASII)ª <70
Abdel-Aziz et al,[68] 2021			*Phase 1 equivalent (30)*	Completed/published	Neonatal outcomes only		No deaths reported				
Rahman et al,[69] 2015	Efficacy Study of Hypothermia Plus Magnesium Sulfate (MgS O₄) in the Management of Term and Near Term Babies With Hypoxic Ischemic Encephalopathy	NCT01646619	*Phase 1 equivalent (60)*	Completed/published	Neonatal outcomes only		6.9% vs 16.1%; P = .426; RR 0.43 (0.10–1.75)				

TH + EPO + MgSO₄

Study	Title	Registration	Phase (n)	Status	Timepoint						Notes
Nonomura et al,[70] 2019	Erythropoietin, magnesium sulfate and hypothermia for hypoxic-ischemic encephalopathy	ISRCTN33604417	Phase 1 equivalent (9)	Completed/published	18 mo	62% (5 of 8 assessed)	Nil	38% (3 of 8 assessed)	38% (3 of 8 assessed)	25% (2 of 8; GMFCS V)	*Kyoto Scale of Psychological Development. Severe neurodevelopmental disability Kyoto Scale of Psychological Development (KPSD) < 70 or an abnormal neurologic finding such as hypotonia or hypertonia with functional impairment. No comparison group.

TH + Melatonin

Study	Title	Registration	Phase (n)	Status	Timepoint						Notes
Tarocco[a,85]	Use of Melatonin for Neuroprotection in Asphyxiated Newborns	NCT03806816		Clinicaltrials.gov: unknown status	Trial registration only						
Aly et al,[71] 2015	Melatonin for Neuroprotection Following Perinatal Asphyxia	NCT02071160	Phase 1/2 (45)	Completed/published	6 mo	n = 10/15 vs n = 3/15 (P<.001)	n = 1 vs n = 4; P = .33 (calculated: 6.7% vs 26.7)	n = 5/15 vs 12/15 (calculated 33.3% vs 80%)	n = 4 vs 8	Not reported	*Neurological assessment and developmental screening with Denver Developmental Screening Test II (DDST-II) (The overall developmental assessment of an infant was considered failed if there were ≥ 2 delays)
Balduini Weiss et al,[72] 2019	Melatonin as a Neuroprotective Therapy in Neonates With HIE Undergoing Hypothermia	NCT02621944	Early phase 1 (5)	Clinicaltrials.gov: recruiting (only pharmacokinetics published in Balduini 2019)	Pharmacokinetics only						

(continued on next page)

Table 2 (continued)

Reference/Trial Registration	Trial Name	Trial Number	Phase (n)	Research Update	Length of Follow-up	Outcomes: Survival Free of Disability	Outcomes: Mortality	Outcomes: Mortality + NDI	Outcomes: NDI Combined	Outcomes: Cerebral Palsy	NDI Measures Used
Jerez-Calero et al,[73] 2020	Whole body hypothermia + melatonin vs whole body hypothermia + placebo in asphyctic newborns	EudraCT No. 2012-000184-24	Phase 2 (25)	Completed/published	18 mo		No deaths reported?		Bayley cognitive score 101.25 ± 21.51 vs 85.56 ± 17.40; P = .05. No significant difference Bayley motor score.	Unclear? No significant difference between groups	aNeurologic and psychomotor development was assessed using the Bayley-III test and by inspection of the scores obtained on the GMFCS and Tardieu scales, at 6 and 18 mo old
TH + Allopurinol											
Rüdiger[A.57]	Effect of Allopurinol for Hypoxic-ischemic Brain Injury on Neurocognitive Outcome	NCT03162653	Phase 3	Clinicaltrials.gov: recruiting (Maiwald et al,[95] 2019; Study protocol published; pharmacokinetics published)	Trial registration only						
TH + Xenon											
Dingley et al,[74] 2014	The CoolXenon Study	ISRCTN7560 2528	Phase 2 equivalent (14)	Completed/published	18-20 mo	n = 6/14 (calculated 42.9%) with normal or mildly delayed outcomes and no visual or hearing impairment	n = 3/14 (calculated 21.4%)	n = 8/14 (calculated 57.1%) 50%	n = 5/14 (calculated 35.7%) if BDI < 70 MDI and/or PDI or sensory impairment	Not reported	aBayley Scales of Infant Development II examination performed at 18-20 mo as a secondary safety analysis. The mental developmental index (MDI) and the psychomotor developmental index (PDI) are classified as mild delay (<1 SD below the mean) if values are <85 and as major delay if <70

Study	Title/Description	Registry No.	Phase (n)	Status	Follow-up	Sample	Mortality	Severe disability	Motor/GMFCS outcome	Assessment tool
Azzopardi et al,[76] 2016; and Azzopardi et al,[75] 2019	Neuroprotective Effects of Hypothermia Combined With Inhaled Xenon Following Perinatal Asphyxia	NCT00934700	Phase 1 and 2 equivalent (92)	Completed/published	2019 paper: 2–3 y	Calculated: n = 21 vs 18	26.08% vs 21.74%; RR 1.2 (0.577–2.498)	Severe: 18.75% vs 13.33%	25% vs 26.05% (RR for GMFCS III–V 1.875 (0.514–6.834)	[a] Bayley Scales of Infant and Toddler Development III
Thoresen[a,86]	Xenon and Cooling Therapy in Babies at High Risk of Brain Injury Following Poor Condition at Birth	NCT02071394	Phase 2 equivalent (82)	Clinicaltrials.gov: completed.	Trial registration only					

TH + Topiramate

Study	Title/Description	Registry No.	Phase (n)	Status	Follow-up	Sample	Mortality	Severe disability	Motor/GMFCS outcome	Assessment tool
Hoffman[a,87]	Topiramate in Neonates Receiving Whole Body Cooling for Hypoxic Ischemic Encephalopathy	NCT01765218	Phase 1/2	Clinicaltrials.gov: terminated	Trial registration only					
Filippi et al,[77] 2018	Safety and Efficacy of Topiramate in Neonates With Hypoxic Ischemic Encephalopathy Treated With Hypothermia	NCT01241019	Phase 2 Equivalent (44)	Completed/published	18–24 mo	n = 3/21 vs 2/23	33.3% vs 30.4% (RR 1.095 (0.46–2.60); $P = .841$ (mortality and severe ND disability)	Severe: n = 4 (of 21) vs n = 5 (of 23)	35.0% vs 27.3%; RR 1.167 (0.476–2.861); $P = .599$	[a] Bayley Scales of Infant and Toddler Development, third edition (BSID III)
Nunez-Ramiro et al,[78] 2019	Multicenter, randomized, blinded clinical study comparing early use of total body moderate hypothermia plus topiramate or placebo in asphyxiated newborn infants evolving to moderate-to-severe hypoxic ischemic encephalopathy	EudraCT No. 2011-005696-17	Phase 2 equivalent (110)	Completed/published	Neonatal outcomes only	9.2% vs 19.2%, $P<.123$				

(continued on next page)

Table 2
(continued)

Reference/Trial Registration	Trial Name	Trial Number	Phase (n)	Research Update	Length of Follow-up	Outcomes: Survival Free of Disability	Outcomes: Mortality	Outcomes: Mortality + NDI	Outcomes: NDI Combined	Outcomes: Cerebral Palsy	NDI Measures Used
TH + hCT-MSC											
Cotten et al,[79] 2023	Study of hCT-MSC in Newborn Infants With Moderate or Severe HIE	NCT03635450	Phase 1 (6)	Completed/published	1 y (12–17 mo)		No deaths reported	All babies survived and developmental assessment scores were within average to low average range for age	All babies' developmental assessment scores were within average to low average range for age	Not reported	[a] Bayley Scales of Infant and Toddler Development 3rd Edition (Bayley III; n = 5; DAYC-II n = 1)
TH + Autologous UCB											
Zhou,[a,88]	Neuroprotective Effect of Autologous Cord Blood Combined With Therapeutic Hypothermia Following Neonatal Encephalopathy	NCT02551003	Phase 1/2	Clinicaltrials.gov: withdrawn	*Trial registration only*						
Geindre C[a,89]	Neonatal Hypoxic Ischemic Encephalopathy: Safety and Feasibility Study of a Curative Treatment With Autologous Cord Blood Stem Cells	NCT02881970	Phase 1/2	Clinicaltrials.gov: recruiting	*Trial registration only*						
Cotten et al,[80] 2014	Cord Blood for Neonatal Hypoxic-ischemic Encephalopathy	NCT00593242	*Phase 1 equivalent* (23)	Completed/published	1 y		Neonatal: 0 of 23 vs 11 of 83 (13%; not significant). At 15 mo: they report as 2/18 vs 11/36; $P = .25$. (3 lost to followup 1 lost but known ot have survived	OR 0.27 (0.08–0.92) (multivariable logistic regression controlling for NICHD score)	Survival with all 3 Bayley scores <85 28% vs 59%, $P = .05$ (p for the inverse proportion: those with survival at/over 85)	Not reported	[a]Bayley Scales of Infant and Toddler Development 3rd Edition (Bayley III)

TH + CL2020						
Matsuyama et al,[90] 2022	The Clinical Trial of CL2020 Cells for Neonatal Hypoxic Ischemic Encephalopathy	NCT0426133 5jRCT2043190112	Phase 1	Protocol published. Clinicaltrials.gov: completed	Protocol only	therefore 2 of 19 died = 10.5% vs 11 of 83 (13.2%)
TH + 2-Iminobiotin						
Favie et al,[81] 2020	2-STEP: A single-center, phase II study to evaluate the safety, tolerability and pharmacokinetics of 2-iminobiotin (2-IB) in neonates with gestational age of ≥36 weeks with moderate to severe perinatal asphyxia treated with therapeutic hypothermia	2014-004265-25 (European)	Phase 1 equivalent (12)	Completed/ published	Neonatal outcomes only	Both groups received 2-iminobiotin (2 doses regimens). 2 of 6 in Group A died vs 0 of 6 in Group B: deaths considered related to severe perinatal asphyxia and not to study medication.
TH + Phenobarbital						
Meyn et al,[82] 2010			Retrospective	Completed/ published	18 mo (range 18–49 mo)	0% vs 14%; $P = .3$; "Multivariate analysis identified prophylactic phenobarbital (0.069; $P = .03$) as associated with improved outcome"
Sarkar et al,[83] 2012			Retrospective: PB loading dose prior to TH	Completed/ published	Neonatal outcomes only	17% vs 12%; $P = .739$ (OR 1.4 [0.35–5.49])

(continued on next page)

Table 2
(continued)

Reference/Trial Registration	Trial Name	Trial Number	Phase (n)	Research Update	Length of Follow-up	Outcomes: Survival Free of Disability	Outcomes: Mortality	Outcomes: Mortality + NDI	Outcomes: NDI Combined	Outcomes: Cerebral Palsy	NDI Measures Used
TH + Dexmedetomidine											
Baserga[a,91]	Dexmedetomidine Use in Infants Undergoing Cooling Due to Neonatal Encephalopathy	NCT04772222	Phase 2	Clinicaltrials.gov: recruiting	*Trial registration only*						
TH + RLS-0071											
Upham[a,92]	A Study to Evaluate the Safety, Tolerability, Pharmacokinetics, and Preliminary Efficacy of RLS-0071 in Newborns With Moderate or Severe Hypoxic-ischemic Encephalopathy Undergoing Therapeutic Hypothermia	NCT05778188	Phase 2	Clinicatrials.gov: recruiting	*Trial registration only*						
TH + Caffeine											
Jackson[a,93]	Caffeine for Hypoxic-Ischemic Encephalopathy	NCT03913221	Phase 1	Clinicaltrials.gov: active (not recruiting)	*Trial registration only*						
TH + Metformin											
Kalish[a,94]	Metformin Treatment in Infants After Perinatal Brain Injury	NCT05590676	Phase 1	Clinicaltrials.gov: not yet recruiting	*Trial registration only*						

Primary outcome bolded.

[a] Trial registration only; chief investigator or contact name included.

preterm HIE or low- or middle-income countries) or to target different mechanisms and time points in the pathway of encephalopathy.

SUMMARY

Long-term outcomes of HIE encompass impairments across all developmental domains. Prospective long-term outcome studies into late childhood are warranted to better understand the prevalence and spectrum of morbidity. In the cooling era, long-term neurodevelopment must be a focus in designing adjuvant therapies. More data are needed on infants with mild HIE. Finally, identifying and defining HIE in the preterm population remain challenging, and outcomes of preterm infants exposed to perinatal HI, especially those less than 32 weeks, warrant further assessment.

Best Practices

What is the current practice?

- Long-term ND follow-up of infants with HIE varies by institution.

What changes in current practice are likely to improve outcomes?

- Infants with HIE experience high rates of impairment across ND domains. Impairments may vary in severity and may present later in childhood. ND surveillance should continue into late childhood to detect impairments and facilitate the implementation of ND therapies and supports.

Major Recommendations

- Long-term ND surveillance of infants with HIE is warranted.

Bibliographic Source(s)

Azzopardi D, Strohm B, Marlow N, Brocklehurst P, Deierl A, Eddama O, et al. Effects of hypothermia for perinatal asphyxia on childhood outcomes. *N Engl J Med.* 2014;371(2):140-149.

Shankaran S, Pappas A, McDonald SA, Vohr BR, Hintz SR, Yolton K, et al. Childhood outcomes after hypothermia for neonatal encephalopathy. *N Engl J Med.* 2012;366(22):2085-2092.

Conway J, Walsh BH, Boylan GB, Murray DM. Mild hypoxic ischaemic encephalopathy and long term neurodevelopmental outcome - A systematic review. *Early Hum Dev.* 2018;120:80-87.

DISCLOSURE

The Neonatal Neurology Fellowship held by Dr S.L. Huntingford is funded by the Cerebral Palsy Alliance.

REFERENCES

1. Shipley L, Gale C, Sharkey D. Trends in the incidence and management of hypoxic-ischaemic encephalopathy in the therapeutic hypothermia era: a national population study. Arch Dis Child Fetal Neonatal Ed 2021;106(5):529–34.
2. McIntyre S, Nelson KB, Mulkey SB, et al. Neonatal encephalopathy: Focus on epidemiology and underexplored aspects of etiology. Semin Fetal Neonatal Med 2021;26(4):101265.
3. Chalak LF, Rollins N, Morriss MC, et al. Perinatal acidosis and hypoxic-ischemic encephalopathy in preterm infants of 33 to 35 weeks' gestation. J Pediatr 2012; 160(3):388–94.

4. Salhab WA, Perlman JM. Severe fetal acidemia and subsequent neonatal encephalopathy in the larger premature infant. Pediatr Neurol 2005;32(1):25–9.
5. Schmidt JW, Walsh WF. Hypoxic-ischemic encephalopathy in preterm infants. J Neonatal Perinat Med 2010;3:277–84.
6. Sarnat HB, Sarnat MS. Neonatal encephalopathy following fetal distress. A clinical and electroencephalographic study. Arch Neurol 1976;33(10):696–705.
7. Jacobs SE, Berg M, Hunt R, et al. Cooling for newborns with hypoxic ischaemic encephalopathy. Cochrane Database Syst Rev 2013;2013(1):Cd003311.
8. Shankaran S, Laptook AR, Ehrenkranz RA, et al. Whole-body hypothermia for neonates with hypoxic-ischemic encephalopathy. N Engl J Med 2005;353(15):1574–84.
9. Gluckman P, Wyatt JS, Azzopardi D, et al. Selective head cooling with mild systemic hypothermia after neonatal encephalopathy: multicentre randomised trial. Lancet 2005;365(9460):663–70.
10. Azzopardi D, Strohm B, Edwards AD, et al. Moderate hypothermia to treat perinatal asphyxial encephalopathy. N Engl J Med 2009;361(14):1349–58.
11. Pedroza-García KA, Calderón-Vallejo D, Quintanar JL. Neonatal hypoxic–ischemic encephalopathy: Perspectives of neuroprotective and neuroregenerative treatments. Neuropediatrics 2022;53(6):402–17.
12. Azzopardi D, Strohm B, Marlow N, et al. Effects of hypothermia for perinatal asphyxia on childhood outcomes. N Engl J Med 2014;371(2):140–9.
13. Shankaran S, Pappas A, McDonald SA, et al. Childhood outcomes after hypothermia for neonatal encephalopathy. N Engl J Med 2012;366(22):2085–92.
14. Robertson C, Finer N. Term infants with hypoxic-ischemic encephalopathy: outcome at 3.5 years. Dev Med Child Neurol 1985;27(4):473–84.
15. Marlow N, Rose AS, Rands CE, et al. Neuropsychological and educational problems at school age associated with neonatal encephalopathy. Arch Dis Child Fetal Neonatal Ed 2005;90(5):F380–7.
16. Barnett A, Mercuri E, Rutherford M, et al. Neurological and perceptual-motor outcome at 5 - 6 years of age in children with neonatal encephalopathy: relationship with neonatal brain MRI. Neuropediatrics 2002;33(5):242–8.
17. Robertson C, Finer NN, Grace MG. School performance of survivors of neonatal encephalopathy associated with birth asphyxia at term. J Pediatr 1989;114(5):753–60.
18. Shankaran S, Woldt E, Toepke T, et al. Acute neonatal morbidity and long-term central nervous system sequelae of perinatal asphyxia in term infants. Early Hum Dev 1991;25(2):135–48.
19. Amiel-Tison C, Ellison P. Birth asphyxia in the fullterm newborn: early assessment and outcome. Dev Med Child Neurol 1986;28(5):671–82.
20. Robertson C, Grace MG. Validation of prediction of kindergarten-age school-readiness scores of nondisabled survivors of moderate neonatal encephalopathy in term infants. Can J Public Health 1992;83:S51–7.
21. Odd D, Whitelaw A, Gunnell D, et al. The association between birth condition and neuropsychological functioning and educational attainment at school age: a cohort study. Arch Dis Child 2011;96(1):30–7.
22. Schreglmann M, Ground A, Vollmer B, et al. Systematic review: long-term cognitive and behavioural outcomes of neonatal hypoxic-ischaemic encephalopathy in children without cerebral palsy. Acta Paediatr 2020;109(1):20–30.
23. Jary S, Lee-Kelland R, Tonks J, et al. Motor performance and cognitive correlates in children cooled for neonatal encephalopathy without cerebral palsy at school age. Acta Paediatr 2019;108(10):1773–80.

24. Lee-Kelland R, Jary S, Tonks J, et al. School-age outcomes of children without cerebral palsy cooled for neonatal hypoxic-ischaemic encephalopathy in 2008-2010. Arch Dis Child Fetal Neonatal Ed 2020;105(1):8–13.

25. Coimbra C, Wieloch T. Moderate hypothermia mitigates neuronal damage in the rat brain when initiated several hours following transient cerebral ischemia. Acta Neuropathol 1994;87(4):325–31.

26. Thoresen M, Bågenholm R, Løberg EM, et al. Kjellmer. Posthypoxic cooling of neonatal rats provides protection against brain injury. Arch Dis Child Fetal Neonatal Ed 1996;74(1):F3–9.

27. Gunn A, Gunn TR, Gunning MI, et al. Neuroprotection with prolonged head cooling started before postischemic seizures in fetal sheep. Pediatrics 1998;102(5):1098–106.

28. Zhou W, Cheng G, Shao X, et al. Selective head cooling with mild systemic hypothermia after neonatal hypoxic-ischemic encephalopathy: a multicenter randomized controlled trial in China. J Pediatr 2010;157(3):367–72.

29. Simbruner G, Mittal RA, Rohlmann F, et al. neon.nEURO.network Trial Participants. Systemic hypothermia after neonatal encephalopathy: outcomes of neo.nEURO.network RCT. Pediatrics 2010;126(4):e771–8.

30. Jacobs S, Morley CJ, Inder TE, et al. Whole-body hypothermia for term and near-term newborns with hypoxic-ischemic encephalopathy: a randomized controlled trial. Arch Pediatr Adolesc Med 2011;165(8):692–700.

31. Thompson C, Puterman AS, Linley LL, et al. The value of a scoring system for hypoxic ischaemic encephalopathy in predicting neurodevelopmental outcome. Acta Paediatr 1997;86(7):757–61.

32. Li Y, Wisnowski JL, Chalak L, et al. Mild hypoxic-ischemic encephalopathy (HIE): timing and pattern of MRI brain injury. Pediatr Res 2022;92(6):1731–6.

33. El-Dib M, Inder TE, Chalak LF, et al. Should therapeutic hypothermia be offered to babies with mild neonatal encephalopathy in the first 6 h after birth? Pediatr Res 2019;85(4):442–8.

34. Yieh L, Lee H, Lu T, et al. Neonates with mild hypoxic-ischaemic encephalopathy receiving supportive care versus therapeutic hypothermia in California. Arch Dis Child Fetal Neonatal Ed 2022;107(3):324–8.

35. Gagne-Loranger M, Sheppard M, Ali N, et al. Newborns referred for therapeutic hypothermia: association between initial degree of encephalopathy and severity of brain injury (what about the newborns with mild encephalopathy on Admission?). Am J Perinatol 2016;33(2):195–202.

36. Oliveira V, Singhvi DP, Montaldo P, et al. Therapeutic hypothermia in mild neonatal encephalopathy: a national survey of practice in the UK. Arch Dis Child Fetal Neonatal Ed 2018;103(4):F388–90.

37. Walsh B, Neil J, Morey J, et al. The frequency and severity of Magnetic Resonance imaging abnormalities in infants with mild neonatal encephalopathy. J Pediatr 2017;187:26–33.e21.

38. Thiim K, Garvey AA, Singh E, et al. Brain injury in infants evaluated for, but not treated with, therapeutic hypothermia. J Pediatr 2023;253:304–9.

39. Chalak L, Nguyen K-A, Prempunpong C, et al. Prospective research in infants with mild encephalopathy identified in the first six hours of life: neurodevelopmental outcomes at 18-22 months. Pediatr Res 2018;84(6):861–8.

40. Finder M, Boylan GB, Twomey D, et al. Two-year neurodevelopmental outcomes after mild hypoxic ischemic encephalopathy in the era of therapeutic hypothermia. JAMA Pediatr 2020;174(1):48–55.

41. Törn A, Hesselman S, Johansen K, et al. Outcomes in children after mild neonatal hypoxic ischaemic encephalopathy: a population-based cohort study. BJOG 2023;130(13):1602–9.

42. Murray D, O'Connor CM, Ryan CA, et al. Early EEG Grade and outcome at 5 Years after mild neonatal hypoxic ischemic encephalopathy. Pediatrics 2016; 138(4):e20160659.

43. Van Handel M, Swaab H, de Vries LS, et al. Behavioral outcome in children with a history of neonatal encephalopathy following perinatal asphyxia. J Pediatr Psychol 2010;35(3):286–95.

44. Conway J, Walsh BH, Boylan GB, et al. Mild hypoxic ischaemic encephalopathy and long term neurodevelopmental outcome - a systematic review. Early Hum Dev 2018;120:80–7.

45. Kariholu U, Montaldo P, Markati T, et al. Therapeutic hypothermia for mild neonatal encephalopathy: a systematic review and meta-analysis. Arch Dis Child Fetal Neonatal Ed 2020;105(2):225–8.

46. Bonifacio S., TIME study: therapeutic hypothermia for infants with mild encephalopathy (TIME), Available at: https://clinicaltrials.gov/study/NCT041764712020. Accessed January 24, 2024.

47. Chalak L., Cool Prime Comparative effectiveness study for mild HIE (COOL-PRIME), Available at: https://clinicaltrials.gov/study/NCT04621279. Accessed January 24, 2024.

48. Thayyil S., Optimising the duration of cooling in mild encephalopathy (COMET), Available at: https://clinicaltrials.gov/study/NCT03409770. Accessed January 24, 2024.

49. Volpe JJ, Inder TE, Darras BT, et al. Volpe's neurology of the newborn e-book. Elsevier Health Sciences; 2017.

50. Yates N, Gunn AJ, Bennet L, et al. Preventing brain injury in the preterm infant-Current Controversies and potential therapies. Int J Mol Sci 2021;22(4).

51. Back SA, Luo NL, Mallinson RA, et al. Selective vulnerability of preterm white matter to oxidative damage defined by F2-isoprostanes. Ann Neurol 2005;58(1):108–20.

52. Pavageau L, Sanchez PJ, Steven Brown L, et al. Inter-rater reliability of the modified Sarnat examination in preterm infants at 32-36 weeks' gestation. Pediatr Res 2020;87(4):697–702.

53. Pisani F, Facini C, Pelosi A, et al. Neonatal seizures in preterm newborns: a predictive model for outcome. Eur J Paediatr Neurol 2016;20(2):243–51.

54. Glass HC, Shellhaas RA, Tsuchida TN, et al. Seizures in preterm neonates: a multicenter observational cohort study. Pediatr Neurol 2017;72:19–24.

55. Logitharajah P, Rutherford MA, Cowan FM. Hypoxic-ischemic encephalopathy in preterm infants: antecedent factors, brain imaging, and outcome. Pediatr Res 2009;66(2):222–9.

56. Wu YW, Comstock BA, Gonzalez FF, et al. Trial of erythropoietin for hypoxic-ischemic encephalopathy in newborns. N Engl J Med 2022;387(2):148–59.

57. Rüdiger M., Effect of Allopurinol for hypoxic-ischemic brain injury on Neurocognitive outcome (ALBINO), Available at: https://clinicaltrials.gov/study/NCT03162653. Accessed January 24, 2024.

58. Liley H., Paean - erythropoietin for hypoxic ischaemic encephalopathy in newborns (PAEAN), Available at: https://clinicaltrials.gov/study/NCT03079167. Accessed January 24, 2024.

59. Patkai J., Efficacy of erythropoietin to improve survival and neurological outcome in hypoxic ischemic encephalopathy (Neurepo), Available at: https://clinicaltrials.gov/study/NCT01732146. Accessed January 24, 2024.

60. Mohamed S.A., Erythropoietin in management of neonatal hypoxic ischemic en-cephalopathy, Available at: https://clinicaltrials.gov/study/NCT03163589. Accessed January 24, 2024.

61. Baserga MC, Beachy JC, Roberts JK, et al. Darbepoetin administration to neo-ates undergoing cooling for encephalopathy: a safety and pharmacokinetic trial. Pediatr Res 2015;78(3):315–22.

62. Roberts JK, Stockmann C, Ward RM, et al. Population pharmacokinetics of dar-bepoetin Alfa in Conjunction with hypothermia for the treatment of neonatal hypoxic-ischemic encephalopathy. Clin Pharmacokinet 2015;54(12):1237–44.

63. Wu YW, Mathur AM, Chang T, et al. High-Dose erythropoietin and hypothermia for hypoxic-ischemic encephalopathy: a phase II trial. Pediatrics 2016;137(6).

64. Mulkey SB, Ramakrishnaiah RH, McKinstry RC, et al. Erythropoietin and brain Magnetic Resonance imaging findings in hypoxic-ischemic encephalopathy: Vol-ume of acute brain injury and 1-year neurodevelopmental outcome. J Pediatr 2017;186:196–9.

65. Wu YW, Bauer LA, Ballard RA, et al. Erythropoietin for neuroprotection in neonatal encephalopathy: safety and pharmacokinetics. Pediatrics 2012;130(4):683–91.

66. Lv HY, Wu SJ, Wang QL, et al. Effect of erythropoietin combined with hypothermia on serum tau protein levels and neurodevelopmental outcome in neonates with hypoxic-ischemic encephalopathy. Neural Regen Res 2017;12(10):1655–63.

67. Kumar C, Adhisivam B, Bobby Z, et al. Magnesium sulfate as an Adjunct to ther-apeutic hypothermia in the management of term infants with hypoxic-ischemic encephalopathy: a randomized, Parallel-group, controlled trial. Indian J Pediatr 2023;90(9):886–92.

68. Abdel-Aziz SM, Rahman MSMA, Shoreit AH, et al. Outcome of infants with hypoxic-ischemic encephalopathy treated by whole body cooling and magne-sium sulfate. Journal of Child Science 2021;11(01):e280–6.

69. Rahman SU, Canpolat FE, Oncel MY, et al. Multicenter randomized controlled trial of therapeutic hypothermia plus magnesium sulfate versus therapeutic hypother-mia plus Placebo in the management of term and near-term infants with hypoxic ischemic encephalopathy (the Mag Cool study): a pilot study. Journal of Clinical Neonatology 2015;4(3):158–63.

70. Nonomura M, Harada S, Asada Y, et al. Combination therapy with erythropoietin, magnesium sulfate and hypothermia for hypoxic-ischemic encephalopathy: an open-label pilot study to assess the safety and feasibility. BMC Pediatr 2019; 19(1):13.

71. Aly H, Elmahdy H, El-Dib M, et al. Melatonin use for neuroprotection in perinatal asphyxia: a randomized controlled pilot study. J Perinatol 2015;35(3):186–91.

72. Balduini W, Weiss MD, Carloni S, et al. Melatonin pharmacokinetics and dose extrapolation after enteral infusion in neonates subjected to hypothermia. J Pineal Res 2019;66(4):e12565.

73. Jerez-Calero A, Salvatierra-Cuenca MT, Benitez-Feliponi Á, et al. Hypothermia plus melatonin in Asphyctic newborns: a randomized-controlled pilot study. Pe-diatr Crit Care Med 2020;21(7):647–55.

74. Dingley J, Tooley J, Liu X, et al. Xenon ventilation during therapeutic hypothermia in neonatal encephalopathy: a feasibility study. Pediatrics 2014;133(5):809–18.

75. Azzopardi D, Chew AT, Deierl A, et al. Prospective qualification of early cerebral biomarkers in a randomised trial of treatment with xenon combined with moderate hypothermia after birth asphyxia. EBioMedicine 2019;47:484–91.

76. Azzopardi D, Robertson NJ, Bainbridge A, et al. Moderate hypothermia within 6 h of birth plus inhaled xenon versus moderate hypothermia alone after birth

asphyxia (TOBY-Xe): a proof-of-concept, open-label, randomised controlled trial. Lancet Neurol 2016;15(2):145–53.

77. Filippi L, Fiorini P, Catarzi S, et al. Safety and efficacy of topiramate in neonates with hypoxic ischemic encephalopathy treated with hypothermia (NeoNATI): a feasibility study. J Matern Fetal Neonatal Med 2018;31(8):973–80.

78. Nuñez-Ramiro A, Benavente-Fernández I, Valverde E, et al. Topiramate plus cooling for hypoxic-ischemic encephalopathy: a randomized, controlled, multicenter, Double-Blinded trial. Neonatology 2019;116(1):76–84.

79. Cotten CM, Fisher K, Malcolm W, et al. A pilot phase I trial of Allogeneic Umbilical cord Tissue-Derived Mesenchymal Stromal cells in neonates with hypoxic-ischemic encephalopathy. Stem Cells Transl Med 2023;12(6):355–64.

80. Cotten CM, Murtha AP, Goldberg RN, et al. Feasibility of autologous cord blood cells for infants with hypoxic-ischemic encephalopathy. J Pediatr 2014;164(5):973–9.e971.

81. Favié LMA, Peeters-Scholte C, Bakker A, et al. Pharmacokinetics and short-term safety of the selective NOS inhibitor 2-iminobiotin in asphyxiated neonates treated with therapeutic hypothermia. Pediatr Res 2020;87(4):689–96.

82. Meyn DF Jr, Ness J, Ambalavanan N, et al. Prophylactic phenobarbital and whole-body cooling for neonatal hypoxic-ischemic encephalopathy. J Pediatr 2010;157(2):334–6.

83. Sarkar S, Barks JD, Bapuraj JR, et al. Does phenobarbital improve the effectiveness of therapeutic hypothermia in infants with hypoxic-ischemic encephalopathy? J Perinatol 2012;32(1):15–20.

84. Thayyil S., Darbepoetin in neonatal encephalopathy trial (EDEN), Available at: https://clinicaltrials.gov/study/NCT04432662. Accessed January 24, 2024.

85. Tarocco A., Use of melatonin for neuroprotection in asphyxiated newborns (MELPRO), Available at: https://clinicaltrials.gov/study/NCT03806816. Accessed January 24, 2024.

86. Thoresen M., Xenon and cooling therapy in babies at high risk of brain injury following poor condition at birth (CoolXenon3), Available at: https://clinicaltrials.gov/study/NCT02071394. Accessed January 24, 2024.

87. Hoffman K.R., Topiramate in neonates receiving whole body cooling for hypoxic ischemic encephalopathy, Available at: https://clinicaltrials.gov/study/NCT01765218. Accessed January 24, 2024.

88. Zhou W., Neuroprotective effect of autologous cord blood combined with therapeutic hypothermia following neonatal encephalopathy, Available at: https://clinicaltrials.gov/study/NCT02551003. Accessed January 24, 2024.

89. Geindre C., Neonatal hypoxic ischemic encephalopathy : safety and feasibility study of a Curative treatment with autologous cord blood Stem cells (NEOSTEM), Available at: https://clinicaltrials.gov/study/NCT02881970. Accessed January 24, 2024.

90. Matsuyama N, Shimizu S, Ueda K, et al. Safety and tolerability of a multilineage-differentiating stress-enduring cell-based product in neonatal hypoxic-ischaemic encephalopathy with therapeutic hypothermia (SHIELD trial): a clinical trial protocol open-label, non-randomised, dose-escalation trial. BMJ Open 2022;12(4): e057073.

91. Baserga M., Dexmedetomidine Use in infants undergoing cooling due to neonatal encephalopathy (DICE trial) (DICE), Available at: https://clinicaltrials.gov/study/NCT04772222. Accessed January 24, 2024.

92. Upham L., A study to Evaluate the safety, tolerability, pharmacokinetics, and Preliminary efficacy of RLS-0071 in newborns with moderate or severe hypoxic-

ischemic encephalopathy undergoing therapeutic hypothermia (STAR), Available at: https://clinicaltrials.gov/study/NCT05778188. Accessed January 24, 2024.

93. Jackson W.M., Caffeine for hypoxic-ischemic encephalopathy, Available at: https://clinicaltrials.gov/study/NCT03913221. Accessed January 24, 2024.
94. Kalish B., Metformin treatment in infants after perinatal brain injury, Available at: https://clinicaltrials.gov/study/NCT05590676. Accessed January 24, 2024.
95. Maiwald CA, Annink KV, Rüdiger M, et al. Effect of allopurinol in addition to hypothermia treatment in neonates for hypoxic-ischemic brain injury on neurocognitive outcome (ALBINO): study protocol of a blinded randomized placebo-controlled parallel group multicenter trial for superiority (phase III). BMC Pediatr 2019; 19(1):210.

Communicating with Parents About Therapeutic Hypothermia and Hypoxic Ischemic Encephalopathy

Integrating a Palliative Care Approach into Practice

Alexa K. Craig, MD[a,b,*], Sara Munoz-Blanco, MD[c,d,e],
Betsy Pilon, BA[f], Monica Lemmon, MD[g,h]

KEYWORDS

- Therapeutic hypothermia • Neonatal encephalopathy
- Hypoxic ischemic encephalopathy • Parent communication • Trauma informed care
- Pediatric palliative care

KEY POINTS

- Neonatal Neurocritical care programs benefit from a robust partnership with specialty palliative care teams. All clinicians caring for infants with serious neurologic conditions should additionally develop a suite of primary palliative care skills.
- Many parents of infants treated with hypothermia describe traumatic experiences associated with their child's hospitalization; principles of trauma-informed care can inform best practices in parent-clinician communication.
- Communication of prognosis and associated uncertainty can be challenging for both clinicians and families. The ALIGN framework offers a parent-informed strategy to support prognostic communication.

Continued

[a] Division of Pediatric Neurology, Department of Pediatrics, The Barbara Bush Children's Hospital at Maine Medical Center, Portland; [b] Department of Pediatrics, Tufts University School of Medicine, Boston, MA, USA; [c] Department of Pediatrics, Johns Hopkins School of Medicine; [d] Division of Perinatal-Neonatal Medicine, Department of Pediatrics, Johns Hopkins Children's Center, 1800 Orleans Street, Baltimore, MD 21287, USA; [e] Division of Pediatric Palliative Care, Department of Pediatrics, Johns Hopkins Children's Center, 1800 Orleans Street, Baltimore, MD 21287, USA; [f] Hope for HIE, West Bloomfield, MI, USA; [g] Division of Pediatric Neurology and Developmental Medicine, Department of Pediatrics, Duke University School of Medicine, DUMC 3936, Durham 27710, USA; [h] Division of Pediatric Neurology and Developmental Medicine, Department of Population Health Sciences, Duke University School of Medicine, DUMC 3936, Durham 27710, USA
* Corresponding author. 92 Campus Drive, Scarborough, ME 04074.
E-mail address: alexa.craig@mainehealth.org

Clin Perinatol 51 (2024) 711–724
https://doi.org/10.1016/j.clp.2024.04.009

Continued

- Parents of infants treated with hypothermia are at increased risk of poor psychosocial well-being. Strategies to improve support include facilitating parent holding during hypothermia, mental health screening and treatment, and peer support programs.

INTRODUCTION

Parents of children with hypoxic ischemic encephalopathy (HIE) describe a variety of challenges in the neonatal intensive care unit, including fragmented communication,[1,2] the strain of prognostic uncertainty,[3] and the trauma[4] associated with medical and family crisis.[2] How clinicians communicate amidst this trauma has the potential to improve parent well-being, facilitate effective decision making, and build a foundation for sustained therapeutic alliance.[5,6] Intentional integration of evidence-based strategies from the discipline of palliative care offers an opportunity for Neonatal Neurocritical care programs to enhance support for patients, families, and teams.

Pediatric Palliative Care (PPC) is a medical subspecialty that provides an added layer of support for patients with a serious illness. Neonatal serious illness is defined as an illness that: "(1) carries a high risk of short-term mortality or lifelong medical complexity with probable shortened lifespan, (2) may involve substantial prognostic uncertainty (especially in regard to neurodevelopment) that complicates medical decision-making, and (3) significantly impacts the patient and family's life now or in the future with strain related to treatments and care".[7] PPC uses a holistic approach, with a focus on personhood, getting to know patients and families beyond their serious illness diagnosis. Palliative medicine trained clinicians receive specialized training in communication skills, facilitating shared decision making, bereavement support, and symptom management. These advanced skills are highly relevant to the care of infants receiving therapeutic hypothermia, as clinicians are often tasked with sharing complex diagnoses, navigating prognostic uncertainty, and engaging in goal-concordant shared decision-making.

PPC refers to basic skills and competencies that ideally all clinicians who care for patients with serious illness should have, including communication skills to facilitate goals of care discussions and shared decision-making, and knowledge of trauma-informed care. Specialty Palliative Care refers to subspecialist-trained clinicians who provide consultation and specialty care. PPC teams are interdisciplinary by nature (eg, physicians, advanced practice providers, nurses, social workers, chaplains, and child life specialists) and PPC team composition and availability varies by institution.[8] Neonatal Neurocritical care programs benefit from robust partnership with specialty palliative care teams.[9] In addition, all clinicians caring for infants with serious neurologic conditions should develop a suite of PPC skills.

In this article, the authors will highlight challenges that arise in communicating information about therapeutic hypothermia and HIE, provide recommendations for practicing clinicians, and offer strategies to integrate a palliative care approach into practice. The authors will use a fictional case to highlight 4 key phases in the care trajectory: the day of birth, a day during hypothermia treatment, MRI day (when prognosis is often communicated to families), and preparing for discharge. At each of these time points, the authors highlight circumstances where communication challenges can arise and provide recommendations to improve communication. While the critical role of and need for specialty palliative care support is well-described in the literature,[10–12] in this article the authors will primarily focus on how non-palliative care trained clinicians can improve their PPC skillset.[9,13] Key topics will include communicating amidst trauma, supporting the parent experience, navigating prognostic uncertainty, and facilitating shared decision making and the transition home.

DAY OF BIRTH: COMMUNICATING AMIDST TRAUMA

Case part 1: Kai was born in a small community hospital via stat C-section to a G1 P1 birth parent, who presented with symptoms of uterine rupture. He required intubation and chest compressions in the delivery room. His Apgar scores were 0, 2, and 4 and cord gases could not be obtained, however, a capillary gas around 90 minutes was 7.14/63/-9. His neurologic examination demonstrated moderate neonatal encephalopathy (NE) and the decision were made to initiate therapeutic hypothermia. Kai was transferred to the tertiary care center and his non-birth parent followed the ambulance by car while the birth parent remained at the community hospital.

Parents are unprepared for the suddenness with which a healthy pregnancy and labor can transition from routine to traumatic.[4,14] For many parents, this day of birth is characterized by trauma that is then exacerbated by separation from their newborn. Amidst the trauma, parents often express feelings of guilt.[15,16] Awareness and implementation of the 6 principles of trauma informed care (TIC) is a key element of PPC and can aid clinicians in their ability to communicate well with traumatized parents.[5] Use of TIC relies on clinicians to *realize* the profound adverse impacts of trauma, *recognize* the signs and symptoms of trauma, *respond* to this trauma in an informed manner, and *resist re-traumatizing* those made vulnerable by their initial trauma experience.[17] The definitions of the 6 TIC principles along with strategies to resist re-traumatization and sample statements can be found in **Tables 1** and **2**.

When implemented successfully, the first 3 TIC principles inherently foster a trusting relationship between the clinician and the traumatized person. The *first* principle of TIC is the principle of safety and applies to both physical safety (the setting where communication occurs) and psychological safety (safe interpersonal interactions-refer to principle 6).[17] A safe setting for communication is private and maintains confidentiality.[6] The *second* principle of TIC is trustworthiness and transparency[17] and applies to communication through the use of layman's terms to describe complex medical issues[2,5,6,18] and the provision of written supplemental information.[1,16] The use of layman's terms not only improves parental understanding, but also improves trust in the clinician or clinical team. The *third* principle of TIC is peer support, a principle that can contribute to safety, further build trust and cultivate hope.[17] Peer support can be achieved through connecting those with lived experience to new parents with experts recommending this occur within 72 hours of admission.[6] Specialty palliative care teams and national organizations such as Hope for HIE, Courageous Parents Network, Child Neurology Foundation, Hand to Hold or regional support groups can provide families with both information and support.

The remaining 3 principles of TIC focus on ways to encourage autonomy and empowerment. The *fourth* principle of TIC is collaboration and mutuality, which identifies the importance of minimizing or eliminating the power differential that can exist between the care team and parents.[17] Implementation of the fourth principle involves respecting families as integral members of the care team and ensuring their involvement with all decisions.[5,6] The *fifth* principle of TIC is voice and choice and encourages parents to be actively involved in shared decision making.[17] Parents should be viewed as key members of the team, not as visitors in the neonatal intensive care unit (NICU).[5] The *sixth* principle of TIC is cultural, historical, and gender issues and focuses on the

Table 1
Trauma informed care principles, strategies to resist re-traumatization and sample statements

Principle	Strategy to Resist Retraumatization	Sample Statement
SAFETY	• Promote physical safety: private location for important discussions • Promote psychological safety: see TIC principle 6	"I have an update about Kai's condition that I would like to share with you. Where would you like to have this conversation? (suggestions can include Kai's hospital room or conference room)"
PEER SUPPORT	• Ensure that difficult conversations occur with parents together • Connect families with peer supports	"Who would you like to be there during the conversation? I know (insert birth parent's name) has not yet been transferred. Can we try to get them to virtually join us for this discussion?"
COLLABORATION AND MUTUALITY	• Minimize power differential between clinical care team and parents	"Thank you for joining us for this conversation. Kai's care team is centered with his parents, so let's begin there."
EMPOWERMENT, VOICE AND CHOICE	• Empower parents as members of the care team	"What would you like to talk about first? Is there anything you want to make sure we address?"
TRUSTWORTHINESS AND TRANSPARENCY	• Explain complex medical information using layman's terminology	"We have had some difficulty overnight maintaining IV access for Kai. As you probably know, an IV is a tiny tube that we place in a vein to allow us to give fluids, nutrition and medication to Kai. We want to ask for your permission to place a different type of IV into Kai's belly button. This is called an umbilical line...."
CULTURAL, HISTORICAL AND GENDER ISSUES	• Avoid sterotypes and biases that may arise from differences in spoken language, culture, ethnicity, race, socio-economic status, substance use, immigration status, sexual orientation, gender or disability	Use the child's and parent's name in conversations. Use non-gendered references to parent roles such as birth parent and non-birth parent rather than mother and father. If unsure, ask the family member what their preferred terminology and pronouns are.

importance of an appropriate response to the racial, ethnic, and cultural needs of the individuals or families for whom care is provided.[17] Studies have identified structural, institutional, and interpersonal racism that adversely impacts care.[19,20] The embodiment of the sixth TIC principle involves confronting and dismantling existing stereotypes and biases and welcoming all equally to the NICU.[6]

VITAL talk© is a training organization for healthcare workers that teaches skills to facilitate effective and empathetic conversations with patients and families and can also build PPC skills. NURSE statements (Naming, Understanding, Respecting, Supporting, Exploring) are an integral part of the VITAL talk methodology and serve to

Table 2
Communication pearls: day of birth

PEARL	WHAT IT MAY SOUND LIKE
BIG PICTURE BEFORE DETAILS - DEVELOP A HEADLINE: Concise, accurate, jargon-free statement about the status and concern of the baby *Based on parental feedback, we recommend using the term "brain injury" instead of "brain damage"*	"In the initial hours to days, this may look like: "We are concerned your baby did not receive enough oxygen to their brain/organs during the labor/delivery process which means they may have suffered a brain injury. The next 72 hours to 1 week will be filled with uncertainty which is usually hard to navigate and cope with for most families who are going through therapeutic hypothermia."
CREATE OPPORTUNITY FOR FAMILY TO VERBALIZE WHAT THEY ARE MOST WORRIED ABOUT	*Many families will share they are most worried about survival. Perhaps offer that baby is either likely or unlikely to survive.* "What worries you the most right now?
ATTENDING TO EMOTION: Naming, Understanding, Respecting, Supporting, Exploring. Let the statement land --> PAUSE *May use VitalTalk NURSE Statements*	**N**aming: It must be so scary to see your baby like this. **U**nderstanding: I can't imagine what you're going through. **R**especting: I can see what a loving and caring parent you are. **S**upporting: Our team will be here every step of the way to support you and your family. **E**xploring: Can you tell me more about what you mean when you say...
ADDRESSING GUILT	"I work with many families in the NICU, and some of the common feelings include guilt, anxiety, and fear." <<PAUSE>> *If parent expresses guilt...* "You made the right decisions to get care for your baby and make sure they are getting what they need right now."
PATIENT NAME AND FAMILY IDENTITY: Be sure to use the baby's name, and ask what the parents prefer being called: first names vs. parental label: Mom, Dad, etc.	"Tell me about your baby's name. What do you prefer I call you?"
AVOID THE INFORMATION VOID	"Each day we will learn some information that will help us with long-term prognosis. For example, the EEG, the baby's exam, and finally the MRI."

articulate empathy and establish rapport.[21] These statements convey understanding, demonstrate respect, validate experiences, and foster connections all factors that also align with a TIC approach. Examples of NURSE statements are provided in the tables for each section of this article (**Table 3**).

DURING HYPOTHERMIA TREATMENT: SUPPORTING THE PARENT EXPERIENCE

Case part 2: Kai remained stable but developed seizures that resolved after treatment with phenobarbital and Fosphenytoin. He extubated to room air on day of life 2 and his

Table 3
Communication pearls: during hypothermia treatment

PEARL	WHAT IT MAY SOUND LIKE
WHAT BABY MIGHT LOOK LIKE DURING COOLING	"We will be closely monitoring your baby for comfort and pain during cooling. It can feel overwhelming looking at your baby with these interventions. Most babies tolerate cooling fairly well. However, you may notice your baby shivering from being cold."
IMPACT OF MEDICATIONS: Sedation, anti-seizure medications, pain medications	"Many medications used during therapeutic hypothermia (or control seizures) can cause them to be extra sleepy. This is to let the brain and body rest."
FAMILY-CENTERED CARE: Partner with nursing and neonatal therapy to encourage families to participate in: • Routine cares: diaper changes, pulse ox changes etc. • Learn about baby cues and signals • Look at the safety and feasibility of holding • Look at the safety and feasibility of feeding or use of other oral stimuli led by parents • Encourage parents to talk, sing and read to their baby • Encourage use of family scented items. • Implement family-centered, multidisciplinary rounds.	*Family-centered, multidisciplinary rounds with neonatology and neurology bring consistency to decrease confusing, inconsistent messaging to families. If neurology is unavailable in person, consider use of teleconferencing software.* "While your baby is in therapeutic hypothermia, typical parenting is interrupted, but there are many things you can do to be close with your baby like participating in their care, reading, talking and singing to them, and we'll evaluate when it's safest to start holding your baby. Working with the nursing staff and even the neonatal therapists can be a way you can feel closer to your baby."
NAMING THE DIAGNOSIS: Parents have a fundamental right to accurate medical information and using words like "probable" or "suspected" tied to Hypoxic Ischemic Encephalopathy when you can accurately rule out other etiology is essential care.	"When baby's brains don't get enough oxygen, they can develop something called hypoxic ischemic encephalopathy or HIE. We do not yet know that Kai has HIE, but we suspect this and will learn more once he has had his MRI."
ATTENDING TO EMOTION: Parents may express significant emotional turmoil, or appear in shock and coping well during therapeutic hypothermia.	Working through the "Naming, Understanding, Respecting, Supporting, Exploring" VitalTalk NURSE statements to validate feelings and complexities in potential maternal health impacts, impacts of trauma (fight, flight, freeze).
INTRODUCTION OF THE PALLIATIVE CARE TEAM IN APPLICABLE SITUATIONS: Share how palliative care is a resource for families whose children may have some medical complexities and different than hospice.	"We have a resource team that many families have found helpful with medical decision-making and bringing your values and beliefs to your child's medical care. This is different than hospice which focuses on end of life care."

parents were able to hold him on day 2 and 3 of cooling. They participated in daily bedside rounds, changed his diaper often, and read aloud to him in the afternoons.

Employing PPC skills, clinicians can help alleviate the re-traumatized parents experience while their newborn is hypothermic (see **Table 3**). This trauma can occur if the skin color is very pale or bluish or if the newborn is shivering.[4,22] Parents may also note that their newborn is moving very infrequently and be frightened. Clinicians should explain how medications are or are not used to treat shivering and how anti-seizure medications can cause excessive sedation. Parents also often mention the loss of the expected skin to skin time after the birth.[4] In interviews and surveys about the experience of therapeutic hypothermia, parents repeatedly expressed frustration over the lack of physical contact with their newborn, specifically the inability to hold during therapeutic hypothermia.[4,15,22,23] Some parents referred to the moment of holding after hypothermia treatment completed as a "moment of rebirth".[23] A pilot study demonstrated feasibility of holding during therapeutic hypothermia without temperature changes outside the goal range of 33 to 34°.[24] A larger study of 70 occurrences of holding in 27 newborns, noted stable vital signs for holding durations of up to 2 hours.[25] Holding during hypothermia can help parents restore normalcy and recover from trauma.

There have been conflicting recommendations regarding use of the term "HIE" with families, particularly given the existing medicolegal environment, which may contribute to avoidance of the term.[26] Some clinicians prefer to use "newborn or neonatal encephalopathy (NE)" as a broader term more inclusive of etiologies other than hypoxia and ischemia.[27] Use of the correct terminology, including HIE when appropriate, is important to families as the experience of having a newborn with HIE can be life altering.[28] One challenge with use of broader terms like NE is the resulting disconnection that can occur between the family and the clinical team. Families may do their own research or discover the term HIE in the medical record and then develop a sense of mistrust in their clinical team feeling as if valuable information that connects them to peer support has been withheld.[16] Some have recommended use of the term "probable HIE" as a way to both use terminology that resonates with families and acknowledge other potential etiologies.[29] Authors from the Definition of Neonatal Encephalopathy Group (DEFiNE) are working on a Delphi consensus approach to develop a subclassification system, in which the various etiologies and timings of NE can be further refined.[30] We recommend that clinicians employ the TIC principles of trustworthiness and transparency, as well as collaboration and mutuality and provisionally name the diagnosis they suspect is present.[5,16]

MRI DAY: NAVIGATING PROGNOSTIC UNCERTAINTY

Case part 3: Kai had an MRI of the brain on day 5 that revealed bilateral moderate basal ganglia injury, bilateral involvement of the posterior limb of the internal capsule with diffusion signal abnormality extending into the cerebral peduncles, as well as injury to the bilateral hippocampi. The NICU team sets up a family meeting to discuss the results and invites Pediatric Neurology, the Palliative Care Team, the bedside nurse, and extended family members.

Prognostication for newborns treated with therapeutic hypothermia is complex and relies on incorporation of the clinical history, neurologic exam, electroencephalography, and neuroimaging. Despite a robust literature around prognostication, the ability to predict an individual outcome remains challenging. The etiology, duration, and severity of the neurologic insult are often incompletely known, and neuroplasticity mediates outcome. Additionally, the composite outcomes used in the landmark trials[31–33] effectively lump together neonates who die with others who have isolated visual impairment and limit the ability of clinicians to extrapolate these clinical trial outcomes to individual experience.

Intensive communication skills trainings, which build the PPC skill set address content relevant to prognostic discussion, have been developed in many disciplines, including neonatology, palliative care, and oncology.[34–36] The authors recommend clinicians familiarize themselves with this literature and adopt strategies that feel authentic to their practice (see Table 4). Physicians, who have had formal education in communication skills, report more comfort and satisfaction with serious news or conversations.[37] Data support that communication skill simulation training leads to changes in clinician's behavior during serious conversations and is an effective method of education grounded in adult learning principles.[37] Neonatal Neurocritical care clinicians, who typically have additional training in estimating and communicating neurologic prognosis, are an important resource to use when available.[38]

Prognostic uncertainty is a short- and a long-term challenge for families and can cause significant distress during and beyond the neonatal period.[1,3,4,14] The ALIGN framework is a parent-informed strategy that employs PPC skills and helps guide discussion of neurologic prognosis relying on 5 key communication phases: Approach,

Table 4
Communication pearls: MRI day

PEARL	WHAT IT MAY SOUND LIKE
PRE-MEETING HUDDLE WITH ALL TEAMS	**WHAT THIS MAY LOOK LIKE:** Designate a lead communicator, develop headline and secondary information bullet points, practice.
REFLECT ON POTENTIAL BIASES BEFORE PROGONSIS CONVERSATION **Example of ouR-HOPE tool:** *How am I...* *... aware of my values and personal experience and how these inform my prognosis and discussion of outcomes?*	**WHAT THIS MAY LOOK LIKE:** Discuss what you know about the family's values and beliefs. Consider using a tool like the ALIGN framework (Lemmon et al) to facilitate prognostic discussion and ouR-HOPE tool to attend to biases as a team. Avoid decision-making/goals of care the same day as disclosing MRI results and prognosis discussion.
HEADLINE: Concise, accurate, jargon-free statement about the status and concern of the baby	"We reviewed the MRI and it showed injury to different parts of your baby's brain and we want to talk about what this may mean for Kai as he grows up."
SECONDARY INFORMATION: Concise, accurate information with **DIAGNOSTIC NAMING and PROGNOSIS GUIDANCE**	"The injured parts of the brain can tell us some things that may or may not happen in the future. Kai is at risk for developing something called cerebral palsy, which occurs due to injury to the brain around the time of birth from lack of oxygen. For some children, cerebral palsy can effect the arms and the legs. This type of CP is called quadriplegic CP."
ATTENDING TO EMOTION: Naming, Understanding, Respecting, Supporting, Exploring. Let the statement land --> PAUSE *May use VitalTalk NURSE Statements*	**Naming:** You may feel overwhelmed with all of this information. **Understanding:** I know this is so much to take in. **Respecting:** Let us know how you need to process this, like if you'd like to come back to this information later, or would like this written down so it's easier to read through. **Supporting:** As questions come up, or if you need to go over this information again, we are happy to do so. We are here to help Kai and your family. **Exploring:** Can you tell me more about what you mean when you say...
INTRODUCTION OF THE PALLIATIVE CARE TEAM IN APPLICABLE SITUATIONS: Share how palliative care is a resource for families whose children may have some medical complexities and different than hospice.	"We have a resource team that many families have found helpful with medical decision-making and bringing your values and beliefs to your child's medical care. This is different than hospice which focuses on end of life care."

Learn, Inform, Give Support, and Next Steps.[39] In the Approach phase, parents value communication from clinicians familiar with the newborn and family. In the Learn phase, parents value being asked how they want to hear information and being offered the opportunity to summarize what they already know. In the Inform phase, parents emphasize the importance of leaving space for hope. In the Give Support and Next Steps phases, parents value real emotional support from clinicians and connection to peer support.

There is a tension between providing direct and transparent information about outcome and the provision of hope. Clinicians may worry that offering concrete information about the potential for poor outcome risks undermining a family's ability to hope for the future. The ouR-HOPE framework is a self-assessment tool designed to help front-line clinicians critically evaluate their approach to estimation and communication of prognosis in neonatal neurologic conditions.[40,41] The authors recommend use of this tool for all clinicians caring for newborns treated with therapeutic hypothermia. For clinicians offering prognostication regularly, routinely revisiting this tool offers a way to refine and improve PPC communication skills. The ouR-HOPE framework relies on 5 key principles: Reflection, Humility, Open-Mindedness, Partnership, and Engagement. Each principle is accompanied by a set of reflective questions that prompt the reader to critically self-reflect helping to avoid unconscious biases **(Table 4)**.[41]

PLANNING FOR DISCHARGE: FACILITATING SHARED DECISION MAKING AND THE TRANSITION HOME

Case part 4: Kai has been able to orally feed small amounts about 2 to 3 times per day averaging 5 to 10 cc per feed and is gavage fed the remainder through a nasogastric tube. He remains on room air with intermittent stridor related to suspected laryngomalacia. His parents are feeling optimistic that he is waking up more as the phenobarbital wears off and eating more each day. The NICU team is worried that he will not achieve full oral feeding.

For the sickest neonates, clinicians and families face decisions about withdrawal or withholding life-sustaining treatment. Most neonates who die during their admission to the NICU do so after life-sustaining treatment is not initiated or is withdrawn.[42] Parents likely rely on a range of values and medical facts as they make these decisions, including considerations about quality of life, spirituality, and future outcome. In many settings, including the United States, a shared decision-making approach is the preferred model of decision making for preference-sensitive decisions and is a cornerstone principle of Palliative Care. A shared decision-making approach is one in which clinicians and parents share decision-making roles, with clinicians providing decision-relevant medical information and helping parents integrate medical information with their values.[43] Existing data suggest that clinicians do not uniformly elicit values in conversations about decisions. Further, data suggest that parents and clinicians may hold different values about the importance of functional outcome in decision making and how to weigh outcomes of death and significant disability.[44–46] These cases can be challenging and can cause significant moral distress to parents and clinicians. It is not uncommon for clinicians to misperceive a family's discussion of hope as an indication of lack of awareness of illness severity. Existing data suggest that families can simultaneously hold devastating information about outcome concurrently with hope for the future.[45,47,48] Palliative care clinicians offer expertise in facilitating shared decision making and communicating about goals of care. All clinicians caring for neonates treated with therapeutic hypothermia should be trained in basic

PPC skills, including facilitating shared decision making, prognostic communication, and symptom management.[49] When available, specialty palliative care services should be engaged to offer both team and family support.

Families of newborns treated with therapeutic hypothermia often share a feeling of being unprepared for discharge home (**Table 5**). Until discharge, their parenting journey has been highly medicalized, and associated with a wide range of emotions, even if their child is getting discharged without any additional medical interventions such as a tracheostomy or feeding tube. While outside the scope of this article, guidelines to support discharge and transition planning exist.[50] Programs to support the transition home, including transitional medical home programs, have demonstrated reductions in re-

Table 5 Communication pearls: planning for discharge	
PEARL	**WHAT IT MAY SOUND LIKE**
UPDATED HEADLINE: As clinical course continues, address updated concerns	"While Kai is making some progress with oral feedings, he is still requiring significant support. We worry he may not be able to take enough by mouth to support his growth."
SECONDARY INFORMATION: Concise, accurate information with potential decision-making introduction	"Kai may need a g-tube to help him get his feeding needs met. This is a decision that you will want to discuss with the different members of the team for their perspectives, including the surgical team."
ATTENDING TO EMOTION: Naming, Understanding, Respecting, Supporting, Exploring. Let the statement land --> PAUSE *May use VitalTalk NURSE Statements*	**Naming:** You may feel like a feeding tube is a failure or a step back. **Understanding:** Many parents share similar feelings. **Respecting:** You are doing a great job working with him on all of this. **Supporting:** Our team will be here every step of the way to support you and your family. **Exploring:** Can you tell me more about what you mean when you say...
TRANSITIONING HOME: Supporting with education and reassurance	Families often feel like they are ill-prepared for the transition home. **WHAT IT MAY LOOK LIKE:** **Education:** Diagnosis-specific information including seizure and medication status, risk of Infantile Spasms, training on using applicable medical equipment, teaching families about early intervention services, with the goal to build health literacy. **Mental Health Screening:** All parents should be screened for mental health conditions prior to discharge, and if identified at risk, outpatient referrals and care should be made to professional and diagnosis-specific, longitudinal peer support. **Longitudinal Healthcare Needs:** Connect families to any applicable outpatient services their child may need, including continuing palliative care. Parents should exit the NICU with an understanding of who to elevate immediate concerns to and how they should elevate them, as they transition home.

admissions[51] and emergency visits[52] for high-risk infants.[53] Parents and caregivers are vulnerable to post-traumatic stress disorder, anxiety, and depression.[54,55] While the sources of these symptoms are multifactorial, multiple studies highlight the value of peer support and connection for parents.[39,56] In addition to screening for mental health sequelae, diagnosis-specific education (eg, discussion of seizures, infantile spasms, and how to contact neurology) is necessary to help families during the transition from NICU to home to outpatient care.

SUMMARY

Families and clinicians who care for infants treated with hypothermia face communication challenges throughout the care continuum. In this article, the authors highlight opportunities to support communication and build PPC skills. The authors propose that employing PPC principles can improve communication. The authors have provided sample statements that can be adapted for use during 4 critical time points during an admission for therapeutic hypothermia: day of birth with the focus on trauma, during hypothermia treatment with the focus on involving the family in the care of the newborn, MRI day with the focus on prognostic uncertainty, and planning for discharge with a focus on shared decision making. As the field of Neonatal Neurocritical Care advances, there must be sustained investment to guide the development of effective communication skills.

DISCLOSURE

None.

Best Practices

What is the current practice for communication during therapeutic hypothermia?

- Parents often wait for the MRI of the brain to be performed after therapeutic hypothermia is complete before they get information about the diagnosis and prognosis.

Best Practice

- Employ PPC principles to communicate at regular intervals with parents and provide them with a provisional HIE diagnosis before the MRI has been performed.

What changes in current practice are likely to improve outcomes?

- Clinicians in the NICU can develop their PPC skills and involve specialty palliative care teams when they are available to assist with discussions surrounding prognostic uncertainty and shared-decision making.

Pearls/Pitfalls at the point-of-care

- Avoid retraumatizing parents through inconsistent or poor-quality communication or by being insensitive to their lived experience.

Major Recommendations

- The authors recommend that:
  - All clinicians caring for infants with HIE should receive training in prognostic communication and facilitating shared decision making.
  - Clinicians should familiarize themselves with evidence-based tools to support effective communication, including the NURSE, ALIGN, and ouR-HOPE frameworks.

> ○ Neonatal neurocritical care programs should promote parent well-being through peer support.
>
> **Bibliographic Source(s)**
>
> ---
>
> Vital Talk Responding to emotion: articulating empathy using NURSE statements. Accessed February 19, 2024. https://www.vitaltalk.org/guides/responding-to-emotion-respecting/

REFERENCES

1. Craig AK, Gerwin R, Bainter J, et al. Exploring parent experience of communication about therapeutic hypothermia in the neonatal intensive care Unit. Adv Neonatal Care : official journal of the National Association of Neonatal Nurses 2018;18(2):136–43.
2. Lemmon ME, Donohue PK, Parkinson C, et al. Communication challenges in neonatal encephalopathy. Pediatrics 2016;138(3). https://doi.org/10.1542/peds.2016-1234.
3. Craig AK, Gerwin R, Bainter J, et al. Exploring parent expectations of neonatal therapeutic hypothermia. J Perinatol 2018;38(7):857–64.
4. Craig AK, James C, Bainter J, et al. Parental perceptions of neonatal therapeutic hypothermia; emotional and healing experiences. J Matern Fetal Neonatal Med 2020;33(17):2889–96.
5. Sagaser A, Pilon B, Goeller A, et al. Parent experience of hypoxic-ischemic encephalopathy and hypothermia: a Call for trauma informed care. Am J Perinatol 2022. https://doi.org/10.1055/a-1739-3388.
6. Sanders MR, Hall SL. Trauma-informed care in the newborn intensive care unit: promoting safety, security and connectedness. J Perinatol 2018;38(1):3–10.
7. Guttmann K, Kelley A, Weintraub A, et al. Defining neonatal serious illness. J Palliat Med 2022;25(11):1655–60.
8. Rogers MM, Friebert S, Williams CSP, et al. Pediatric palliative care programs in US hospitals. Pediatrics 2021;148(1). https://doi.org/10.1542/peds.2020-021634.
9. Quill TE, Abernethy AP. Generalist plus specialist palliative care–creating a more sustainable model. N Engl J Med 2013;368(13):1173–5.
10. Lemmon ME, Bidegain M, Boss RD. Palliative care in neonatal neurology: robust support for infants, families and clinicians. J Perinatol 2016;36(5):331–7.
11. Rent S, Bidegain M, Lemmon ME. Neonatal neuropalliative care. Handb Clin Neurol 2023;191:185–99.
12. Rent S, Bidegain M, Bost MH, et al. Neuropalliative care for neonates. J Child Neurol 2021;36(12):1120–7.
13. Ito K, George N, Wilson J, et al. Primary palliative care recommendations for critical care clinicians. J Intensive Care 2022;10(1):20.
14. Lemmon ME, Donohue PK, Parkinson C, et al. Parent experience of neonatal encephalopathy. J Child Neurol 2017;32(3):286–92.
15. Nassef SK, Blennow M, Jirwe M. Experiences of parents whose newborns undergo hypothermia treatment following perinatal asphyxia. J Obstet Gynecol Neonatal Nurs 2013;42(1):38–47.
16. Pilon B, Craig AK, Lemmon ME, et al. Supporting families in their child's journey with neonatal encephalopathy and therapeutic hypothermia. Semin Fetal Neonatal Med 2021;26(5):101278.
17. SAMHSA's conceptof trauma and guidance for a trauma-informed approach. Available at: https://ncsacw.acf.hhs.gov/userfiles/files/SAMHSA_Trauma.pdf. [Accessed 31 January 2024].

18. Craig A, James C, Bainter J, et al. Survey of neonatal intensive care Unit nurse Attitudes toward therapeutic hypothermia treatment. Adv Neonatal Care : official journal of the National Association of Neonatal Nurses 2017;17(2):123–30.
19. Witt RE, Malcolm M, Colvin BN, et al. Racism and quality of neonatal intensive care: Voices of Black Mothers. Pediatrics 2022;150(3). https://doi.org/10.1542/peds.2022-056971.
20. Sigurdson K, Morton C, Mitchell B, et al. Disparities in NICU quality of care: a qualitative study of family and clinician accounts. J Perinatol 2018;38(5):600–7.
21. Vital Talk Responding to emotion: articulating empathy using NURSE statements. Available at: https://www.vitaltalk.org/guides/responding-to-emotion-respecting/. [Accessed 19 February 2024].
22. Thyagarajan B, Baral V, Gunda R, et al. Parental perceptions of hypothermia treatment for neonatal hypoxic-ischaemic encephalopathy. J Matern Fetal Neonatal Med 2018;31(19):2527–33.
23. Heringhaus A, Blom MD, Wigert H. Becoming a parent to a child with birth asphyxia-From a traumatic delivery to living with the experience at home. Int J Qual Stud Health Well-Being 2013;8:1–13.
24. Craig A, Deerwester K, Fox L, et al. Maternal holding during therapeutic hypothermia for infants with neonatal encephalopathy is feasible. Acta Paediatr 2019;108(9):1597–602.
25. Odd D, Okano S, Ingram J, et al. Physiological responses to cuddling babies with hypoxic-ischaemic encephalopathy during therapeutic hypothermia: an observational study. BMJ Paediatr Open 2021;5(1). https://doi.org/10.1136/bmjpo-2021-001280.
26. Donn SM, Chiswick ML, Fanaroff JM. Medico-legal implications of hypoxic-ischemic birth injury. Semin Fetal Neonatal Med 2014;19(5):317–21.
27. Leviton A. Why the term neonatal encephalopathy should be preferred over neonatal hypoxic-ischemic encephalopathy. Am J Obstet Gynecol 2013;208(3):176–80.
28. Pilon B. Family reflections: hope for HIE. Pediatr Res 2019;86(5):672–3.
29. Gunn AJ, Soul JS, Vesoulis ZA, et al. The importance of not increasing confusion around neonatal encephalopathy and hypoxic-ischemic encephalopathy. Pediatr Res 2023. https://doi.org/10.1038/s41390-023-03001-6.
30. Molloy EJ, Branagan A, Hurley T, et al. Neonatal encephalopathy and hypoxic-ischemic encephalopathy: moving from controversy to consensus definitions and subclassification. Pediatr Res 2023;94(6):1860–3.
31. Lally PJ, Montaldo P, Oliveira V, et al. Residual brain injury after early discontinuation of cooling therapy in mild neonatal encephalopathy. Arch Dis Child Fetal Neonatal Ed 2018;103(4):F383–7.
32. Shankaran S, Laptook AR, Ehrenkranz RA, et al. Whole-body hypothermia for neonates with hypoxic-ischemic encephalopathy. N Engl J Med 2005;353(15):1574–84.
33. Azzopardi DV, Strohm B, Edwards AD, et al. Moderate hypothermia to treat perinatal asphyxial encephalopathy. N Engl J Med 2009;361(14):1349–58.
34. Boss RD, Urban A, Barnett MD, et al. Neonatal Critical Care Communication (NC3): training NICU physicians and nurse practitioners. J Perinatol 2013;33(8):642–6.
35. Taylor LJ, Nabozny MJ, Steffens NM, et al. A framework to improve Surgeon communication in high-Stakes Surgical decisions: best case/Worst case. JAMA Surg 2017;152(6):531–8.
36. Back AL, Arnold RM, Tulsky JA, et al. Teaching communication skills to medical oncology fellows. J Clin Oncol 2003;21(12):2433–6.

37. Munoz-Blanco S, Boss R. Simulation for communication training in neonatology. Semin Perinatol 2023;47(7):151821.
38. Smyser CD, Tam EWY, Chang T, et al. Fellowship training in the emerging fields of Fetal-neonatal neurology and neonatal neurocritical care. Pediatr Neurol 2016;63: 39–44 e3.
39. Lemmon ME, Barks MC, Bansal S, et al. The align framework: a parent-informed approach to prognostic communication for infants with neurologic conditions. Neurology 2023;100(8):e800–7.
40. Bracken-Roche D, Shevell M, Racine E. Understanding and addressing barriers to communication in the context of neonatal neurologic injury: Exploring the ouR-HOPE approach. Handb Clin Neurol 2019;162:511–28.
41. Racine E, Bell E, Farlow B, et al. The 'ouR-HOPE' approach for ethics and communication about neonatal neurological injury. Dev Med Child Neurol 2017; 59(2):125–35.
42. Weiner J, Sharma J, Lantos J, et al. How infants die in the neonatal intensive care unit: trends from 1999 through 2008. Arch Pediatr Adolesc Med 2011;165(7):630–4.
43. Lantos JD. Ethical Problems in decision making in the neonatal ICU. N Engl J Med 2018;379(19):1851–60.
44. Gerrity C, Farley S, Barks MC, et al. Decision making for infants with neurologic conditions. J Child Neurol 2022;37(3):202–9.
45. Lemmon ME, Huffstetler H, Barks MC, et al. Neurologic outcome after Prematurity: Perspectives of parents and clinicians. Pediatrics 2019;144(1). https://doi.org/10.1542/peds.2018-3819.
46. Lam HS, Wong SP, Liu FY, et al. Attitudes toward neonatal intensive care treatment of preterm infants with a high risk of developing long-term disabilities. Pediatrics 2009;123(6):1501–8.
47. Kamihara J, Nyborn JA, Olcese ME, et al. Parental hope for children with advanced cancer. Pediatrics 2015;135(5):868–74.
48. Arnolds M, Xu L, Hughes P, et al. Worth a Try? Describing the experiences of families during the Course of care in the neonatal intensive care Unit when the prognosis is poor. J Pediatr 2018;196:116–122 e3.
49. Creutzfeldt CJ, Kluger B, Kelly AG, et al. Neuropalliative care: Priorities to move the field forward. Neurology 2018;91(5):217–26.
50. Smith VC, Love K, Goyer E. NICU discharge preparation and transition planning: guidelines and recommendations. J Perinatol 2022;42(Suppl 1):7–21.
51. Vohr B, McGowan E, Keszler L, et al. Impact of a transition home program on Rehospitalization Rates of preterm infants. J Pediatr 2017;181:86–92 e1.
52. Vohr B, McGowan E, Keszler L, et al. Effects of a transition home program on preterm infant emergency room visits within 90 days of discharge. J Perinatol 2018; 38(2):185–90.
53. Liu Y, McGowan E, Tucker R, et al. Transition home plus program Reduces Medicaid Spending and health care Use for high-risk infants Admitted to the neonatal intensive care Unit for 5 or more Days. J Pediatr 2018;200:91–97 e3.
54. Franck LS, Shellhaas RA, Lemmon ME, et al. Parent mental health and family Coping over two Years after the birth of a child with Acute neonatal seizures. Children 2021;9(1). https://doi.org/10.3390/children9010002.
55. Grunberg VA, Geller PA, Hoffman C, et al. Parental mental health screening in the NICU: a psychosocial team initiative. J Perinatol 2022;42(3):401–9.
56. Bansal S, Willis R, Barks MC, et al. Supporting Disclosure of Unmet mental health needs among parents of critically Ill infants. J Pediatr 2023;262:113596.

Ethical and Legal Perspectives on the Treatment of Hypoxic Ischemic Encephalopathy in the Newborn

Alice C. Baker, MD, MPH[a], Mark R. Mercurio, MD, MA[b],
Steven M. Donn, MD, FAARC[c], Jonathan M. Fanaroff, MD, JD[d,e],*

KEYWORDS

- Bioethics • Medicolegal • Medical malpractice • Perinatal asphyxia
- Therapeutic hypothermia • Hypoxic Ischemic Encephalopathy • HIE

KEY POINTS

- The severe outcomes that can be associated with neonatal encephalopathy and hypoxic ischemic encephalopathy including death or life-long functional impairments give rise to complex ethical and legal implications.
- For some babies, it is ethically permissible to offer parents limitations on life-sustaining medical therapy based on anticipated severe or profound disability.
- Physicians should understand the legal environment in which they practice and be aware of the medical–legal issues commonly associated with therapeutic hypothermia.

INTRODUCTION

Hypoxic ischemic encephalopathy (HIE) in neonates can cause severe, life-long functional impairments or death. The prospect of significant limitations in neurologic function can raise concerns about anticipated quality of life (QOL) which can lead to decisions to limit life-sustaining medical treatment (LSMT). Deciding if, when, and how to limit LSMT can be ethically challenging and cause significant distress among

[a] Department of Pediatrics, Yale University School of Medicine, PO Box 208064, 333 Cedar Street, New Haven, CT 06519, USA; [b] Program for Biomedical Ethics, Department of Pediatrics, Yale University School of Medicine, PO Box 208064, 333 Cedar Street, New Haven, CT 06519, USA; [c] Division of Neonatal-Perinatal Medicine, Department of Pediatrics, C.S. Mott Children's Hospital, Michigan Medicine, 1540 East Hospital Drive, Ann Arbor, MI 48109, USA; [d] Department of Pediatrics, Case Western Reserve University School of Medicine, 11100 Euclid Avenue, Cleveland, OH 44106, USA; [e] Rainbow Center for Pediatric Ethics, Rainbow Babies & Children's Hospital, Cleveland, OH, USA
* Corresponding author. Department of Pediatrics, Case Western Reserve University School of Medicine, 11100 Euclid Avenue, Cleveland, OH 44106.
E-mail address: jmf20@case.edu

Clin Perinatol 51 (2024) 725–734
https://doi.org/10.1016/j.clp.2024.04.010
0095-5108/24/© 2024 Elsevier Inc. All rights reserved.
perinatology.theclinics.com

parents and medical staff. While the interests of the neonate are paramount, the rights and obligations of all involved must be considered. In addition to ethical challenges, babies with HIE may be the subject of a medical malpractice lawsuit. The following hypothetical cases highlight important ethical and legal aspects of clinical decision making for infants with HIE.

DISCUSSION: ETHICAL CONSIDERATIONS
Case 1

Baby A is a 7 days old who was delivered emergently for placental abruption, required extensive resuscitation in the Delivery Room, and underwent cooling for HIE. He has made no respiratory effort or spontaneous movements since birth. Though not dead by neurologic criteria, based on his physical examination, brain imaging, and electroencephalogram, he is expected to be profoundly neurologically disabled. The pediatric resident, based on experience with older children with HIE, questions whether LSMT should be withdrawn.

Approaching Decisions Regarding Limitation of Life-Sustaining Medical Treatment

Decisions regarding withholding or withdrawing LSMT, such as mechanical ventilation or medically administered nutrition and hydration (MANH), require understanding of the relevant outcome data, as well as basic ethical principles and relevant rights involved in pediatric decision making. While infants have a right to receive treatments expected to prevent significant harm, suffering, or death, they also have a right not to be subjected to painful or invasive therapies not expected to provide benefit.[1,2] These rights must be considered when weighing the benefits and burdens to the patient of LSMT.

If survival is extremely unlikely despite provision of LSMT, the balance of benefits and burdens is likely such that it would be reasonable to withdraw those interventions to allow natural death. In HIE, when survival with LSMT is likely, this requires careful consideration of the benefits and burdens of not only each individual therapy, but also of survival itself. In many cases, treatments are withdrawn not because survival is unlikely, but because of concern that an infant will survive with a degree of impairment the family finds unacceptable.[3,4] Some may consider survival sufficiently important or beneficial regardless of anticipated disability. However, many believe that there is a point at which, based on anticipated disability, the QOL will be so poor that survival would not benefit the patient.[5] When estimating the benefits of survival, people place varying degrees of importance on factors such as the presence of pain, ability to experience pleasure, capacity to form relationships, or cognitive ability.[5–7] Individual values and religious or cultural factors have a large impact on this determination, and assessing QOL is, at best, a highly subjective undertaking. Despite the high degree of subjectivity in the assessment, the degree of anticipated disability may reach a point where many would consider ongoing LSMT to no longer be in the patient's best interest or the best course of action.

Generally, parents are believed to have the right to make decisions for their children and are well poised to do so based on their unique understanding of, and responsibility to protect their children's and family's interests.[8] The American Academy of Pediatrics (AAP) recognizes the important role of parental judgment in decisions regarding LSMT when QOL is expected to be poor.[9] Recognizing the impact of significant disability on the entire family, the AAP and others acknowledge parents' right to consider the whole family's interests.[7,9] However, decisions should primarily be driven by consideration of the patient's welfare. Moreover, parental authority is not unlimited. When a parental request would result in unjustified harm to the patient, physicians should seek to override parental authority.

The impermissible–permissible–obligatory framework can be helpful in defining the limits of parental authority. Any intervention under consideration may be viewed as ethically impermissible (wherein it should not be provided), ethically permissible (wherein parents should have wide latitude regarding its use), or ethically obligatory (wherein the treatment should be provided regardless of parental preference). Location of a treatment within one of these categories is based largely on the prognosis with and without the proposed treatment, feasibility of providing it, and the relevant rights of all involved.[1] The most difficult cases from a decisional standpoint will lie in that middle zone of ethical permissibility, which has also been described as the zone of parental discretion. While one treatment approach might be highly recommended for a given patient, there may be a range of interventions that would be ethically permissible, including some that the physician might not recommend. Here, as always, clear and respectful communication with parents is essential. Parents should be made aware of all ethically permissible options, including ones that the physician does not recommend. Moreover, physicians should be aware that parents may have questions about limitation of treatment that they are reluctant to verbalize, but nevertheless deserve to have addressed in an open and nonjudgmental manner. Physicians might therefore need to initiate these discussions. Such discussions may occur over several meetings, often beginning before 7 days of age.[8,10–14]

Consideration of Specific Limitations

When the burdens of treatment are low and survival is not expected to be associated with significant morbidity, LSMT is typically considered ethically obligatory and limitations of LSMT should not be offered.[12] For Baby A, the neurologic prognosis makes the benefit of survival less clear, and it would be ethically permissible to limit LSMT. Decisions to either withdraw or withhold certain interventions should be made at the parents' discretion after open and honest discussion of all ethically permissible treatment options.[9] In this case, following a lengthy discussion, the parents expressed their desire to avoid painful interventions, and a do-not-attempt-resuscitation order was placed.

Given the anticipated burdens associated with survival, withdrawal of other therapies should be considered.[9,15] Interventions such as mechanical ventilation and provision of MANH are ethically permissible options in this case, and decisions to either continue or withdraw such therapies fall in the zone of parental discretion. Withdrawing an intervention that has already been initiated, such as mechanical ventilation, might be emotionally and psychologically more difficult for families than withholding that same treatment initially. Clinicians must be cognizant of that possibility, but from an ethical standpoint withdrawing and withholding are widely considered equivalent.[9] That is, if it was ethically permissible not to initiate a given treatment, it would be ethically permissible to withdraw it unless there has been a significant change in clinical status and/or prognosis.

Withdrawal of mechanical ventilation for patients such as Baby A is an accepted practice in neonatology. In fact, most deaths in neonates with HIE occur in physiologically stable infants following elective extubation when neurologic outcomes are anticipated to be poor.[3,4] Withdrawing MANH (eg, intravenous fluids and/or nasogastric tube feedings) is more controversial, perhaps due to the symbolic meaning of feeding as a basic component of the care of infants.[16] As with any medical intervention, the benefits and burdens of MANH should be carefully considered. Many professional societies, including the AAP, as well as the authors of this essay, acknowledge that in limited circumstances it can be appropriate to withdraw MANH at parents' discretion.[9,17–19] Discussion of options with parents should include the likely outcome of each option, and the range of possible outcomes. For example, survival beyond minutes or hours might not be expected after withdrawal of mechanical ventilation, but it nevertheless could rarely occur. Also, after withdrawal of MANH, survival could potentially continue for 1 to 2 weeks, and possibly longer.

Once a decision has been made to forgo LSMT, some consider active euthanasia a compassionate approach to end suffering and allow a more dignified death. Many others consider this practice ethically impermissible, noting a distinction between *permitting* and *actively causing* death.[7] While neonatal euthanasia has been legalized for rare extreme circumstances in the Netherlands, it is very rarely done there, remains illegal in the United States, and is not a practical option within the current legal environment.[15,20] Nevertheless, parental requests for measures to expedite the dying process should be met with empathy and understanding.[15]

After careful discussions with the clinical team and close family advisors, Baby A's parents elected to continue LSMT. Given the devastating neurologic injury, some questioned whether continuation of LSMT was ethically permissible. However, consideration of the benefits and burdens of prolonging life are intrinsically linked to subjective value judgments about disability, QOL, and well-being. The AAP and others emphasize the important role parents play in making these judgments, and decisions to limit LSMT based solely on anticipated disability should be deferred to them.[9,21] Baby A survived and was eventually discharged with tracheostomy, ventilator support, and feeding via gastrostomy tube.

Case 2

Baby B is a 2 day old term infant who was born via emergency cesarean section for a nonreassuring fetal heart rate tracing. He required intubation and initiation of mechanical ventilation in the delivery room. Cooling was initiated shortly thereafter for a poor neurologic examination and significant acidemia. He has shown inconsistent respiratory effort, and his neurologic examination has not significantly improved. Based on history, physical examination, and other diagnostic studies, the clinical team explains to the family that he may have suffered significant neurologic injury and could develop significant neurologic deficits. They are told that his course over the next few days and further brain imaging might give them helpful prognostic information, though that is not certain.

Prognostic Uncertainty

The prognosis is much more ambiguous for Baby B than it was for Baby A. Though prognostication in HIE has improved, there is no single biomarker that allows physicians to definitively tell parents, in most cases, whether their child will be able to perform basic acts such as eat on their own, communicate verbally, or interact meaningfully with their environment. Composite outcomes of "death or disability" that do not delineate various neurologic deficits, and the paucity of data regarding which outcomes are most important to parents, further limit meaningful prognostication.[17,22] In addition to the already difficult process of deciding how neurologic deficits impact QOL, parents must often make decisions without knowing exactly what deficits their children will have. It is important for physicians to be open with parents about these uncertainties, but uncertainty should not preclude honest discussion of the most likely outcome when prognosis is poor.

Before discussing treatment options with the parents, the medical team must determine whether the injury is significant enough that limiting LSMT would be ethically permissible. AAP guidance recommends weighing the benefits and burdens of LSMT to determine when treatment limitations are in the best interests of a child.[9] This is consistent with the concept of a "zero point" at which benefits to the patient of ongoing LSMT are equal to the burdens, which may include the difficulties associated with the treatment course, as well as long-term burdens such as disability. As described by Wilkinson, above the zero point benefits outweigh burdens. Below the zero point, the burdens outweigh benefits, and anticipated QOL may be considered unacceptable by some parents.[6] Without knowing the exact degree of impairment an infant will have, it can be unclear whether this point has been reached. For Baby B, there is a chance that he will have a degree of disability that parents would consider unacceptable, though this is not certain. The "threshold view" advocated by Wilkinson accounts for this uncertainty, and suggests there exists a threshold at which impairments are anticipated to be significant enough that limiting LSMT would be ethically permissible, even when the burdens might not clearly outweigh the benefits.[6] Once this threshold is reached, this view holds, parents should decide whether the risk of severe impairment is high enough to warrant limitations of LSMT.[6]

The threshold approach allows for more parental latitude than a more straightforward, if still difficult, determination that burdens outweigh benefits. Determining where this threshold lies is not simple, and some would suggest that the proper threshold should only be seen to have been reached when anticipated burdens clearly outweigh the benefits, more consistent with the patient's best interest standard. Though the threshold approach would reasonably give parents more latitude than the more widely accepted patient's best interest standard, either approach would require an inevitably subjective assessment of benefits and burdens. When it is unclear whether limitations of LSMT would be an acceptable option, physicians should consult with medical colleagues, such as other neonatologists and neurologists, and consider an ethics consultation. Given that nursing staff could have important insights into both the ethical and practical aspects of these decisions (as well as a better understanding of family dynamics), and may be charged with carrying them out, they should also be included in the discussions.

Timing of Treatment Limitation

For Baby B, time and further testing may help clarify the prognosis. However, infants with HIE often require hemodynamic and respiratory support for the first several days of life, then stabilize to the point of no longer needing LSMT. For infants treated with therapeutic hypothermia, gathering of prognostic data can be delayed for several days.[23] After this time, even if it becomes clear that there will be a high likelihood of severe disability, some infants may have stabilized enough to survive regardless of limitations placed on LSMT.[24] Even if further testing might clarify the prognosis, however, in some cases it might already be clear that the damage is severe enough to meet the threshold of impairment to make treatment limitations ethically permissible. In these cases, when prognosis is sufficiently clear and decisions may be time sensitive, it is reasonable to offer limitation of LSMT to parents before completion of prognostic testing. Parents should understand what information further testing might provide, as well as the risk that delaying treatment limitations could result in survival with a degree of disability they would consider unacceptable.[18] If it is uncertain whether the impairments will have a significant enough impact to justify withholding LSMT, more information should be gathered before this option is offered. For Baby B, LSMT was continued, and further testing indicated the prognosis was better than it initially appeared. His neurologic examination improved, and he was discharged without obvious deficits.

DISCUSSION: LEGAL CONSIDERATIONS

In addition to ethical issues, caring for babies with neonatal encephalopathy raises legal considerations as well. When there is a poor outcome, parents understandably want to seek answers, and may turn to the legal system in an effort to find them. Indeed, a simple Internet search for "hypoxic ischemic encephalopathy" will yield a number of malpractice lawyer web sites advertising their services to stricken families. Additionally, with the introduction of therapeutic hypothermia nearly 2 decades ago, the focus of malpractice lawsuits expanded from obstetric care alone to now include delivery room and early neonatal care. Consequently, pediatric and neonatal health care professionals should have a basic understanding of the legal system. While this article focuses on the United States system, health care professionals should be aware of the legal environment in their own countries. It is also critical to remember that medical malpractice is generally regulated by the states, and laws vary significantly between states.

Disclaimer

The information provided here is for general information only and should not be taken as substantive legal advice. Clinicians are strongly advised to consult a qualified attorney for any issues that arise from the care of patients.

Case 3

Baby C is a 39 week gestational age male. The pregnancy had been complicated by sonographically suspected intrauterine growth restriction and a small placenta. Labor was unremarkable until the electronic fetal heart rate monitoring pattern changed from Category I to Category II 20 minutes prior to delivery. Following an uncomplicated vaginal delivery, Apgar scores were 3 at 1 minute (2 for heart rate and 1 for tone) and 8 at 5 minutes after brief positive pressure ventilation. The umbilical cord gases were 7.12/P_{CO_2} 59/P_{O_2} 22/HCO_3 18.4/BD -9.3 (arterial) and 7.15/P_{CO_2} 52/P_{O_2} 28/ HCO_3 17.5/BD -9.9 (venous). The baby weighed 1450 g, had a head circumference of 29.5 cm, and was noted to have mild arthrogryposis and a cleft palate. The attending neonatologist did not offer hypothermic neuroprotection and was sued after the infant developed significant neurologic deficits.

Case 4

Baby D is a 37 week gestational age female. The mother was a 19 year old primigravida who presented to the Labor and Delivery with complaints of decreased fetal movement for several days. Sonography displayed polyhydramnios. Mom was noted to have preeclampsia and was started on magnesium sulfate therapy. The electronic fetal heart rate monitor pattern was always Category I. A primary Cesarean section was performed for failure to progress, and the infant was unexpectedly depressed and required resuscitation. Umbilical cord blood gases were normal, Apgar scores were 2 (heart rate) at 1 minute and 7 at 5 minutes. The baby displayed generalized lethargy and hypotonia and underwent hypothermic neuroprotection. A serum magnesium level was 6.6. The infant later developed spastic quadriplegic cerebral palsy and the mother sued, alleging intrapartum hypoxic ischemic brain injury.

The Tort System

The United States Constitution, written in 1787, sets up the framework for the government and the court system which oversees medical malpractice lawsuits. Medical malpractice is part of a larger area of civil law known as *negligence*. Physicians, advanced practice providers, nurses, and other health care professionals are held to a certain level of expected conduct. When an injured party (plaintiff) believes that the medical care provided was substandard, they may file a lawsuit seeking compensation for their injuries. The ultimate decision-maker is usually a jury, a right set out in the Constitution. Should the jury find that negligence occurred they can then award damages to the plaintiff as compensation. For this to occur, the plaintiff has the "burden of proof" for each of the following 4 elements. In most cases, the level of burden is "more likely than not," a much lower threshold than the "beyond a reasonable doubt" burden in criminal cases.

Duty

In order to be held liable for medical malpractice, the health care professional must have a *duty* to care for the patient. This is not generally an issue in most cases. The neonatologist on service will clearly have a physician–patient relationship and duty toward a baby in the neonatal intensive care unit (NICU). Note that a duty may be created even when the neonatologist has never actually seen the patient. This can occur when supervising others, such as advanced practice providers or trainees. Additionally, a legal duty may attach, for example, when a tertiary care center provides specific care advice to a smaller community hospital, while directing a transport, or through telemedicine care. All of these situations, however, will be highly fact-dependent and may vary based on state law as well.

Breach

Once a duty is established, the next element that must be proven is that the defendant health care professional *breached* the duty to the patient to meet the standard of care. This is generally a highly disputed area of the lawsuit. Two important points. First, "standard of care" is not a medical term, but rather a legal term that must be shown, taking into account the circumstances of each individual case. Second, the standard of care does not require a health care professional to be perfect, but rather is defined by Black's legal dictionary as that "[d]egree of care a prudent and reasonable person will exercise under the circumstances."[25] Medicine, of course, is a complex and inexact blend of art and science, and 2 health care professionals could reasonably make different care decisions. Judges and juries do not usually have medical training, and consequently the courts rely on expert witnesses to explain both the medicine at issue as well as the way the care did or did not breach the standard or care.

When Did Therapeutic Hypothermia Become Standard of Care?

Neonatology as a field has made remarkable progress over the last several decades. Unfortunately, however, along with the development of life-saving beneficial therapies such as surfactant and infant ventilators, have come nonbeneficial and even harmful treatment including the Bloxsom air lock and Epsom salts enemas.[26] Consequently, changes in clinical care in the NICU generally occur gradually as neonatologists wait for multiple studies to confirm efficacy and safety before adapting newer therapies.

The question sometimes arises in birth injury lawsuits concerning exactly when therapeutic hypothermia became standard practice. There is no clear-cut answer. Animal trials were followed by small human pilot studies confirming safety. While the first larger human trial was published in 2005, a meta-analysis confirming efficacy only came 5 years later in 2010. A year later, in 2011, therapeutic hypothermia was incorporated into the neonatal resuscitation program. Keep in mind that standard of care is a legal term, so there is not and never will be an exact answer to this question.

Causation

The third element of a malpractice lawsuit is causation. As with breach, this element is often vigorously disputed by both plaintiff and defense. It is not enough to show that a health care professional violated the standard of care, that violation must also have caused an injury. This is not always a simple task in cases of neonatal encephalopathy. The AAP and the American College of Obstetricians and Gynecologists have recognized that there are "multiple potential causal pathways that lead to cerebral palsy in term infants."[27] This could occur during the pregnancy prior to labor, during labor, or after delivery. The complete answer, when it can be determined, often requires examination of both the maternal and neonatal medical course and laboratory results, imaging studies including MRI, and placental pathology (and where possible, a postmortem examination). A multitude of experts including obstetricians, neonatologists, pediatric neurologists, neuroradiologists, and placental pathologists may provide causation opinions in a malpractice lawsuit involving neonatal encephalopathy.

Damages

The fourth and final element of a malpractice lawsuit is damages. Damages are intended to compensate the injured party for their injuries. There are 2 types of damages. Economic damages include the costs that have been or will be incurred, such as medical bills or lost wages. Noneconomic damages are intended to compensate for more subjective losses such as pain and suffering. In rare cases involving egregious behavior a third type of damages known as punitive damages may be awarded. Because infants with severe encephalopathy who end up with a poor neurologic outcome require a lifetime (decades) of round the clock care, the damages can be significant. Indeed, many of the largest medical malpractice awards in history involve birth injury cases, including an April 2023 jury verdict in Philadelphia, Pennsylvania, for $183 million dollars.[28]

Case 3 and 4 Analyses

Cases 3 and 4 are illustrative of medico-legal issues frequently associated with hypothermic neuroprotection. In Case 3, the plaintiff argued that failure to provide cooling contributed to the child's poor neurologic outcome. The defendant argued that the baby did not qualify under most clinical guidelines. First, the symmetric intrauterine growth restriction was not an acute event, but was a longstanding problem that was most likely of placental etiology. The arthrogryposis was indicative of chronically decreased fetal movement, the cord gases were nonqualifying, and there was no evidence of an intrauterine sentinel event.

In Case 4, the plaintiff argued that because the infant underwent cooling, there must have been intrapartum hypoxia-ischemia, since this is the *only* indication for hypothermic neuroprotection. The defendant argued that although a decision was made to cool the baby, in reality the baby did not qualify once all of the data were available. There was no sentinel event, the cord gases were normal, and the baby's hypotonia and lethargy were the result of significant hypermagnesemia secondary to maternal treatment. Furthermore, the mother presented with a history of decreased fetal movement, and the polyhydramnios was suggestive of decreased fetal swallowing and pre-existent neurologic dysfunction.

SUMMARY

The severe outcomes that can be associated with neonatal encephalopathy and HIE, including death or life-long functional impairments, give rise to many complex ethical and legal implications. Health care professionals should have a basic understanding of the ethical principles and legal system and environment where they practice, and must recognize the importance of keeping up to date in their practice and documenting properly. From both an ethical and legal standpoint, good communication and involvement of parents in decision-making are essential when caring for these critically ill patients.

Best Practices

- Parents should be informed about, and have the right to decide among, all ethically permissible treatment options.

- It is ethically permissible, but not obligatory, to continue or to withdraw LSMT based on anticipated profound disability.

- Withholding or withdrawing CPR, mechanical ventilation, and/or MANH is ethically permissible in newborns with severe HIE when parents and physicians agree that ongoing provision would not be in the child's best interest.

- In the setting of prognostic uncertainty, it is ethically permissible to forgo LSMT once a threshold of anticipated impairment is reached, even when additional testing might further clarify the prognosis.

- Physicians should consult with colleagues and consider ethics consultation when it is not clear whether limiting LSMT would be ethically permissible.

- Physicians should understand the legal environment in which they practice and be aware of the medical–legal issues commonly associated with therapeutic hypothermia.

DISCLOSURE

The authors have nothing to disclose.

REFERENCES

1. Mercurio MR, Cummings CL. Critical decision-making in neonatology and pediatrics: the I-P-O framework. J Perinatol 2021;41(1):173–8.
2. Religious objections to medical care. American academy of pediatrics committee on bioethics. Pediatrics 1997;99(2):279–81.
3. Lemmon ME, Boss RD, Bonifacio SL, et al. Characterization of death in neonatal encephalopathy in the hypothermia era. J Child Neurol 2017;32(4):360–5.
4. Natarajan G, Mathur A, Zaniletti I, et al. Withdrawal of life-support in neonatal hypoxic-ischemic encephalopathy. Pediatr Neurol 2019;91:20–6.
5. Brick C, Kahane G, Wilkinson D, et al. Worth living or worth dying? The views of the general public about allowing disabled children to die. J Med Ethics 2020; 46(1):7–15.
6. Wilkinson DJ. A life worth giving? The threshold for permissible withdrawal of life support from disabled newborn infants. Am J Bioeth 2011;11(2):20–32.
7. Racine E, Shevell MI. Ethics in neonatal neurology: when is enough, enough? Pediatr Neurol 2009;40(3):147–55.
8. Salter EK, Hester DM, Vinarcsik L, et al. Pediatric decision making: consensus recommendations. Pediatrics 2023;152(3). https://doi.org/10.1542/peds.2023-061832.
9. Weise KL, Okun AL, Carter BS, et al, COMMITTEE ON BIOETHICS, SECTION ON HOSPICE AND PALLIATIVE MEDICINE, COMMITTEE ON CHILD ABUSE AND

NEGLECT. Guidance on forgoing life-sustaining medical treatment. Pediatrics 2017;140(3). https://doi.org/10.1542/peds.2017-1905.

10. Sullivan A, Cummings C. Historical perspectives: shared decision making in the NICU. NeoReviews 2020;21(4):e217–25.

11. Bell EF, Bell EF. Noninitiation or withdrawal of intensive care for high-risk newborns. Pediatrics 2007;119(2):401–3.

12. Cummings J, COMMITTEE ON FETUS AND NEWBORN. Antenatal counseling regarding resuscitation and intensive care before 25 weeks of gestation. Pediatrics 2015;136(3):588–95.

13. Adams RC, Levy SE, COUNCIL ON CHILDREN WITH DISABILITIES. Shared decision-making and children with disabilities: pathways to consensus. Pediatrics 2017;139(6). https://doi.org/10.1542/peds.2017-0956.

14. Gillam L. Children's bioethics and the zone of parental discretion. Monash Bioeth Rev 2010;20(2):09.1–3.

15. Mercurio MR, Gillam L. Ethics at the end of life in the newborn intensive care unit: conversations and decisions. Semin Fetal Neonatal Med 2023;28(3):101438.

16. Diekema DS, Botkin JR, Committee on Bioethics. Clinical report–Forgoing medically provided nutrition and hydration in children. Pediatrics 2009;124(2):813–22.

17. Lemmon ME. Deciding when a life is not worth living: animperative to measure what matters. J Med Ethics 2020;46(1):18–9.

18. Lemmon ME, Wusthoff CJ, Boss RD, et al, Newborn Brain Society Guidelines and Publications Committee. Ethical considerations in the care of encephalopathic neonates treated with therapeutic hypothermia. Semin Fetal Neonatal Med 2021;26(5):101258.

19. Tsai E. Withholding and withdrawing artificial nutrition and hydration. Paediatr Child Health 2011;16(4):241–4.

20. Verhagen AAE. Neonatal euthanasia in the context of palliative and EoL care. Semin Fetal Neonatal Med 2023;28(3):101439.

21. Koogler TK, Wilfond BS, Ross LF. Lethal language, lethal decisions. Hastings Cent Rep Mar-Apr 2003;33(2):37–41.

22. Janvier A, Farlow B, Baardsnes J, et al. Measuring and communicating meaningful outcomes in neonatology: a family perspective. Semin Perinatol 2016;40(8): 571–7.

23. Wilkinson D. The window of opportunity for treatment withdrawal. Arch Pediatr Adolesc Med 2011;165(3):211–5.

24. Shevell M. Ethical perspectives in cooling for term infants with intrapartum asphyxia. Dev Med Child Neurol 2012;54(3):197–9.

25. Blacks law dictionary, 2nd edition. Standard of care. Available at: https://thelawdictionary.org/?s=standard+of+care.

26. Robertson AF. Reflections on errors in neonatology: II. The "Heroic" years, 1950 to 1970. J Perinatol 2003 Mar;23(2):154–61.

27. Neonatal encephalopathy and neurologic outcome, 2nd edition. Pediatrics 2014; 133(5):e1482–8.

28. Cass A. Jury awards $183 million for birth injury at Penn Medicine hospital. Becker's Hospital Review 2023. Available at: www.beckershospitalreview.com/legal-regulatory-issues/jury-awards-183m-for-birth-injury-at-penn-medicine-hospital.html.

Pipeline to Neonatal Clinical Transformation

The Importance of Preclinical Data

Sandra E. Juul, MD, PhD[a,b], Thomas R. Wood, BM BCh, PhD[a,b],*

KEYWORDS

- Hypoxia-ischemia • Neonatal • Animal models • Hypoxic-ischemic encephalopathy
- Therapeutic hypothermia • Erythropoietin

KEY POINTS

- The preclinical pipeline of therapies for hypoxic-ischemic encephalopathy (HIE) faces challenges related to i) adjuncts for therapeutic hypothermia, and ii) therapies for HIE in lower resource settings.
- The field must expand beyond its reliance on rodent and large animal models of single acute asphyxial events in order to address the heterogenous clinical presentations of HIE worldwide.
- To minimize the risk of further failed clinical trials, the most promising therapies should be reproducibly tested in multiple laboratories using both the same and different species, as well as models specific to the target clinical scenario, before clinical testing.

INTRODUCTION

We live in a time of incredible scientific and medical break throughs, ranging from new protective vaccines for respiratory syncytial virus and other diseases, to gene editing treatments for sickle cell disease. Despite these and other scientific advances throughout medicine, improvements in the development and implementation of novel therapeutic strategies to improve the care and outcomes of sick newborns continue to lag behind achievements in many other fields. This is particularly the case for neonatal brain injuries, for which the last major therapeutic advance was therapeutic hypothermia (TH) for neonatal hypoxic-ischemic encephalopathy (HIE) nearly 2 decades ago. Other than TH, there have been few transformational breakthroughs in neonatal care over the past decades. This is reflected in epidemiologic studies which show

[a] Institute on Human Development and Disability, University of Washington, Box 357920, 1701 Northeast Columbia Road, Seattle, WA 98195-7920, USA; [b] Division of Neonatology, Department of Pediatrics, University of Washington, Box 356320, 1959 Northeast Pacific Street, RR451 HSB, Seattle, WA 98195-6320, USA
* Corresponding author.
E-mail address: tommyrw@uw.edu

Clin Perinatol 51 (2024) 735–748
https://doi.org/10.1016/j.clp.2024.04.011
0095-5108/24/© 2024 Elsevier Inc. All rights reserved.
perinatology.theclinics.com

that under-5 pediatric deaths decreased by 12% from 2015 to 2021, while neonatal mortality remained relatively stable, only decreasing from 20 to 18 deaths per 1000 live births globally.

NATURE OF THE PROBLEM

As complications around birth are not entirely predictable or preventable, the perinatal period remains the time of greatest potential risk of permanent brain injury or death in the otherwise healthy neonate. The 2 most prevalent causes of neonatal death and disability globally are prematurity and intrapartum-related complications.[1] For the purposes of this article, however, we will focus on intrapartum-related complications, with ensuing HIE after presumed hypoxia-ischemia.

EPIDEMIOLOGY OF HYPOXIC-ISCHEMIC ENCEPHALOPATHY AND GAPS IN KNOWLEDGE

Historically, approximately 60% of infants diagnosed with moderate or severe HIE died or developed severe developmental impairments.[2] Several randomized controlled trials (RCT) of infants with moderate or severe HIE then clearly established that TH significantly reduces death or disability when started within 6 hours of birth (RR 0.75, 95% CI 0.68–0.83), with a number needed to treat of 6 to 7.[3] However, 30% to 50% of treated infants still have poor outcomes in high-resource settings.[4,5] In low-income and middle-income countries (LMICs), TH may not be available or appropriate as was confirmed by the recent phase-III "hypothermia for moderate or severe neonatal encephalopathy in low-income and middle-income countries" (HELIX) trial,[6] where TH did not reduce the combined outcome of death or disability and significantly increased death alone. Neonates in the HELIX trial tended to be of lower birth weight than their counterparts in the original cooling trials, and early seizures were more common at the time of presentation, suggesting a subacute or more protracted injury period in addition to poorer nutritional status.[6] Transcriptomic analyses and the pattern of brain injury also suggest that the mechanisms of injury seen in HELIX were different from those described as a result of acute asphyxia events in the high-resource settings used to develop TH as standard of care.[6,7] A more recent prospective study in Vietnam confirmed the high mortality rate and poorer outcomes of infants treated with TH in lower resource settings.[8] In order to address HIE globally, condition-specific therapies must therefore be developed, and these must be inexpensive, shelf-stable, and present few barriers to delivery and monitoring at scale to be applicable to regions of the world where HIE is most common. Such a precision medicine approach may also benefit the 30% to 50% of Western patients who do not respond to TH.

Thus, despite some success in decreasing death and disability due to HIE in some settings, we have 2 main therapeutic dilemmas that we consider: (1) how to further improve outcomes for infants with moderate or severe HIE treated with TH, and (2) how to improve outcomes for infants with HIE where TH is not available or not indicated. Using information gleaned from recent multi-center clinical trials of erythropoietin (Epo) therapy for neonatal injury, the authors will discuss the promise and potential pitfalls of preclinical research in the search for answers to these pressing dilemmas.

ERYTHROPOIETIN AS A POTENTIAL NEUROTHERAPEUTIC

Interest in Epo as a neurotherapeutic began in 1993, with a preclinical study demonstrating the presence of Epo receptors on a cultured neuronal cell line.[9] It was then determined that Epo was produced by astrocytes in the human brain, and that the cell surface receptor was present on a variety of brain cells including neuronal progenitor cells,[10] and subsets of mature neurons,[11] astrocytes,[12] oligodendrocytes,[12–14] microglia,[15] and endothelial cells.[10] Follow-up studies showed that Epo decreased neuronal apoptotic cell death,[15,16] decreased inflammation,[17,18] increased antioxidant activity,[19] reduced excitotoxic cell injury,[20] and protected neuronal progenitor cells from inflammatory and hypoxic ischemic (HI) injury.[13,14,21] As neurons in the developing brain are more likely than adult neurons to undergo apoptosis if exposed to injurious stimuli, and antioxidant systems are immature, these functions seemed particularly relevant to neonatal brain injury.[22,23] Epo was also found to stimulate growth factors such as brain-derived neurotrophic factor and glial cell-derived neurotrophic factor, increasing newly-generated neuronal precursor cells and directing stem cells to differentiate into neurons.[12,24–26] In acute injury models, Epo results in a 49% to 79% decrease in size of infarction when appropriate dosing is used.[27] These promising studies were done using Epo as a monotherapy. However, preclinical data combining TH and Epo showed variable results, likely due to variability in approach (ie, timing and duration of TH and Epo dosing) and limitations in the models.[28–30] The majority of all these studies were also done in rodents, and there are, of course, many important differences between the developing rodent and human brain.[31]

Subsequently, in a nonhuman primate model of perinatal asphyxia, the combination of TH plus multiple doses of Epo resulted in a significantly lower rate of death or moderate/severe cerebral palsy (CP) than did treatment with saline vehicle (0% vs 43%, $P<.05$), with no benefit from TH alone.[32] Animals who received Epo + TH demonstrated improved long-term motor and cognitive function.[33] This study suggested an additive effect of Epo when combined with TH; however, the numbers in the study were small.

Based on these preclinical results, phase I and II clinical trials of Epo were undertaken in both preterm infants and term infants with HIE.[34–38] For *HIE in term infants*, Epo monotherapy improved neurodevelopmental outcomes in 2 trials in China and Egypt.[37,38] In a *phase I* dose-response trial in 24 infants receiving TH,[39] Epo 1000 U/kg IV provided optimal plasma levels consistent with animal studies of neuroprotection, with encouraging neurodevelopmental outcomes at mean age 22 months,[40] and a lower rate of death or moderate/severe disability (4.5%) than that reported in infants with similar study entry criteria who received TH only in large trials (44%–51%).[41–44] Only 12.5% with moderate or severe MRI brain injury in this study died or developed a significant neurodevelopmental disability; in contrast, 70% to 80% of cooled infants with moderate/severe MRI brain injury in the National Institute of Child Health and Human Development (NICHD) TH trial exhibited this outcome.[45] In a subsequent *phase II* trial of Epo for moderate or severe HIE undergoing TH, 50 infants were randomized to Epo 1000 U/kg/dose or placebo. Deaths were less common in the Epo group (8% vs 19%), MRIs done at 5 days after birth showed less brain injury in Epo-treated infants, and developmental testing at 6 and 12 months showed improved motor outcomes.[40]

Many large RCTs using Epo in neonatal populations have now been published. Both the Swiss Neuroprotection Trial and The Preterm Epo neuroprotection (PENUT) Trial in (extremely) preterm infants found no reduction in death of neurodevelopmental impairment.[46–48] Studies in term infants with HIE have been equally disappointing, as the recently published High Dose Epo for Asphyxia and Encephalopathy (HEAL) Trial (N = 500) also showed no difference in death or neurodevelopment at 2 years of age.[49] Of potential concern, Epo-treated children in the HEAL Trial showed a nonspecific increase in serious adverse events and in externalizing behaviors on the Child Behavior Check List.[50] Across both the PENUT and HEAL trials, extensive biomarker analyses found that the robust anti-inflammatory effects of Epo demonstrated in rodents were not replicated in humans.[51,52]

What can we learn from this history? First, it highlights the importance of adequately powered phase III RCTs. Meta-analyses of smaller phase II trials cannot substitute for well-conducted phase III trials and may lead to false conclusions. Second, they highlight the importance of preclinical trials in the development of future neuroprotective agents.

PRECLINICAL MODELS AT A CROSSROADS

With the development of TH as a neuroprotective strategy for infants with moderate-severe HIE, neonatal neuroscience could previously boast one of the most successful preclinical-to-clinical therapeutic pipelines due to the robust and repeatable effects of TH across multiple laboratories using multiple animal models.[53–56] The current protocol for TH was initially developed in sheep, and appears to be an optimal single cooling strategy for use in high-resource settings after acute asphyxial events.[57] Despite this successful pipeline, several therapies that showed success in those same models have failed to translate clinically, including Epo as the most high-profile "failure," but also therapies such as xenon gas.[48,49,58] Though there are several promising therapies in current or planned Phase-III clinical trials, such as melatonin and sildenafil, there are several potential reasons why the current preclinical approach may not be adequate for identifying and translating the most impactful therapies for HIE.

Rodent Models

The rat is useful in determining broad strokes of whether a therapy might be useful or not. They are abundant, relatively inexpensive, and mature quickly, so experiments evaluating therapies with short-term and long-term anatomic and developmental outcomes can be done quickly with multiple replicates. However, there are many drawbacks to using rats as experimental models of human newborn disease. Rats are lissencephalic, with only approximately 12% white matter compared to greater than 50% in humans (**Fig. 1**). Thus, they lack many of the structures that are at particular risk of injury to the developing brain, which may contribute to difficulties in translating therapies from rodents to larger animals and humans.[59,60] Comparison of developmental stage with humans is context-dependent between rats and humans and varies with anatomic, neurophysiological, electrophysiological, or metabolic development, all of which occur on different time scales.[59,61] Developmental stage is of critical

	Rat	Ferret	Piglet	Fetal Sheep	Macaque	Human
Term-equivalent animal models	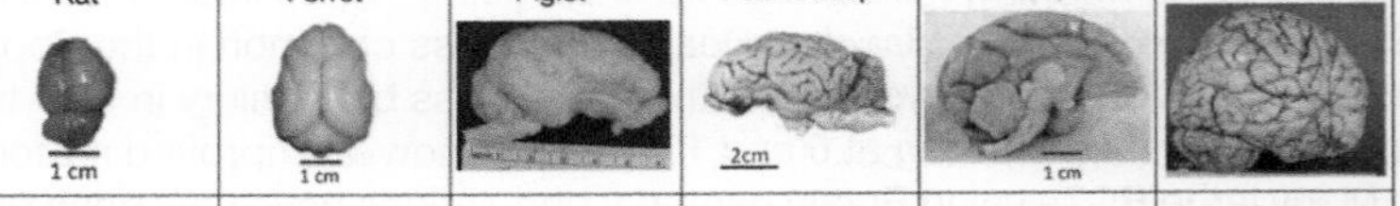 1 cm	1 cm		2cm	1 cm	
Brain weight	0.5-1g	3-5g	25-35g	40-50g	50-70g	350-400g
White matter	<12%	>50%	>60%	>60%	>60%	>60%
Gyrified?	No	Yes	Yes	Yes	Yes	Yes
Amenable to testing TH adjuncts?	Partially (TH paradigms are short <6h)	No (TH not protective in current model)	Yes	Yes	Yes	N/A
Amenable to modeling LMIC HIE?	Uncertain (may require further model development)	Yes	Uncertain (may require further model development)	Yes (acute on chronic/intermittent hypoxia models)	Yes (acute on chronic/intermittent hypoxia models)	N/A

Fig. 1. Comparison of animal models and their relationship to the ongoing challenges for preclinical hypoxic-ischemic encephalopathy research. (Adapted with necessary permissions from Empie et al. (2015),[75] Koehler et al. (2018),[71] Murray et al. (2022),[88] and Howell et al. (2010).[89]

importance when modeling neonatal disease, as preterm and term infants have very different vulnerabilities. Furthermore, the rat inflammatory response may be quite different from humans as was well demonstrated by the differences in response to Epo in the context of HIE.

Over the past 2 decades, the workhorse model of early preclinical HIE research has been the Vannucci model, where carotid artery ligation is followed by prolonged hypoxia to induce a largely unilateral brain injury.[62] Though all therapies closest to translation for HIE showed benefit in the Vannucci model, many have argued that the model produces more of a large unilateral stroke than the deep grey-matter injuries commonly seen with acute perinatal asphyxia, or the white matter injuries described with prolonged partial or acute-on-chronic hypoxia-ischemia.[60,63] Another issue with the Vannucci model is the heterogeneity of injury.[64,65] Most highly-powered studies in the model show a bimodal (non-normal) and wide distribution of injury, with sex differences in response to injury and neurotherapeutics. Most studies in the model are therefore hugely underpowered, and often use inappropriate statistics used to analyze the resulting data.[64] These hurdles are not insurmountable, but require very large group sizes and multiple rounds of experiments in order to aggregate the data and examine true treatment effects over and above random variability in injury.[64,65] For instance, the authors have previously shown that treatment effects of TH are similar in magnitude in the Vannucci rat model as they are in human clinical trials, but only once hundreds of animals per group were analyzed.[64] This issue of translating from the rat to the human has been well-described in the adult stroke literature as well. Nearly 20 years ago, O'Collins *and colleagues* described in their seminal paper that 1026 treatments were described to treat acute experimental stroke in the rat, but that there was no relationship between efficacy in animal models and successful translation to the clinic.[66] The mouse has increasingly been used instead of the rat when using the Vannucci model, but it is not clear whether that cerebral anatomy of the mouse is similar enough to the human or even the rat to produce translationally meaningful results, an issue that is also still hotly debated in the field. Similarly, sex responses to hypoxia-ischemia and to treatment differ by species.[28,67] Mice also have very strain-specific responses to hypoxia-ischemia and inflammation that may or may not correspond to human responses.[68]

Thus, it remains to be seen whether rodent models can remain the mainstay of preclinical HIE research. As rodent work has generally failed to result in translation to impactful treatments across both pediatric and adult neurology, their use in preclinical neuroscience is increasingly questioned. With that said, some groups have developed alternative or refined models to improve translation. For example, new models of alternating short periods of deeper and lighter hypoxia (eg, 5% and 9% oxygen) with concurrent hypercapnia (20% CO_2) have recently been developed.[69,70] These models result in a more clinically-relevant total hypoxia period (30 minutes rather than 1–3 hours), and better recapitulate other aspects of clinical HIE such as seizure development in the hours after hypoxia, presumably in line with the timing of secondary energy failure. The injury is also global and bilateral, with much less variability than the Vannucci model. Therefore, though questions remain about how well rodent models can translate to humans due to differences in biology and brain structure, newer models provide some promise for the role of rodents as part of the preclinical pipeline of therapeutic development for HIE.

Large Animal Models

In general, large animals with gyrified brains can more closely model human brain development and disease (see **Fig. 1**). However, they are expensive to buy and house, which leads to experiments with fewer animals that are evaluated for shorter time periods than rodents. The 2 primary large animal models employed in therapeutic studies for HIE are the 0.85 gestation fetal sheep and the newborn piglet, with additional contributions from nonhuman primates.[60,63,71] These animals have a gyrified brain and are developmentally and structurally much more similar to the human than is the rodent, with injury models also more similar to what is thought to occur in the human—a relatively short/acute severe global hypoxia/asphyxia event. The animals can be instrumented and treated in a manner that is very similar to what is done in the neonatal intensive care unit (NICU), including continuous monitoring of physiology and biochemistry.[72] After injury, the fetal sheep model includes ongoing physiologic support from the ewe, umbilical cord, and placenta. This allows for easier longer term survival but removes some of the difficulties and physiologic derangement associated with maintaining and caring for a sick human newborn. By comparison, piglet models, especially those that employ global asphyxia rather than focal cerebral HI, more accurately replicate the multi-organ derangements seen in moderate-severe HIE but are incredibly time-intensive. As a result, survival after injury and treatment in piglet models is generally very short, often less than 48 hours.[73,74] As injuries in HIE are known to evolve over days and weeks, if not years, it is possible that early neuroprotective signals in large animals do not translate to meaningful neurologic outcomes in early childhood, when most HIE clinical trials are assessed.

As a potential bridge between the rodent and larger animal models, the authors have recently proposed the ferret as a species in which to model longer term outcomes of HI in the gyrified brain[75] as it is amenable to long-term behavioral assessments.[76] In addition, the ferret brain has a similar white matter content to the human brain, and includes critical developmental structures such as the cortical subplate that the rodent does not, though others have argued that the ferret still displays critical differences in neuronal architecture and physiology compared to the human.[77] This may partly explain why the ferret is particularly resilient to single acute brain injuries, requiring more prolonged, intermittent, and inflammation-sensitized insults in order to develop long-term neuropathological and behavioral deficits. One potential upside of this is that these insults may more closely mimic the etiologic processes and resulting injury pattern associated with HIE in LMICs. For instance, in the authors' near-term equivalent model of inflammation-sensitized HI, significant white matter injury is seen in addition to cortical dysmaturation, which responds to Epo monotherapy but not TH.[76] However, it must be acknowledged that further evidence showing that therapies can successfully translate from the ferret model to the human are still required.

When considering comparisons between treatment effects in large animal models versus humans, it is possible to find examples both for and against these models depending on the particular experimental parameters used. These include injury model, drug dose and dosing intervals, duration of follow-up, and type of outcome assessment. With respect to the efficacy of Epo as an adjunct to TH, in the nonhuman primate model of HIE, adding Epo to TH was significantly more neuroprotective than TH alone, including long-term improvement in behavioral outcomes and reductions in cerebral palsy.[32] By comparison, however, more recent sheep and piglet studies showed only modest benefit of Epo, particularly when paired with TH.[72,74] It is not clear whether the lack of synergy of TH with Epo is due to an overlap in neuroprotective mechanisms, or whether there are other species-related factors that will continue to make it difficult to translate therapies from large animals to the clinic. The studies in most larger animals have better modeled the results from HEAL, where no benefit was noted with the addition of Epo to TH. The negative results may also be a reflection of the greater heterogeneity of injury seen in clinical trials compared to the highly controlled experimental situation.

Issues Relevant to all Models

In addition to model-specific issues, there are some commonalities across methodologies that are worth considering as potential hurdles to translation.

As TH is currently standard of care for infants with moderate-severe HIE in high-resource countries, any therapy to be used in this context should show robust treatment effects across multiple models when provided in conjunction with TH before being considered for clinical trials. This presents several challenges, in particular that (i) outcomes of infants with HIE in high-resource settings have generally improved since TH was made standard of care, largely due to improvements in general management,[49,57,78,79] and (ii) finding an additional benefit on top of a successful therapy would require either a large effect size of the adjunctive therapy or very large treatment groups. The timing will also be very specific to the therapy, as different therapies have different optimal windows of action based on their mechanism of action. Furthermore, the mechanism of neuroprotection between combined therapies may be additive, synergistic, or mutually inhibiting. A detailed mechanistic exploration of complementary or synergistic protection is therefore warranted, ideally replicated in multiple species. A final, though potentially more difficult issue to deal with in the research setting is the large role that postnatal environment plays in development. Many studies, including the HEAL and PENUT trials, have shown that maternal education, family environment, and socioeconomic status are the most important predictors of neurodevelopmental outcome.[48,49,80,81] These drivers of neurodevelopment can easily overshadow the beneficial effects of treatments administered years prior to outcome assessment. This will likely remain an ongoing tension between preclinical work and clinical outcomes in the patients whose lives we hope to improve.

Related to improving outcomes for infants with HIE with differing mechanisms of injury, it is clear from the HELIX trial that many infants with HIE in middle-resource NICUs have a different pathophysiology underlying their brain injury compared to those in the original cooling trials.[6,7] Since most preclinical animal models employ an acute asphyxia event that more accurately reflects HIE in high-resource settings, work must be done to develop LMIC-specific models of HIE. Historical data from nonhuman primates and the fetal sheep suggest that the white matter injury and seizures seen in the HELIX trial can be replicated with acute-on-chronic or intermittent partial hypoxia,[82] but few laboratories are employing these models currently. An additional contributor to differences in the mechanisms of injury may be the presence of inflammation, as both the HELIX trial and earlier trials had approximately 6% of infants who presented with infection.[4,6,78] We and others have shown that sensitizing the rodent, sheep, and piglet brain with E coli lipopolysaccharide prior to HI mitigates the benefits of subsequent TH treatment,[83–85] whereas presensitization with a TLR 1/2 agonist that more accurately mimics a gram-positive infection does not prevent neuroprotection by TH in the Vannucci model.[86] Clearly, development of a precision medicine approach to the different presentations of HIE, including those seen in lower resource settings, is essential. We must therefore invest in the development and validation of models that more accurately reflect both acute injury such as those seen with sentinel events (25%–30% of cases), and more chronic processes such as intermittent hypoxia, and hypoxia-ischemia associated with infections. Both monotherapies and TH with adjuvant therapies should be considered. With this approach, there is significant promise for developing therapies for more infants with HIE, including those in low-resource settings, but a more coordinated and rigorous condition-specific approach in preclinical work will be required.

Two more areas should be considered, both of which are relevant to all the current therapeutic dilemmas for HIE. The first is replication and collaboration across laboratories. Currently, each expert group in this field has its own therapies of interest that are tested in their own highly complex models. This is particularly the case for the large animal models, which are routinely used by only a small handful of groups. To increase the likelihood of translation, successful therapeutic strategies, including the same drug, dose, and dosing strategy, should be replicated in multiple laboratories using the same and different species. This will require significant effort and investment, but can be performed with collaborative consortia, as has recently been attempted by funders such as the Bill and Melinda Gates Foundation. Related to this, the Stroke Therapy Academic Industry Roundtable (STAIR) criteria were previously developed by adult neurologists investigating experimental treatments for acute stroke.[66] These criteria included recommendations that a brain injury model should be tested in 2 or more laboratories, in 2 or more species, in male and female animals with drug administered at least 1 hour after brain injury with at least 2 doses tested, and behavioral and histologic outcomes measured at both short-term and long-term end points. These are valid recommendations that are relevant to studies of neonatal brain injury. O'Collins and colleagues state: "A good animal model should be both reliable and valid, that is, produce consistent, replicable outcomes, have sound theoretic underpinnings, and have the ability to predict the effect of an intervention on clinical outcome."[66] However, nearly 2 decades after the STAIR criteria were developed, there is little evidence that they are being routinely applied in the stroke literature or any other related field. This is relevant to the final area the authors wish to discuss, which is ensuring that adequate evidence is available from preclinical studies before embarking on clinical trials. Limited resources and limited numbers of patients should dictate that only the most promising therapies are deployed in large clinical trials, and this should require the levels of evidence outlined earlier. As an example, the authors have adapted the STAIR criteria to develop a suggested framework for preclinical HIE studies to ensure that only those therapies that have undergone full and thorough assessment to ensure both internal and external validity are tested clinically (**Table 1**). Failure to do this will result in further wasted resources and failed trials.

POTENTIAL REMEDIES AND FUTURE DIRECTIONS

After 2 decades of promise from a world-leading preclinical pipeline that resulted in the development of TH for HIE, the field has recently been faced with 2 high profile failures—the absence of detectable benefit of TH in LMICs, and Epo as an adjunct to TH in higher resource settings. While disheartening, the authors believe that several potential remedies exist, with the field being well-placed to implement them in the coming years. These include.

- More targeted preclinical models that mimic a specific clinical scenario, particularly more chronic or intermittent HI events on the background of nutrient insufficiency or infection/inflammation. In order to successfully translate these, ongoing focus on phenotyping clinical cases of HIE shortly after birth will be needed.
- Acknowledging the critical contribution of the home environment, this may overshadow any small neuroprotective benefit of novel therapies. This should involve including maternal and neonatal chronic stress or environmental enrichment as

Table 1
Best practice recommendations for preclinical research to maximize the likelihood of successful neurotherapeutic translation

Item*	Description
1. Animal Model	Model specifically designed to recapitulate a specific clinical scenario, for example, encompassing variables beyond a single acute asphyxia event
2. Laboratory setting	The same therapy assessed in the same model employed in 2 or more laboratories
3. Animal species	The same therapy assessed in models in multiple species
4. Sex of animals	Studies powered to detect sex-specific effects or interactions between therapy and outcome by sex
5. Group sizes	Employing group sizes that overcome the inherent variability of the model employed. This may involve dozens of animals per group in rodent studies.
6. Time window	Therapy tested at least 1 h but ideally 2–3 h or longer after injury to ensure pragmatic translation to clinical trials
7. Dose response	Multiple doses assessed in multiple models
8. Route of delivery	Therapy assessed using a route of therapy that is amenable to the target population and setting
9. Endpoint	Assessment of neuropathology, imaging (eg, MRI), and behavioral outcomes
10. Long-term effect	Long-term outcome studies, ideally in gyrencephalic animal models

*Not given in order of priority.
Adapted from the STAIR criteria for acute adult stroke.[66]

part of preclinical injury models in addition to more important efforts to address social determinants of health at the population level.
- Leveraging variability in animal models by including large enough group sizes and powering to detect sex-specific effects. For example, embracing rather than avoiding experimental heterogeneity is now increasingly being encouraged in the adult stroke literature.[87]
- Enacting HIE-specific STAIR criteria that require any potential therapy to be tested in multiple species across multiple laboratories using clinically relevant models and dosing schedules. A suggested framework is provided in **Table 1**.
- Increasing collaboration across groups to enable larger studies to be conducted with greater external validity.

As a field, if we embrace the challenges facing us and adapt and work together to do so, neonatal neuroscience can remain a leading light in preclinical research and ensure the long-term betterment of infants with HIE worldwide.

DISCLOSURE

The authors have nothing to disclose.

REFERENCES

1. Villavicencio F, Perin, Eilerts-Spinelli, et al. Global, regional, and national causes of death in children and adolescents younger than 20 years: an open data portal with estimates for 2000-21. Lancet Glob Health 2024;12(1):e16–7.

2. Mwaniki MK, Atieno, Lawn, et al. Long-term neurodevelopmental outcomes after intrauterine and neonatal insults: a systematic review. Lancet 2012;379(9814): 445–52.

3. Jacobs SE, Berg, Hunt, et al. Cooling for newborns with hypoxic ischaemic encephalopathy. Cochrane Database Syst Rev 2013;1:Cd003311.

4. Tagin MA, Woolcott, Vincer, et al. Hypothermia for neonatal hypoxic ischemic encephalopathy: an Updated systematic review and meta-analysis. Arch Pediatr Adolesc Med 2012;166(6):558–66.

5. Edwards AD, Brocklehurst, Gunn, et al. Neurological outcomes at 18 months of age after moderate hypothermia for perinatal hypoxic ischaemic encephalopathy: synthesis and meta-analysis of trial data. BMJ 2010;340:c363.

6. Thayyil S, Pant, Montaldo, et al. Hypothermia for moderate or severe neonatal encephalopathy in low-income and middle-income countries (HELIX): a randomised controlled trial in India, Sri Lanka, and Bangladesh. Lancet Glob Health 2021; 9(9):e1273–85.

7. Montaldo P, Burgod, Herberg, et al. Whole-blood gene Expression profile after hypoxic-ischemic encephalopathy. JAMA Netw Open 2024;7(2):e2354433.

8. Tran HTT, Le, Tran, et al. Therapeutic hypothermia after perinatal asphyxia in Vietnam: medium-term outcomes at 18 months - a prospective cohort study. BMJ Paediatr Open 2024;8(1).

9. Masuda S, Nagao, Takahata, et al. Functional erythropoietin receptor of the cells with neural characteristics. Comparison with receptor properties of erythroid cells. J Biol Chem 1993;268(15):11208–16.

10. Wang L, Zhang, Wang, et al. Treatment of stroke with erythropoietin enhances neurogenesis and angiogenesis and improves neurological function in rats. Stroke 2004;35(7):1732–7.

11. Wallach I, Zhang, Hartmann, et al. Erythropoietin-receptor gene regulation in neuronal cells. Pediatr Res 2009;65(6):619–24.

12. Sugawa M, Sakurai, Ishikawa-Ieda, et al. Effects of erythropoietin on glial cell development; oligodendrocyte maturation and astrocyte proliferation. Neurosci Res 2002;44(4):391–403.

13. Genc K, Genc, Baskin, et al. Erythropoietin decreases cytotoxicity and nitric oxide formation induced by inflammatory stimuli in rat oligodendrocytes. Physiol Res 2006;55(1):33–8.

14. Iwai M, Stetler, Xing, et al. Enhanced oligodendrogenesis and recovery of neurological function by erythropoietin after neonatal hypoxic/ischemic brain injury. Stroke 2010;41(5):1032–7.

15. Chong ZZ, Kang, Maiese. Erythropoietin fosters both intrinsic and extrinsic neuronal protection through modulation of microglia, Akt1, Bad, and caspase-mediated pathways. Br J Pharmacol 2003;138(6):1107–18.

16. Wei L, Han, Li, et al. Cell death mechanism and protective effect of erythropoietin after focal ischemia in the whisker-barrel cortex of neonatal rats. J Pharmacol Exp Ther 2006;317(1):109–16.

17. Sun Y, Calvert, Zhang. Neonatal hypoxia/ischemia is associated with decreased inflammatory mediators after erythropoietin administration. Stroke 2005;36(8): 1672–8.

18. Juul SE, Beyer, Bammler, et al. Microarray analysis of high-dose recombinant erythropoietin treatment of unilateral brain injury in neonatal mouse hippocampus. Pediatr Res 2009;65(5):485–92.

19. Kumral A, Tugyan, Gonenc, et al. Protective effects of erythropoietin against ethanol-induced apoptotic neurodegenaration and oxidative stress in the developing C57BL/6 mouse brain. Brain Res Dev Brain Res 2005;160(2):146–56.
20. Zacharias R, Schmidt, Kny, et al. Dose-dependent effects of erythropoietin in propofol anesthetized neonatal rats. Brain Res 2010;1343:14–9.
21. Mizuno K, Hida, Masuda, et al. Pretreatment with low doses of erythropoietin ameliorates brain damage in periventricular leukomalacia by targeting late oligodendrocyte progenitors: a rat model. Neonatology 2008;94(4):255–66.
22. Oppenheim RW. Cell death during development of the nervous system. Annu Rev Neurosci 1991;14:453–501.
23. McDonald JW, Behrens, Chung, et al. Susceptibility to apoptosis is enhanced in immature cortical neurons. Brain Res 1997;759(2):228–32.
24. Iwai M, Cao, Yin, et al. Erythropoietin promotes neuronal replacement through revascularization and neurogenesis after neonatal hypoxia/ischemia in rats. Stroke 2007;38:2795–803.
25. Osredkar D, Sall, Bickler, et al. Erythropoietin promotes hippocampal neurogenesis in in vitro models of neonatal stroke. Neurobiol Dis 2010;38(2):259–65.
26. Gonzalez FF, Larpthaveesarp, McQuillen, et al. Erythropoietin increases neurogenesis and oligodendrogliosis of subventricular zone precursor cells after neonatal stroke. Stroke 2013;44(3):753–8.
27. van der Kooij MA, Groenendaal, Kavelaars, et al. Neuroprotective properties and mechanisms of erythropoietin in in vitro and in vivo experimental models for hypoxia/ischemia. Brain Res Rev 2008;59(1):22–33.
28. Fan X, van Bel, van der Kooij, et al. Hypothermia and erythropoietin for neuroprotection after neonatal brain damage. Pediatr Res 2013;73(1):18–23.
29. Fang AY, Gonzalez, Sheldon, et al. Effects of combination therapy using hypothermia and erythropoietin in a rat model of neonatal hypoxia-ischemia. Pediatr Res 2013;73(1):12–7.
30. Juul SE. Hypothermia plus erythropoietin for neonatal neuroprotection? Commentary on Fan et al. and Fang et al. Pediatr Res 2013;73(1):10–1.
31. Semple BD, Blomgren, Gimlin, et al. Brain development in rodents and humans: identifying benchmarks of maturation and vulnerability to injury across species. Prog Neurobiol 2013;106-107:1–16.
32. Traudt CM, McPherson, Bauer, et al. Concurrent erythropoietin and hypothermia treatment improve outcomes in a term nonhuman primate model of perinatal asphyxia. Dev Neurosci 2013;35(6):491–503.
33. McAdams RM, Fleiss, Traudt, et al. Long-term neuropathological Changes associated with cerebral palsy in a nonhuman primate model of hypoxic-ischemic encephalopathy. Dev Neurosci 2017;39(1–4):124–40.
34. Ohls RK, Kamath-Rayne, Christensen, et al. Cognitive outcomes of preterm infants randomized to darbepoetin, erythropoietin, or placebo. Pediatrics 2014; 133(6):1023–30.
35. McAdams RM, McPherson, Mayock, et al. Outcomes of extremely low birth weight infants given early high-dose erythropoietin. J Perinatol 2013;33(3): 226–30.
36. Leuchter RH, Gui, Poncet, et al. Association between early administration of high-dose erythropoietin in preterm infants and brain MRI abnormality at term-equivalent age. JAMA 2014;312(8):817–24.
37. Zhu C, Kang, Xu, et al. Erythropoietin improved neurologic outcomes in newborns with hypoxic-ischemic encephalopathy. Pediatrics 2009;124(2):e218–26.

38. Elmahdy H, El-Mashad, El-Bahrawy, et al. Human recombinant erythropoietin in asphyxia neonatorum: pilot trial. Pediatrics 2010;125(5):e1135–42.
39. Wu YW, Bauer, Ballard, et al. Erythropoietin for neuroprotection in neonatal encephalopathy: safety and pharmacokinetics. Pediatrics 2012;130(4):683–91.
40. Rogers EE, Bonifacio, Glass, et al. Erythropoietin and hypothermia for hypoxic-ischemic encephalopathy. Pediatr Neurol 2014;51(5):657–62.
41. Shankaran S, Laptook, Ehrenkranz, et al. Whole-body hypothermia for neonates with hypoxic-ischemic encephalopathy. N Engl J Med 2005;353(15):1574–84.
42. Gluckman PD, Wyatt, Azzopardi, et al. Selective head cooling with mild systemic hypothermia after neonatal encephalopathy: multicentre randomised trial. Lancet 2005;365(9460):663–70.
43. Azzopardi DV, Strohm, Edwards, et al. Moderate hypothermia to treat perinatal asphyxial encephalopathy. N Engl J Med 2009;361(14):1349–58.
44. Jacobs SE, Morley, Inder, et al. Whole-Body hypothermia for term and near-term newborns with hypoxic-ischemic encephalopathy: a randomized controlled trial. Arch Pediatr Adolesc Med 2011;165(8):692–700.
45. Shankaran S, Barnes, Hintz, et al. Brain injury following trial of hypothermia for neonatal hypoxic-ischaemic encephalopathy. Arch Dis Child Fetal Neonatal Ed 2012;97(6):F398–404.
46. Fauchère JC, Koller, Tschopp, et al. Safety of early high-dose recombinant erythropoietin for neuroprotection in very preterm infants. J Pediatr 2015;167(1):52–3.
47. Natalucci G, Latal, Koller, et al. Neurodevelopmental outcomes at age 5 Years after Prophylactic early high-dose recombinant human erythropoietin for neuroprotection in very preterm infants. JAMA 2020;324(22):2324–7.
48. Juul SE, Comstock, Wadhawan, et al. A randomized trial of erythropoietin for neuroprotection in preterm infants. N Engl J Med 2020;382(3):233–43.
49. Wu YW, Comstock, Gonzalez, et al. Trial of erythropoietin for hypoxic–ischemic encephalopathy in newborns. N Engl J Med 2022;387(2):148–59.
50. Juul SE, Comstock, Cornet, et al. Safety of high dose erythropoietin used with therapeutic hypothermia as treatment for newborn hypoxic-ischemic encephalopathy: secondary analysis of the HEAL randomized controlled trial. J Pediatr 2023;258:113400.
51. Juul SE, Voldal, Comstock, et al. Association of high-dose erythropoietin with Circulating biomarkers and neurodevelopmental outcomes Among neonates with hypoxic ischemic encephalopathy: a secondary analysis of the HEAL randomized clinical trial. JAMA Netw Open 2023;6(7):e2322131.
52. Wood TR, Parikh, Comstock, et al. Early biomarkers of hypoxia and inflammation and two-Year neurodevelopmental outcomes in the preterm erythropoietin neuroprotection (PENUT) trial. EBioMedicine 2021;72:103605.
53. Bennet L, Roelfsema, George, et al. The effect of cerebral hypothermia on white and grey matter injury induced by severe hypoxia in preterm fetal sheep. J Physiol 2007;578(Pt 2):491–506.
54. Thoresen M, Satas, Løberg, et al. Twenty-four hours of mild hypothermia in unsedated newborn pigs starting after a severe global hypoxic-ischemic insult is not neuroprotective. Pediatr Res 2001;50(3):405–11.
55. Haaland K, Løberg, Steen, et al. Posthypoxic hypothermia in newborn piglets. Pediatr Res 1997;41(4 Pt 1):505–12.
56. Gunn AJ, Gunn, Gunning, et al. Neuroprotection with prolonged head cooling started before postischemic seizures in fetal sheep. Pediatrics 1998;102(5):1098–106.

57. Shankaran S, Laptook A, Pappas A, et al. Optimizing hypothermia as neuroprotection at < 6 hours of age for neonatal hypoxic ischemic encephalopathy NICHD neonatal research Network, 2013. Available at: https://www.nichd.nih.gov/sites/default/files/about/Documents/Optimizing_Cooling_Protocol.pdf. (Accessed 8 May 2024).

58. Azzopardi D, Robertson, Bainbridge, et al. Moderate hypothermia within 6 h of birth plus inhaled xenon versus moderate hypothermia alone after birth asphyxia (TOBY-Xe): a proof-of-concept, open-label, randomised controlled trial. Lancet Neurol 2016;15(2):145–53.

59. Hamdy N, Eide, Sun, et al. Animal models for neonatal brain injury induced by hypoxic ischemic conditions in rodents. Exp Neurol 2020;334:113457.

60. Hagberg H, Ichord, Palmer, et al. Animal models of developmental brain injury: relevance to human disease. A summary of the panel discussion from the Third Hershey Conference on Developmental Cerebral Blood Flow and Metabolism. Dev Neurosci 2002;24(5):364–6.

61. Dobbing J, Sands, Gratrix. Cell size and cell number: a reconsideration of organ growth and catch-up potential. Proc Nutr Soc 1979;38(3):99A.

62. Vannucci RC, Vannucci SJ. Perinatal hypoxic-ischemic brain damage: evolution of an animal model. Dev Neurosci 2005;27(2–4):81–6.

63. Roohey T, Raju, Moustogiannis. Animal models for the study of perinatal hypoxic-ischemic encephalopathy: a critical analysis. Early Hum Dev 1997;47(2):115–46.

64. Wood TR, Gundersen, Falck, et al. Variability and sex-dependence of hypothermic neuroprotection in a rat model of neonatal hypoxic-ischaemic brain injury: a single laboratory meta-analysis. Sci Rep 2020;10(1):10833.

65. Sabir H, Maes, Zweyer, et al. Comparing the efficacy in reducing brain injury of different neuroprotective agents following neonatal hypoxia-ischemia in newborn rats: a multi-drug randomized controlled screening trial. Sci Rep 2023;13(1):9467.

66. O'Collins VE, Macleod, Donnan, et al. 1,026 experimental treatments in acute stroke. Ann Neurol 2006;59(3):467–77.

67. Burnsed JC, Chavez-Valdez, Hossain, et al. Hypoxia-ischemia and therapeutic hypothermia in the neonatal mouse brain–a longitudinal study. PLoS One 2015;10(3):e0118889.

68. Sheldon RA, Sedik, Ferriero. Strain-related brain injury in neonatal mice subjected to hypoxia-ischemia. Brain Res 1998;810(1–2):114–22.

69. Ala-Kurikka T, Pospelov, Summanen, et al. A physiologically validated rat model of term birth asphyxia with seizure generation after, not during, brain hypoxia. Epilepsia 2021;62(4):908–19.

70. Welzel B, Schmidt, Johne, et al. Midazolam prevents the adverse outcome of neonatal asphyxia. Ann Neurol 2023;93(2):226–43.

71. Koehler RC, Yang, Lee, et al. Perinatal hypoxic-ischemic brain injury in large animal models: relevance to human neonatal encephalopathy. J Cereb Blood Flow Metab 2018;38(12):2092–111.

72. Wassink G, Davidson, Fraser, et al. Non-additive effects of adjunct erythropoietin therapy with therapeutic hypothermia after global cerebral ischaemia in near-term fetal sheep. J Physiol 2020;598(5):999–1015.

73. Arduini A, Escobar, Vento, et al. Metabolic adaptation and neuroprotection differ in the retina and choroid in a piglet model of acute postnatal hypoxia. Pediatr Res 2014;76(2):127–34.

74. Pang R, Avdic-Belltheus, Meehan, et al. Melatonin and/or erythropoietin combined with hypothermia in a piglet model of perinatal asphyxia. Brain Commun 2021;3(1):fcaa211.
75. Empie K, Rangarajan, Juul. Is the ferret a suitable species for studying perinatal brain injury? Int J Dev Neurosci 2015;45:2–10.
76. Corry KA, White, Shearlock, et al. Evaluating neuroprotective effects of Uridine, erythropoietin, and therapeutic hypothermia in a ferret model of inflammation-sensitized hypoxic-ischemic encephalopathy. Int J Mol Sci 2021;22(18).
77. Primiani CT, Lee, O'Brien, et al. Hypothermic protection in Neocortex is Topographic and Laminar, seizure Unmitigating, and partially Rescues neurons Depleted of RNA Splicing Protein Rbfox3/NeuN in neonatal hypoxic-ischemic male piglets. Cells 2023;12(20).
78. Azzopardi D, Brocklehurst, Edwards, et al. The TOBY Study. Whole body hypothermia for the treatment of perinatal asphyxial encephalopathy: a randomised controlled trial. BMC Pediatr 2008;8:17.
79. Shankaran S, Pappas, Laptook, et al. Outcomes of safety and effectiveness in a multicenter randomized, controlled trial of whole-body hypothermia for neonatal hypoxic-ischemic encephalopathy. Pediatrics 2008;122(4):e791–8.
80. Bush NR, Wakschlag, LeWinn, et al. Family environment, neurodevelopmental risk, and the environmental Influences on Child health outcomes (ECHO) Initiative: Looking Back and Moving Forward. Front Psychiatry 2020;11:547.
81. Benavente-Fernández I, Synnes A, Grunau RE, et al. Association of socioeconomic status and brain injury with neurodevelopmental outcomes of very preterm children. JAMA Netw Open 2019;2(5):e192914.
82. De Haan HH, Gunn, Williams, et al. Brief repeated umbilical cord occlusions cause sustained cytotoxic cerebral edema and focal infarcts in near-term fetal lambs. Pediatr Res 1997;41(1):96–104.
83. Falck M, Osredkar, Maes, et al. Hypothermic neuronal Rescue from infection-Sensitised hypoxic-ischaemic brain injury is Pathogen dependent. Dev Neurosci 2017;39(1–4):238–47.
84. Dhillon SK, Gunn, Jung, et al. Lipopolysaccharide-Induced Preconditioning Attenuates apoptosis and Differentially Regulates TLR4 and TLR7 gene Expression after ischemia in the preterm ovine fetal brain. Dev Neurosci 2015;37(6):497–514.
85. Martinello KA, Meehan, Avdic-Belltheus, et al. Acute LPS sensitization and continuous infusion exacerbates hypoxic brain injury in a piglet model of neonatal encephalopathy. Sci Rep 2019;9(1):10184.
86. Falck M, Osredkar, Maes, et al. Hypothermia is neuroprotective after severe hypoxic-ischaemic brain injury in neonatal rats Pre-exposed to PAM3CSK4. Dev Neurosci 2018;40(3):189–97.
87. Usui T, Macleod, McCann, et al. Meta-analysis of variation suggests that embracing variability improves both replicability and generalizability in preclinical research. PLoS Biol 2021;19(5):e3001009.
88. Murray SJ, Mitchell NL. The translational benefits of sheep as large animal models of human neurological Disorders. Front Vet Sci 2022;9:831838.
89. Howells DW, Porritt, Rewell, et al. Different strokes for different folks: the rich diversity of animal models of focal cerebral ischemia. J Cereb Blood Flow Metab 2010;30(8):1412–31.

Moving?

Make sure your subscription moves with you!

To notify us of your new address, find your **Clinics Account Number** (located on your mailing label above your name), and contact customer service at:

Email: journalscustomerservice-usa@elsevier.com

800-654-2452 (subscribers in the U.S. & Canada)
314-447-8871 (subscribers outside of the U.S. & Canada)

Fax number: 314-447-8029

Elsevier Health Sciences Division
Subscription Customer Service
3251 Riverport Lane
Maryland Heights, MO 63043

*To ensure uninterrupted delivery of your subscription, please notify us at least 4 weeks in advance of move.

Printed and bound by CPI Group (UK) Ltd, Croydon, CR0 4YY

08/05/2025

01864747-0003